Multiperspective Case Formulation

A Step Towards Treatment Integration

Multiperspective Case Formulation

A Step Towards Treatment Integration

by
Priyanthy Weerasekera

KRIEGER PUBLISHING COMPANY
MALABAR, FLORIDA
1996

Original Edition 1996

Printed and Published by
KRIEGER PUBLISHING COMPANY
KRIEGER DRIVE
MALABAR, FLORIDA 32950

Printed in the United States of America.

Library of Congress Cataloging-In-Publication Data

Weerasekera, Priyanthy.
Multiperspective case formulation : a step towards treatment integration / by Priyanthy Weerasekera. — Original ed. 1996.
p. cm.
Includes bibliographical references and index.
ISBN 0-89464-814-4 (alk. paper) (cloth)
ISBN 0-89464-976-0 (alk. paper) (paperback)
1. Psychiatry — Case formulation. I. Title.
[DNLM: 1. Mental Disorders—diagnosis. 2. Mental Disorders—therapy. 3. Cognition. 4. Behavior. 5. Psychophysiology. WM 100 W398m 1996]
RC473.C37W44 1996
616.89--dc20 93-36572
DNLM/DLC CIP
for Library of Congress

10 9 8 7 6 5 4 3 2

Dedicated with love to
my husband Bruce
our daughter Rachel

and my parents Walter & Charlotte

CONTENTS

FOREWORD

I am one among many who has struggled to integrate the different concepts to which psychiatric residents are exposed. Meeting this objective enables us to answer that frequently posed question, "so how would you formulate this patient?"

Although there is literature which focuses on the various biological, psychological, and social factors to which our educators refer, this book provides the psychiatric learner with a new and refreshing approach to formulation.

The ideas in this book are exciting because they unite the many diverse schools of thought in a clear, comprehensive, and readable way. This enables the reader to become familiar with all aspects relevant to understanding why a person is presenting with particular symptoms at a given time. The development of an effective therapeutic plan is dependent on this understanding.

Dr. Weerasekera's ability to increase the reader's awareness of the various elements affecting a person's ability to function fully is timely and much needed.

Dr. Weerasekera's approach, for example, is to subdivide the broad concept of individual factors into biological, behavioral, cognitive, and dynamic components. These factors she then describes in terms of predisposing, precipitating, perpetuating, and protective factors, and also includes an approach for understanding a particular patient's coping-response style and a manner in which to explore effective possible modes of treatment.

Using her newly-developed multiperspective grid, she presents many of these ideas side by side. This allows psychiatric residents to increase their awareness and understanding of the inter-relationship of the elements contributing to a patient's less than optimal functioning.

My colleagues and I have found this new approach to be extremely useful in our work with patients. Dr. Weerasekera has not merely presented an academic exercise; she has introduced a new approach to understanding patients which should prove very helpful to all learners in the psychiatric field.

Carolynne D. Darby (M.B.B.Ch.)
Psychiatry Resident
McMaster University,
Hamilton, Ontario
Canada

ACKNOWLEDGMENTS

The idea to write this book originated after several years of attending Formulation Rounds at McMaster University as a psychiatry resident. At these rounds residents were expected to present a formulation of a clinical case. Needless to say, this generated much anxiety, especially if one was a junior resident. In my first presentation I considered three individual models in an attempt to formulate the case: biological, cognitive-behavioral, and psychodynamic. Previous training in psychology and a then brief exposure to psychiatry enabled me to understand and formulate the case from these perspectives. After the presentation, I was encouraged to write up the case by the then chairman of the department, Dr. Edward Kingstone. Although his suggestion was appreciated I did not actually pursue this task until much later.

After completing my residency, I had additional training to enhance my ability to formulate systemically. A Fellowship year at the Hincks Institute, University of Toronto, provided a rich experience in family therapy that offered an alternative perspective to understanding behavioral problems. Additional training in couple therapy, child therapy, and psychotherapy research was also pursued during this year, and provided a more expansive outlook on psychological problems. It was during this Fellowship year that the original manuscript that provided the skeleton for the current book was written. Observing psychiatry residents, psychology interns, and social work fellows struggle with a comprehensive formulation, motivated me to develop a model that could integrate the variety of perspectives represented by these disciplines.

Writing a book to present such a model has been a very difficult yet challenging task. There are several individuals I would like to acknowledge who assisted me at various stages during the writing of this book. First, I would like to thank Drs. Elsa Marziali, Marshall Korenbloom, Roy Muir, and the late Dr. Jock Cleghorn for their encouraging comments on the original Fellowship paper. For reading selected chapters and providing constructive feedback I wish to acknowledge Drs. Peter Elder, Patricia Rosebush, and Nick Kates. For their helpful comments on several chapters, I would like to express appreciation to Mr. Ron Dolson, Dr. Stephen Allnutt, and Dr. Les Greenberg. I am especially grateful to Dr. Peter Szatmari and Ms. Nancy Wynnyk for their time, effort, and excellent feedback on the entire manuscript. A special thank you to Dr. Carolynne Darby for all her time in reviewing the original document and for her comments in the foreword.

To Mrs. Claire Kostyshyn a very special thanks for all her long hours and hard work in getting the manuscript to its final form. Her support and encouragement are also appreciated.

To Dr. Anthony Bellissimo I would like to express deep appreciation for all his helpful comments and encouragement through all phases of writing this book.

And finally, to my husband Bruce, for his excellent feedback on selected chapters and tolerance of my unavailability during the writing of this book, and especially for all the support and confidence he gave me through my years of training and beyond, my deepest gratitude and affection.

CHAPTER 1

INTRODUCTION

A 38-year-old married lawyer visits her family physician after a four- to six-week period of feeling unwell. She complains of chronic fatigue, poor sleep and appetite, and a loss of interest in previously enjoyed activities. She has been married for eight years, has two children, ages 3 and 5, and works full-time as a lawyer in a well known firm in a large city. On further questioning she reports experiencing marital tension over the past six months, and feeling socially isolated from most of her friends. She is becoming more and more distressed about her feelings of sadness and emptiness, that have been worsening over the past three months. Significant events in her life include the death of her mother six months ago, and the loss of a close friend, who recently moved to a city considerably distant from hers. She is still able to work at home and in her profession but is worried about how long she can continue to do this successfully. She is confused and puzzled about her symptoms, unsure as to why she feels depressed, and is requesting that her family physician help her.

This presentation is commonly seen by family physicians and mental health professionals, including psychiatrists, psychologists, and social workers. Family physicians treat many of these individuals themselves, but on some occasions they refer their patients to mental health professionals. If referred to any one of these professionals the understanding and treatment of the case will likely differ, depending on the orientation and professional background of the therapist. After further assessment a psychiatrist may diagnose this woman's symptoms as a major depressive episode. Prior to making this diagnosis, the psychiatrist may carry out medical investigations to ensure that this patient's symptoms are not attributable to an underlying medical illness. Some of these investigations may have already been carried out by the family physician prior to the referral. Once a specific medical illness is ruled out that indicates an alternate treatment, the psychiatrist may consider prescribing an antidepressant medication. If the woman is suicidal and having difficulty functioning, an admission to a hospital may be considered.

If admission is unnecessary, the patient may be given a prescription and followed as an outpatient. There will be an expectation that these symptoms will begin to improve over a three to four week period after a therapeutic blood level is attained. Once her symptoms improve the patient may be followed less frequently until she has returned to her previous level of functioning. When recovery is established, the patient will be either referred back to her family physician or she will be followed infrequently for a few months and then discharged. She will be told that she has a depressive illness, a disorder that results from a chemical imbalance in the brain. She will be informed that she is at risk of developing a future episode, and should this occur, similar treatment should be considered.

The approach described above is common practice in psychiatry. It is based on the biological model of human behavior that understands disturbances in mood to be a result of chemical imbalances in the brain. The treatment then, is aimed at correcting these imbalances; however, there is great variability among psychiatrists in how they practice. Some may have chosen not to administer medications immediately, and would have carefully monitored this woman's symptoms while conducting psychotherapy. Medications may or may not be integrated with whatever form of psychotherapy is utilized. If she had seen a psychoanalyst, medications might not have been prescribed, and analysis may have been recommended to help her uncover the unconscious mechanisms responsible for her depression. What becomes evident is that the treatment prescribed depends on the psychiatrist's orientation and adherence to a particular model of human behavior.

If the "client" is referred to a psychologist, once again opinions will vary with respect to the understanding and treatment of the case. A psychologist who is trained as a psychoanalyst may view the client in a similar fashion to the psychoanalytically oriented psychiatrist. However, psychoanalytic treatment also varies according to the theoretical model adhered to by the analyst. Alternatively, the client could receive cognitive-behavioral therapy, a form of psychotherapy that is practiced more frequently by psychologists than other mental health professionals. A variety of therapies could be offered by a number of psychologists because the training received in graduate school is quite variable. These include psychodynamic therapy, cognitive-behavioral therapy, client-centered therapy, rational-emotive therapy, gestalt therapy, and many others. In addition to offering a form of psychotherapy, a psychologist may administer various instruments such as personality inventories and other psychological tests. The administration and interpretation of these tests are carried out primarily by psychologists who receive special training in this area. A clinical psychologist although sensitive to the biological model would be less likely to use this model given that medications are prescribed by physicians. Although physiological psychologists study brain and behavior, they tend to work in academic settings and are not usually involved in clinical work.

The client could also be referred to a social worker. Clinical social workers usually have a master's degree and work in a variety of social and health care settings. Social workers with Ph.D's tend to work in academic settings teaching and conducting research, although some may be clinically active. Social work training emphasizes the importance of the individual's social system. Therefore, this profession gives more emphasis to systemic factors such as marriage, family, social networks, and social support. If this client is referred to a social worker, the treatment may involve the family, or, at least attention would be given to this area. More attention may be given to how this woman is experiencing her social role as wife, mother, and professional. Her marital problems may also be addressed through marital therapy. Her depression may be understood in terms of her difficulty maintaining all these roles in the absence of any social support. Weekly appointments to deal with all these factors may be organized through individual, couple, or family therapy.

The form of therapy chosen will once again differ according to the training and orientation of the social worker. Similar to other mental health professionals, social workers practice a wide variety of therapies including psychoanalysis, psychodynamic psychotherapy, cognitive-behavioral therapy, interpersonal therapy, supportive therapy, couple, family, and group therapy. All these therapies may be practiced in a variety of settings where social workers tend to work, including mental health clinics, general hospitals, child and family centers and a variety of other institutions. The training, orientation, and setting will likely determine the treatment that is offered.

The preceding discussion of the multiple approaches that can be taken with one patient across mental health professionals illustrates one point: variability across disciplines and within disciplines is dependent upon beliefs and or training in a particular model or perspective in understanding human emotional and behavioral problems. There are, of course, certain standards of practice that are consistent across individuals adhering to a particular model (e.g., biological model-medications). However, wide differences are evident across groups that maintain subjective biases towards particular models, with different models being emphasized in different training programs. Trainees are known to leave programs with knowledge in one or two perspectives of human behavior, with limited skills in one or possibly two therapies. One attempt to motivate trainees to consider multiple factors in understanding a case is to request a "formulation."

The teaching of formulation likely varies across disciplines and within disciplines. Although there have been articles devoted to the subject, the idea of formulating has not been accepted by all. Those who practice from a purely biological model may be less likely to pay attention to nonbiological variables in the understanding and treatment of psychological problems. Those from a purely psychodynamic perspective may give great importance to the dynamic formulation to the exclusion of nondynamic variables. One who takes a comprehensive approach sees the importance of multiple factors in understanding the etiology and treatment of psychological problems.

There has been some difficulty defining the term formulation. The Royal College of Physicians and Surgeons, the national governing body of the medical specialities in Canada, has replaced the term formulation in the psychiatric Fellowship Oral Examination, with the word "understanding" (R.C.P.S.C., 1990). This has made it difficult for psychiatry residents to develop a clear idea of what formulation in psychiatry really means. Even in psychology and social work this term has different meanings and is either not pursued in some areas, such as the client-centered and humanistic perspectives, or is focused on at length in the psychodynamic school.

Any discussion on formulation must deal with a definition of the term. Although many discuss various types of formulation models, few define the term. Cleghorn (1985) defined a formulation as "a description and hypothetical explanation of data that the diagnostic system ignores or cannot explain" (p. 505). He recommended supplementing DSM-III diagnoses with a formulation due to the inadequacy of DSM-III to infer pathogenesis or predict course of illness. This view is supported by this book and Cleghorn's definition is expanded.

In this book, "formulation" is defined as a provisional explanation or hypothesis of how an individual comes to present with a certain disorder or circumstance at a particular point in time. A number of factors may be involved in understanding the etiology of the disorder or condition. These include biological, psychological, and systemic factors. All these variables interact under certain conditions to produce a specific condition or phenomenon. This phenomenon can be expressed biologically, psychologically, and systemically, and the mode of expression does not infer a specific etiology related to that mode. A comprehensive formulation then needs to examine all three modes carefully.

The purpose of developing a more comprehensive formulation is multifold. First, it will teach students to examine common phenomena (such as depression, anxiety, child and family problems, etc.) from different theoretical perspectives, and it will prevent a telescopic view of psychological problems as being entirely of biological or psychodynamic origin. Second, individual differences in the expression of clinical disorders need to be considered in understanding etiology, and managing treatment. A comprehensive formulation should pay attention to these important differences. Third, such an approach should integrate pharmacotherapy with various psychotherapies, as well as integrate the different psychotherapies, a direction in which the mental health and psychotherapy fields are heading (Karasu, 1990; Beitman, Goldfried, & Norcross, 1989; Norcross & Newman, 1992; Mohl, Lomax, Tasman, Chan, Sledge, Summergard & Notman, 1990). Fourth, if educators create an expectation for a more comprehensive formulation, this will encourage students to become more aware of areas that they may not otherwise pursue. For example, a comprehensive formulation may encourage the examination of behavioral principles and therapies, cognitive therapies, marital and family therapies, and others. And fifth and most importantly, one might predict that a comprehensive assessment and formulation may lead to a more comprehensive treatment plan that can only benefit the patient. This of course needs to be empirically demonstrated.

This book will first review the existing literature on formulation and then examine its ability to deal with the issues described above. Second, a multiperspective model will be presented that provides students with a visual aid and method to assessment and formulation. This model is an elaboration of the existing grid used by psychiatry residents today. This grid is depicted in Figure 1.1, and although its origins are unclear, it has been extensively used by residents and is the model more commonly used to formulate. This grid consists of three variables on the x-axis: biological, psychological, and social. The four Ps; predisposing, precipitating, perpetuating, and protective factors on the y-axis are incorporated within the three x-axis variables to arrive at a formulation. The biological column contains the physical or organic factors important in the etiology of the disorder. The second and third columns have created difficulties in that they have included all other nonbiological factors, with no real method being provided to assist the organization of complex data included under these columns. Another model is presented to help deal with these problems.

This book presents a multiperspective model of formulation (see Figure 1.2) that is an expansion of the original grid described above. The major expansion is in the "psychosocial" area, which has been divided to give separate consideration to individual and systemic factors. Specific psychological models which include the behavioral, cognitive, and psy-

Table 1.1 Standard grid

	Biological	Psychological	Social
Predisposing			
Precipitating			
Perpetuating			
Protective			

chodynamic model are given separate columns. The social section, renamed "systemic," has also been expanded and divided to include couple, family, occupational/school, and social factors. Therefore, this new model provides a clearer format for exploring specific theoretical perspectives, and separates the important systemic areas so that they can each be explored independently.

This model has been briefly discussed elsewhere (Weerasekera, 1993) and is described in detail in chapter 3. A separate chapter is devoted to each column on the grid (chapters 5–12). The purpose of each chapter is to introduce the learner to the perspective discussed in each column. Each chapter will follow a similar format and will include a discussion of (1) the *perspective,* or point of view represented by that particular model, (2) a *brief history* on the development of the perspective, (3) *basic principles,* (4) *assessment,* (5) *coping-response style* related to that perspective, (6) the *four Ps,* and (7) various *treatments* associated with the perspective. Chapter 13 presents an actual case in which this model was utilized in all three phases of management: assessment, formulation and treatment. The case will be presented in detail to illustrate the clinical application of this model. Chapter 14 will focus on how this model can assist the process of treatment integration, since formulation is considered a first step toward this process. And finally, appendix I provides a guide to assist the learner in writing an integrated formulation, considered the most difficult task by mental health students. An empty grid is provided in appendix II for easy photocopying and use in each case.

This model is a first step. It is a beginning. It is an attempt to try to integrate the different ways in which mental health professionals under-

Table 1.2. Multiperspective Grid

	INDIVIDUAL FACTORS				SYSTEMIC FACTORS			
	BIOLOGICAL	BEHAVIORAL	COGNITIVE	PSYCHO-DYNAMIC	COUPLE	FAMILY	OCCUPATIONAL/ SCHOOL	SOCIAL
PREDISPOSING								
PRECIPITATING								
PERPETUATING								
PROTECTIVE								
COPING-RESPONSE STYLE								
TREATMENT								

stand and treat their patients. I hope this new grid can be utilized from the first year to the final year of training and can also be used to assess deficiencies in a trainee's knowledge base. This book does not advocate that mental health students become experts in all theoretical orientations and therapies, but that they become *aware* of their existence. An ideal training program should strive toward providing its trainees with a variety of resources to explore these areas. Supervision in different modalities can provide a broader understanding of different theoretical frameworks. Once these perspectives are learned, empirical research and good clinical judgment should aid the clinician in selecting the best treatment possible in each case.

Sufficient time will be required to learn alternate ways of looking at the same phenomenon. The model discussed in this book, and the ability to use it efficiently, will also take time. It is a model I found helpful in residency training, and thereafter. Initial exposure of this model to a few residents and supervisors was met with great enthusiasm. It was this enthusiasm that motivated the writing of this book.

This book is written primarily for trainees in the mental health field: psychiatry residents, clinical psychology graduate students, and social work students. The purpose of the book is to provide a framework that will guide the student through the process of treatment selection. As research in psychotherapy and pharmacotherapy advances, there is a movement towards treatment integration. It is possible that future research will help us select the best treatment for a particular individual presenting with a specific problem. At the moment we do not have a sophisticated method of doing this. The model presented here is an attempt to begin this process. It is a first step towards treatment integration.

This book is also aimed at bringing together the individuals represented in the mental health field. Although there are many other disciplines under the umbrella "mental health professional" (such as psychiatric nurses, occupational therapists, and others), the main audience referred to in the book is from the three main disciplines described above—psychiatry, psychology, and social work. Although intended for students, clinicians who have finished their training may find the book helpful, in that it offers a model of formulation that is comprehensive, easy to recall, and encourages the exploration of alternative perspectives one may not have previously considered. Educators in the mental health field may also find the model helpful in that it provides students with a framework to understand their clinical cases in a more theoretically sophisticated manner and may increase the possibility that a variety of treatment options will be considered early in training. I hope that use of this method will produce more competent clinicians across all disciplines and increase our ability to communicate with each other, providing us with a much needed common language.

REFERENCES

Beitman, B. D., Goldfried, M. R., & Norcross, J. C. (1989). The Movement Toward Integrating the Psychotherapies: An Overview. *American Journal of Psychiatry, 146,* 138–147.

Cleghorn, J. M. (1985). Formulation: A Pedagogic Antidote to DSM-III. *Comprehensive Psychiatry, 26*(6), 504–512.

Karasu, B. (1990). Toward a Clinical Model of Psychotherapy for Depression: I. Systematic Comparison of Three Psychotherapies. *American Journal of Psychiatry, 147,* 133–147.

Mohl, P., Lomax, J., Tasman, A., Chan, C., Sledge, W., Summergard, P., & Notman, M. (1990). Psychotherapy Training of Psychiatrists of the Future. *American Journal of Psychiatry, 147,* 7–13.

Norcross, J. C. & Newman, C. F. (1992). Psychotherapy Integration: Setting the Context. In J. C. Newman & M. R. Goldfried, (Eds.), *Handbook of Psychotherapy Integration.* New York: Basic Books.

Royal College of Physicians and Surgeons of Canada. (1990). *Guide to the Fellowship Examination in Psychiatry,* Ottawa, ONT: Author.

Weerasekera, P. (1993). Formulation: A Multiperspective Model. *Canadian Journal of Psychiatry, 38,* 351–358.

CHAPTER 2

REVIEW OF THE LITERATURE

A review of the literature over the past 10 years yields about 25 articles depending on the definition of formulation used. Only those papers that discussed a specific approach to formulation or discussed educational issues related to formulation were included in this book. This review can be divided into three areas: (1) survey information about the study of formulation in different programs, (2) formulation studied from a psychodynamic perspective, and (3) broader models of formulation.

A study conducted over a decade ago (Ben-Aron & McCormick, 1980), evaluated the teaching of formulation in psychiatry residency programs in Canada, the United States, United Kingdom, and Ireland. A 70% response rate evaluating 1,300 residents reported using written guidelines in 40% of the centers. In Canada the rate was 40% (outside Toronto) with only 22% of the Toronto units using written guidelines. The United States, United Kingdom, and Ireland showed a 38%, 55%, and 55% rate respectively.

A more recent survey by the Canadian Psychiatric Association revealed that although case formulation is taught formally in most psychiatric departments, less than half of these programs provided written guidelines on how to formulate a case (Fleming & Patterson, 1993). Furthermore, the bio-psychosocial format was preferred by residents and program directors, even though they did not agree on the content of such a formulation. When comparing the Canadian versus the British formulation, Ross and Leicher (1986) found the bio-psychosocial model was favored in Canada, while the biological model was favored in Britain. Canadian opinion also gave greater emphasis to the psychodynamic element of the formulation.

The emphasis given to the psychodynamic component of the formulation is supported by the numerous articles on this subject, and appears to be the predominant focus in United States teaching centers. Most of these articles give guidelines on how to formulate psychodynamically, with more recent papers focusing on psychometric properties of specific models. A variety of psychodynamic constructs have been investigated.

Perry and associates (Perry, Cooper, & Michaels, 1987) discuss central conflicts and themes apparent in three psychodynamic models: (1) ego-psychology, (2) self-psychology, and (3) object-relations theory. In their paper they discussed how various conflicts within these models are played out in major depression and personality disorders. They presented a good discussion of the psychodynamic models through examples that can help students apply these theories to clinical cases.

Mardi Horowitz (1988) described formulating "states of mind" early in insight oriented psychotherapy and referred to three states that deal with the control of inner experiences. He went on to present a Role Relationship Model that examined relationship schemas in formulation. This model looked at internal representations of self and other and is a psychodynamic-cognitive model of formulation.

The search for more reliable and valid measures of psychodynamic constructs in formulation have been furthered by Perry, Luborsky, Silberschatz & Papp (1989), in their comparison of three different methods of psychodynamic case formulation. They compared Luborsky & Crits-Christoph's (1990) Core Conflictual Relationship Theme (CCRT), Silberschatz, Curtis, Fretter & Kelly's (1988) Plan Diagnosis, and Perry et al.'s (1987) Idiographic Conflict Formulation and found three similar themes relating to (1) wishes, (2) intentions, and (3) goals. All these models are attempting to operationalize psychodynamic constructs so that they can be measured and utilized in formulation.

Curtis, Sampson, Weiss, Rosenburg & Silberschatz (1986) have also increased the reliability of the psychodynamic case formulation by describing four specific components: goals, obstacles, insights, and tests, that were reliably rated by independent judges and found to be useful in the psychodynamic case formulation. Other psychodynamic models also give guidelines on "how to" formulate psychodynamically (Melchrode, 1988; Smith, 1987; Shapiro, 1989).

Most of the studies described above have attempted to define the various components important in a psychodynamic formulation. This research developed in response to the poor reliability found in Malan's dynamic change ratings (DeWitt, Kaltreider, Weiss & Horowitz, 1983). Malan used a two stage approach: the first involved judges arriving at a psychodynamic hypothesis based on the core neurotic conflict considered to be central to the patient's presenting problem. The second stage involved setting criteria of maximum improvement. The emphasis was on simple language and observable behavior. Results revealed poor reliability among judges, necessitating further research in this area.

Although psychodynamic formulators are becoming more empirically oriented, few of these authors discuss teaching applications. In addition, none of the authors address formulation in a comprehensive manner, integrating biological and other nondynamic psychological areas.

Only three groups of investigators have provided a more comprehensive formulation guide specifically aimed at educating trainees, in this case psychiatry residents. The first, by Cameron & Kline (1978), described the psychosocial aspects of formulation and emphasized the psychodynamic as well as social and family factors. A developmental longitudinal approach is described which adds a fluid component to the formulation, rather than a "snapshot" presentation. Although social and family factors are discussed, this model is viewed primarily from an individual perspective. Within the individual perspective it does not discuss cognitive or behavioral theories, and omits a discussion of treatment.

Perhaps the most comprehensive analysis of formulation written to date is that of Cleghorn and associates (Cleghorn, Bellissimo, & Will 1983; Cleghorn, 1985; Cleghorn, 1989). In these papers one finds a definition of formulation, a rationale for its utility, and an overinclusion of items from the bio-psychosocial areas. The main goal is to provide the beginning therapist with a language that is understandable, especially in the psychodynamic area. Repetitive patterns that lead to conflict are described without the "metaphysical jargon." Major dynamic components are: key relationships, conflicts, and experience of the self. Other constructs are used such as illness behavior, cognition, gender identity, role, and sense of self. Family aspects are stressed as are social variables. The only criticism is that its over-inclusiveness and presentation do not provide easy access to a cognitive schema that can be visualized and utilized in clinical practice. The various components discussed are vital to a comprehensive formulation but elaborate retrieval cues are necessary for recall. However, this is by far the most scholarly paper one will find in the area of formulation that attempts to integrate biological, psychological and social factors.

A recent source (Sperry, Gudeman, Blackwell, & Faulkner, 1992) also provides a more comprehensive approach to formulation with discussions on the biological, cognitive, behavioral, and dynamic areas. The systemic areas, however, are discussed under the "psychosocial" heading making it difficult to clearly delineate important subfields in therapy. Also missing is a cognitive schema that is easily retrievable for clinical use. Like Cleghorn's model, an easily accessible framework is not provided.

The literature to date has offered some assistance to help trainees formulate. Those who focus primarily on the psychodynamic formulation further the research in this area and help us utilize these concepts when formulating. They do not however, help us with the broader picture of integrating different perspectives and treatments. They missed the importance of the biological, cognitive, behavioral, marital, family, occupational and social factors. The three formulation models discussed above strive to be more complete and include the psychosocial aspects, with only Cleghorn (1985) and Sperry's (et al., 1992) model giving attention to behavioral, cognitive, and systemic issues. However, a more visual representation that integrates individual and systemic areas is needed.

What is more significant is that none of the above papers connect assessment within these domains to formulation, although Cleghorn's model does discuss assessment issues (Cleghorn, 1985). One needs to know how to assess biologically, cognitively, behaviorally, psychodynamically, and systemically before one can formulate within these models. Also missing is a clear link between assessment, formulation, and treatment. Formulation must lead to treatment, otherwise it becomes an intellectual exercise for the therapist that does not benefit the patient. None of the above papers discuss this connection in a clear, constructive manner.

Therefore it is time for a new grid—simple enough to be recalled yet elaborate enough to encompass the relevant variables. A new grid must teach assessment and formulation in a multiperspective manner so that a comprehensive treatment may be considered. The purpose of this book is to present such a model.

REFERENCES

Ben-Aron, M., & McCormick, W. O. (1980). Teaching Formulation. *Canadian Journal of Psychiatry, 25,* 163–166.

Cameron, P. M., & Kline, S. I. (1978). Formulation. *Canadian Psychiatric Association Journal, 23,* 39–42.

Cleghorn, J. M. (1985). Formulation: A Pedagogic Antidote to DSM-III. *Comprehensive Psychiatry, 26*(6), 504–512.

Cleghorn, J. M. (1989). *Formulation: Clinical Relevance and the Biopsychosocial Model.* Unpublished manuscript.

Cleghorn, J. M., Bellissimo, A., & Will, D. (1983). Teaching Some Principles of Individual Psychodynamics Through an Introductory Guide to Formulation. *Canadian Journal of Psychiatry, 28,* 162–172.

Curtis, J. T., Sampson, H., Weiss, J., Rosenburg, S. E., & Silberschatz, G. (1986). A Method of Establishing Reliability of Statements from Psychodynamic Case Formulation. *American Journal of Psychiatry, 143,* 1454–1456.

DeWitt, K. M., Kaltreider, N. B., Weiss, D., & Horowitz, M. (1983). Judging Change in Psychotherapy. *Archives of General Psychiatry, 40,* 1121–1128.

Fleming, J. A. E., & Patterson, P. G. R. (1993). The Teaching of Case Formulation in Canada. *Canadian Journal of Psychiatry. 38*(5), 345–350.

Horowitz, M. (1988). Formulation of States of Mind in Psychotherapy. *American Journal of Psychotherapy, 52,* 514–528.

Luborsky, L., & Crits-Christoph, P. (1990). *Understandıng Transference: The CCRT Method.* New York: Basic Books.

Melchrode, G. A. (1988). The Psychodynamic Formulation: How and Why. *General Hospital Psychiatry, 10,* 40–45.

Perry, J. C., Luborsky, L., Silberschatz, G., & Papp, C. (1989). An Examination of Three Methods of Psychodynamic Formulation Based on the Same Videotaped Interview. *Psychiatry, 52,* 303–323.

Perry, S., Cooper, A. M., & Michaels, R. (1987). The Psychodynamic Formulation: Its Purpose, Structure and Clinical Application. *American Journal of Psychiatry, 144,* 543–550.

Ross, C. A., & Leicher, P. (1986). Canadian and British Opinion in Formulation. *Annals of the Royal College of Physicians and Surgeons of Canada, 19*(1), 49–52.

Shapiro, T. (1989). The Psychodynamic Formulation in Child and Adolescent Psychiatry. *Journal of The American Academy of Child and Adolescent Psychiatry, 28*(5), 675–680.

Silberschatz, G., Curtis, J. T., Fretter, P. B., & Kelly, T. J. (1988). Testing Hypotheses of Psychotherapeutic Change. In H. Dahl, H. Kachele & H. Thoma (Eds.), *Psychoanalytic Process Research Strategies.* New York: Springer-Verlag.

Smith, D. (1987). Formulating and Evaluating in Psychoanalytic Psychotherapy. *British Journal of Medical Psychology, 60,* 313–316.

Sperry, L., Gudeman, J. E., Blackwell, B., & Faulkner, L. R. (1992). *Psychiatric Case Formulation.* Washington: Americn Psychiatric Press.

CHAPTER 3

THE MULTIPERSPECTIVE GRID

THE MODEL

Table 3.1 displays the model proposed in this book. It is an eclectic model in that it attempts to understand phenomena from a multi-perspective view. The grid is similar in construction to the grid already used by psychiatry residents and other students in the mental health field. The new Multiperspective Grid presented in Table 3.1 is divided into two major headings: individual and systemic. Within these headings are subheadings that encompass different perspectives and different systems. Under the individual area are four perspectives: biological, behavioral, cognitive, and psychodynamic. The latter three perspectives were chosen for their theoretical distinctiveness in how they view human behavior. They also represent the major forms of individual psychotherapy relevant in the treatment of psychological and psychiatric disorders. Under the systemic heading are four significant systems in an individual's life, couple, family, occupational/school, and social. Each of these perspectives will be discussed at length in the subsequent chapters.

The y-axis contains six headings, four of which are most familiar to psychiatry residents. The four Ps—predisposing, precipitating, perpetuating, and protective factors—have been used to evaluate biological, psychological, and social factors in the commonly used grid. It is the synthesis of these four factors that comprise the formulation. The items on the y-axis; the four Ps, the coping-response style, and treatment will be briefly discussed below in order to provide an outline of the grid.

THE FOUR PS

Under each perspective one can examine the important predisposing, precipitating, perpetuating, and protective factors. *Predisposing* factors are those factors that make an individual vulnerable to a specific condition or phenomenon. Usually this refers to antecedent conditions that predate the disorder or disturbance. These are usually events that have

Table 3.1
Multiperspective Grid

	INDIVIDUAL FACTORS			
	Biological	Behavioral	Cognitive	Psychodynamic
Predisposing	• fam hx • genetics • prenatal/ postnatal • developmental • temperament	• hx of *R & *P • classical conditioning history • modeling • learned helplessness	• EMS – autonomy – connectedness – worthiness – unrelenting standards • NAT • CD	• developmental arrests/fixations • attachment to bad objects • poor containing environment • ↓ mirror/idealiz functions • defensive style • insecure attachment • trauma/abuse
Precipitating	• trauma • toxins • vascular • metabolic • infectious • neoplastic	• ↓ , □, loss of *R • *P • classical conditioning to novel stimuli	• activ of EMS ↓ • ↑ NAT/CD	• rel'ship losses or diffic/sig events ↓ activate dynamic processes
Perpetuating	• chronic ingestion of mood altering substances • chronic illness • handicaps • disabilities	• chronic low *R • accessing *R • *R of illness behavior • poor variety of R*	• self-perpetuating EMS ↓ chronic NAT	• repetition compulsion • primitive defenses • lack of insight • compulsive attachments to bad objects • ongoing projective identification
Protective	• good health • ↓ risk factor • medications • intelligence	• variety of *R • wide behavioral repertoire • ↓ or ○ *P	• adaptive self-schemas • ↓ NAT/CD • challenges to EMS	• secure attachment • good self/other differentiation • good self-objects • minimal splitting
Coping-Response Style	• somatizer • meds oriented	• activity-oriented • likes "to do"	• introspective • reflects on thoughts	• introspective • search for meaning
Treatment	• Medication • ECT • light • surgery	• behavior tx –SD / relaxation –exposure – ↑ activity – ↑ skills	• cognitive tx –thought stopping –disputing –countering –challenging	• psychodynamic tx • psychoanalysis • humanistic/ experiential • interpersonal

*R=reinforcement; *P=punishment; ↑=increase; ↓=decrease; □=change; sig=significant; hx=history; EMS=early maladaptive schema; CD=cognitive distortion; ○=no; obj=objects; NAT=negative automatic thoughts; tx=therapy; activ=activation

SYSTEMIC FACTORS			
Couple	Family	Occupational/School	Social
• poor communication • dysfunctional interactional style • neg. attributions • lack of intimacy • poor self-other differentiation	• parental psychopathology • poor instrum/affective communication • poor boundaries/ hierarchies • triangulations • enmeshed/disengaged • closed system	• employment hx • learning difficulties • I.Q./school • economic limitations	• Poor social support • Social or geographic isolation • race, gender, class • poor social skills • poor neighborhood
• change in spouse –growth –illness • couple events –children –affairs	• indiv or family crises –illness/death –births –moves –separ/divorce –$	• loss or □ in job • failure at school • □ in school • ↓ $ on job	• loss of social support • loss of spouse • loss or change in social role • immigration
• chronic problems –children, $, in-laws –communication –intimacy –ongoing affair –destructive projective identification	• chronic problems –marital discord –illness –occup.stress –child problems –$	• occup stress • undiagnosed learning disability • ongoing unemployment • lack of leisure/rec	• chronic social isolation • poor living conditions • social anxiety • shyness • frequent moves
• ↑ intimacy • indiv. flexibility • = power • good communication	• open system • intimacy & autonomy • good communication • clear boundaries	• job satisfaction • $ security • high academic achievement	• good social support • good social skills • stable social role
• rel'ship provides major support	• family provides major support	• work provides –support – ↑ self-esteem	• social support network
• couple therapy –dynamic –CBT –systemic	• family therapy –dynamic –systemic –behavioral	• occupationally focused therapy • vocational counseling	• group therapy • social skills training • community resources

indiv=individual; neg=negative; rel'ship=relationship instrum=instrumental; separ=separation; occup=occupational; rec=recreation occurred early in life that "predispose" an individual to a particular condition. It can be referred to as a vulnerability or constitutional factor that increases the probability of a specific condition if the necessary conditions prevail. Examples include family history of psychiatric illness, prenatal or developmental insult and early loss of primary caretaker. A family history of depression and early loss of mother may "predispose" an individual towards depression under certain circumstances.

Precipitating factors are those events that have a temporal relationship with the onset of the disturbance. The difference between a predisposing factor and a precipitating factor is the latency between the event and the disorder. A precipitant occurs just prior to the onset of the disorder, a predisposing factor has been present for a greater period of time prior to any evidence of any difficulties. An example of a precipitant is the loss of a significant relationship that precedes the development of an emotional disorder.

Perpetuating factors are those factors that become pervasive and aggravate or maintain an ongoing disorder or disturbance. Examples include an ongoing stressor such as a medical illness, marital distress, other interpersonal difficulties, and problems in the work place. Perpetuating factors may not always be easy to assess because they are chronic in nature and thus not apparent to the individual. Therefore a careful assessment is necessary in order to ascertain the more common ongoing stressors that can produce psychological distress in most individuals, and severe symptoms in some. A precipitating event may become a perpetuating factor if it takes on a chronic course. In this case selecting the right 'P' may be difficult. For practical purposes this does not matter. These variables although technically distinct are not always mutually exclusive. That is, a variable can be seen initially as a precipitant, and later as a perpetuating factor. An example here is a medical illness that precipitates psychological distress, and then maintains an ongoing level of stress as a result of it becoming a chronic illness.

Protective factors are those that provide the individual with some resilience or protection against developing emotional and other psychological disorders. These could be individual constitutional factors, environmental factors, or the absence of a risk factor. The key feature is that these factors prevent the occurrence of a disorder in situations where the individual may have been vulnerable. Protective factors are important to assess in that they can be utilized to decrease stress and increase recovery. The absence of protective factors may make an individual more vulnerable, and this may become the focus of treatment.

The Four Ps will be discussed at length within each model, and clinical examples will be used to illustrate how these factors are viewed within each perspective. The four Ps provide the basic information necessary for the formulation, and it is the synthesis of these factors that forms the basis of the formulation. Up to now students have struggled with the plethora of "psychosocial" factors, and have found it difficult to draw out the relevant predisposing, precipitating, perpetuating, and protective factors. This new grid has been developed to help the student organize this information in a more coherent and sophisticated manner. The multiperspective model offers two additional dimensions to be explored—coping-response style and treatment. Each of these is discussed below.

COPING-RESPONSE STYLE

Following the four Ps is the coping-response style, a new category for most mental health students, that has been discussed extensively by Lazarus (1966; Lazarus & Folkman, 1991), and Mechanic (1978). The area of stress and coping has advanced considerably following Hans Selye's (1946) original description of the general adaptation response. Stressors that have been investigated include physical illnesses, natural disasters, wars, unemployment, death or loss of a significant other, and hassles of everyday life. Others have focused on the measurement of coping, and have devised various instruments to attempt this difficult yet challenging task.

Research on the measurement of coping is divided into two areas; dispositional and episodic (Cohen & Lazarus, 1973). Dispositional research views coping as an enduring, stable, trait, referred to by some as a style, hence the term "coping-response style." The investigators have attempted to capture this stable pattern of acting or reacting to stress by various methods of assessment. New scales have been developed and assessed for their psychometric properties. In addition, subscales from existing personality inventories such as the Minnesota Multiphasic Personality Inventory, and the California Personality Inventory, have been used to measure coping-response styles (Green, 1980; Gough, 1987). Investigators have used subscales from these scales to measure enduring patterns or styles that will predict future response to stress. Some of these measures include Externalization/Internalization (created from the Pa + Pd subscales of the MMPI), Resistance Potential, and Repression/Sensitization (both from the MMPI) (Beutler, Machado, Engle & Mohr, 1993).

Other dispositional researchers have focused on measuring defensive styles or defense mechanisms. Vaillant (1977), Haan (1969; 1977) and

Menninger (1963) measured various traits or defensive styles that could be followed across the life span to predict differential response to stress. Other more recent scales in this area include Gleser and Ihilevich's (1969) Defense Mechanism Inventory and the Coping-Defense Scale (Joffe & Naditch, 1977). All these instruments have attempted to measure individual differences in coping styles and differential response to stress.

The episodic investigators view coping as a behavior that varies from situation to situation. Given the complex nature of coping behavior, they criticize the trait approach for its view of coping as a stable enduring pattern. According to the episodic view, the term "coping" refers to a wide behavioral repertoire that varies from situation to situation, rather than being consistent across situations. The investigators have attempted to evaluate specific coping strategies in specific situations to understand various coping styles. Examples of episodic measures include the Avoidance-Vigilance Interview (Cohen & Lazarus, 1973), The Hackett and Cassem Denial Scale (Hackett & Cassem, 1974), the Billings and Moos Coping Measure (1981), and the Ways of Coping Questionnaire (Lazarus & Folkman, 1991). These assessment instruments assess situational coping. For example, the Avoidance-Vigilance Interview was originally used to assess coping strategies in an impending surgical operation. The Ways of Coping Questionnaire instructs individuals to answer items according to how they dealt with a recent stressor, thus referring to a specific stressful event rather than a general coping style.

The conclusion made by researchers at this particular time (Lazarus & Folkman, 1991), is that most individuals have a variety of coping styles that are situation specific. Although it has been difficult to demonstrate a stable enduring coping-response style, there have been attempts to look at various clusters of coping-response styles. Whether an individual has a predictable coping-response style has yet to be determined. At the present time the literature indicates two approaches to coping, and further research will be needed to help with this difficult yet intriguing area. It is possible that the term coping reflects a very complex process that involves a "propensity" toward a specific coping style, as well as a variety of "styles" that are utilized in certain situations. Therefore, the greater the repertoire the potentially more adaptive it is for the individual. Although there may be situation specific coping-response styles, it is possible that this response is part of a complicated pattern of interactions. Some have referred to this as coping flexibility and have attempted to measure it through interviews.

In this book coping-response style will simply refer to the specific method of behavior used by the individual to deal with a variety of stressors. There are important reasons to emphasize individual differences in coping. The psychiatric and to some extent psychological approach has focused on the treatment of disorders, and specific therapies have been compared to determine the best treatment for the *disorder.* This has enriched our practice of psychiatry and psychology in that specific treatments have been found to be successful for certain disorders. For example, evidence exists for the usefulness of cognitive therapy for depression, behavioral therapy for anxiety disorders, and psychodynamic therapy for the more "neurotic" disorders, although evidence for the last therapy is controversial. Nevertheless, there are failures in all these therapies, even pharmacotherapy. None of the therapies can boast a 100% success rate, and to suggest such an outcome is unrealistic. However, it is recommended that attention be paid to individual differences in coping-response style, and that it be utilized to match patient to treatment.

The multiperspective grid identifies eight coping-response styles that can be conveniently matched to a specific therapy. These coping-response styles are presented in Table 3.2, and can be described as individually (biological, behavioral, cognitive, or psychodynamic) or systemically (couple, family, occupational, or social) oriented. An individual with a biological coping-response style could be described as someone who "medicalizes" or seeks medical explanations for psychological symptoms, thereby focusing on "the body" to explain current difficulties. Individuals with a behavioral coping-response style can be described as "action oriented" in that they may like "to do" something to overcome their difficulties. A cognitive coper is a problem solver, or someone who "thinks through" the difficulties they are experiencing. They may very quickly see the connection between their thoughts and their feelings. A similar more "inner focused" approach to coping is also evident in the psychodynamic coping-response style. Individuals with this style of coping may be self-reflective, and more interested in self-exploration and self-understanding when dealing with their problems.

Systemically oriented coping-response styles infer the use of an existing system as a buffer during times of stress. A variety of systems may be utilized during the coping process. Individuals who use their significant relationships to cope can be considered to have a dyadic or relationship-oriented coping-response style. A familial coping-response style involves the use of the family as a support system. An occupational coping-response style involves the use of one's occupation as a distraction during times of stress in other areas. A socially oriented

Table 3.2
Coping-Response Styles

Biological	* somatizer * visits M.D. * medication oriented * hypochondriacal
Behavioral	* action oriented * likes "to do" * activity oriented * exercises
Cognitive	* reflects on thoughts * capacity to introspect * problem solver * "thinks through things" * sees connection between thoughts & feelings
Psychodynamic	* introspective * motivated for self-understanding * searches for meaning * connects past with present difficulties * inner focused
Couple	* uses dyadic relationship for support
Family	* uses family for support
Occupational	* work provides: –positive self-esteem needs –interpersonal relationships –distraction from personal problems –sense of mastery & productivity
Social	* social support seeker via –spouse & family –friends & neighbors –community resources, agencies –support group

coping-response style involves the use of friends and other larger support networks to cope during stressful times. All these coping-response styles will be described in more detail in each of the corresponding chapters.

The purpose of matching the treatment to the individual's coping-response style is twofold. First, it may be easier to obtain compliance if patients' perception of their difficulty is congruent with the proposed treatment plan. This may lead to a better therapeutic alliance, which has been considered the fundamental process necessary for any successful therapy (Gomes-Schwartz, 1978; Foreman & Marmar, 1985). A better therapeutic alliance in the beginning of treatment may also increase the patient's trust in the therapist who can then shift to other therapeutic modalities. The second and probably more significant factor is that matching the patient to treatment may also increase the potency of the treatment.

In an intriguing study by Michelson (1986) where the treatment of an anxiety disorder was matched to the individual's coping-response style as opposed to random assignment, significant results favored the matching of patient response style to the specific treatment. That is, individuals with a more cognitive response style did better in cognitive therapy than those with a more behavioral one, who did better in behavior therapy. A more recent study (Beutler et al., 1993) used the internalizing/externalizing coping styles (from the MMPI) to match patients to cognitive or insight-oriented therapy. Results revealed that externalizers and internalizers responded differentially to the two treatments, with the first group faring better with cognitive therapy and the second group showing a better improvement with insight-oriented therapy. Further research in this area will help us take into account individual differences in selecting treatment.

Although not empirically validated, the coping-response styles represented on the grid can be assessed early in the assessment phase. In order to complete this section of the grid attention needs to be paid to individual differences in coping-response style as well as coping systems that are used on a regular basis. Usually individuals seek help when they are no longer able to cope on their own. In some situations this may be due to worsening symptoms of an illness such as major depression or schizophrenia, or it may be due to a change in the usual coping buffer that is offered by a marital or family relationship. Identifying the loss of a coping system has important implications for therapy, for this system may need to be restored in the individual's life so that treatment is not simply disorder focused, but person and system focused.

TREATMENT

The last item on the y-axis and by far the most important is treatment. The purpose of this exercise that involves assessing and synthesizing all this information is to arrive at the bottom of the grid. Unlike the old grid, the new grid includes treatment. This section is filled only after the boxes above are completed. Once the assessment is completed a formulation can be made using the most likely hypothesis or hypotheses. There can be several hypotheses regarding the development of the presenting problem, or several hypotheses can be integrated into one rich, comprehensive formulation. This formulation offers suggestions for treatment. The suggestions should be considered with respect to the available research, and I hope that this information guides the clinician regarding treatment decisions. Before considering a particular treatment, the coping-response style of the individual needs to be examined with respect to how it fits with the recommended treatment. Various treatment options can be considered by following the various columns. Decisions can be made regarding whether to follow a specific individual therapy, systemic therapy, or the integration of a variety of therapies within the individual and systemic categories.

The addition of this section differentiates this model of formulation from others, since it is the first formulation model to include treatment. This emphasizes the point that the purpose of formulation is to arrive at a comprehensive treatment that will hopefully benefit the patient. This section is placed at the bottom of the grid since it follows the formulation and the consideration of the individual's coping-response style.

REFERENCES

Beutler, E. E., Machado, P. P. P., Engle, D., & Mohr, D. (1993). Differential Patient × Treatment Maintenance Among Cognitive, Experiential, and Self-Directed Psychotherapies. *Journal of Psychotherapy Integration, 3*(1), 15–31.

Billings, A. G., & Moos, R. (1981). The Role of Coping Responses and Social Resources in Attenuating the Stress of Life Events. *Journal of Behavioral Medicine, 4,* 139–157.

Cohen, F., & Lazarus, R. S. (1973). Active Coping Processes, Coping Dispositions and Recovery from Surgery. *Psychosomatic Medicine, 35,* 375–389.

Foreman, J. A., & Marmar, C. R. (1985). Therapist Actions that Address Initially Poor Therapeutic Alliances in Psychotherapy. *American Journal of Psychiatry, 142,* 922–926.

Gleser, G. C., & Ihilevich, D. (1969). An Objective Instrument for Measuring

Defense Mechanisms. *Journal of Consulting and Clinical Psychology, 33,* 251–260.

Gomes-Schwartz, B. (1978). Effective Ingredients in Psychotherapy: Prediction of Outcome From Process Variables. *Journal of Consulting and Clinical Psychology, 46,* 1023–1035.

Gough, H. G. (1987). *California Psychological Inventory.* Palo Alto, CA.: Consulting Psychological Press.

Greene, R. L. (1980). *The Minnesota Multiphasic Personality Inventory: An Interpretive Manual.* Stratton, NY: Grunewald.

Haan, N. (1969). A Tripartite Model of Ego-Functioning: Values and Clinical Research Applications. *Journal of Nervous and Mental Disorders, 148,* 14–30.

Haan, N. (1977). *Coping and Defending: Process of Self-Environment Organization.* New York: Academic Press.

Hackett, T. P., & Cassem, N. H. (1974). Development of a Quantitative Rating Scale to Assess Denial. *Journal of Psychosomatic Research, 18,* 93–100.

Joffe, P. E., & Naditch, M. P. (1977). Paper and Pencil Measures of Coping and Defense Processes. In N. Haan, (Ed.), *Coping and Defending: Process of Self-Environment Organization.* New York: Academic Press.

Lazarus, R. J. (1966). *Psychological Stress and the Coping Response.* New York: McGraw-Hill.

Lazarus, R. S., & Folkman, S. (1991). The Concept of Coping. In A. Monat, & R. S. Lazarus, (Eds.), *Stress and Coping. An Anthology* (3rd ed.). New York: Columbia University Press.

Mechanic, D. (1978). *Medical Sociology: A Comprehensive Text* (2nd ed.). New York: Free Press.

Menninger, K. (1963). *The Vital Balance: The Life Process in Mental Health and Illness.* New York: Viking Publications.

Michelson, L. (1986). Treatment Consonance and Response Profiles in Agoraphobia: The Role of Individual Differences in Cognitive, Behavior, and Psychological Therapies. *Behavior Research and Therapy, 24*(3), 263–275.

Selye, H. (1946). The General Adaptation Syndrome and the Disease of Adaptation. *Journal of Clinical Endocrinology, 6,* 117–120.

Vaillant, G. E. (1977). *Adaptation to Life.* Boston: Little, Brown.

CHAPTER 4

INTRODUCTION TO PERSPECTIVES

In order to present a clear description of how to utilize the grid, a separate chapter will be devoted to each perspective represented by each column in Table 3.1 (chapter 3). Each perspective will be discussed under seven headings: (1) perspective, (2) brief history, (3) basic principles, (4) assessment, (5) the four Ps (the components of the formulation), (6) coping-response style, and (7) treatment.

The first heading *perspective* will describe the basic understanding of human behavior adopted by that particular point of view. This explanation will be followed by a brief discussion of the historical development of that perspective. Attention will be given to the significant ideas that have emerged under the perspective and the individuals who have been involved in developing these ideas into a formal theory. Next will be a discussion of the basic principles within each perspective, which will be presented at an introductory level and is not intended to replace comprehensive textbooks on the subject. Included in this section will be a discussion on the various theoretical models present in each perspective. Many perspectives, such as the psychodynamic one, contain several models and the basic ideas of each of these models will be presented. Several models are also prevalent in the couple and family areas. Theoretical models are usually filled with jargon that make comprehension difficult. Every attempt will be made throughout the book to describe these concepts and constructs as simply as possible so that they can be more easily understood and applied in clinical work.

Some terminology must be learned to appreciate the theoretical models of each perspective. Some theories lend themselves to specific therapies, and it is mainly these theories that will be described. Before one can institute a therapy or variety of therapies one needs to *understand* the patient's presenting problem. This understanding is provided by a model that allows us to conceptualize the patient's problem. Therapists may use common-sense models to arrive at an understanding of their patients. Such theories include "he is never happy unless things are perfect," or "he needs to deal with his feelings more." Although at first glance these appear to be atheoretical statements, they are in fact part of various models of human behavior. For example, the first statement suggests that the patient has an irrational belief that creates specific difficulties, according to cognitive therapy. The second may refer to suppressive or repressive defense mechanisms discussed in the psychodynamic model. Therefore, theoretical models offer a common language that can be used by mental health professionals to communicate about various complex human processes. The more theoretical models one can apply to understand suffering, the greater the therapeutic options that can be offered to the patient. It is the aim of this book to describe the various perspectives and the models within these perspectives so that the similarities as well as the differences can be appreciated.

Prior to conceptualizing clinical problems, one needs to be able to obtain the relevant data, and this is done in the assessment phase, usually in the first few sessions. The assessment process will likely differ from discipline to discipline depending on the training provided in this area. A good assessment will likely consider a variety of theoretical perspectives.

Most mental health professionals carry out some form of assessment process prior to recommending therapy. The assessment conducted will vary according to the therapist's background and theoretical affiliation. A psychiatrist may carry out a psychiatric and medical examination to arrive at a diagnosis. A behavioral therapist will focus on obtaining behavioral data which includes a history of reinforcement and punishment. Based on the assessment a behavioral formulation will be arrived at that points to a particular behavioral therapy. A psychodynamic therapist may focus on early relationships with the primary caretakers and subsequent relationships, to arrive at a psychodynamic formulation. The assessment then is already biased toward the theoretical orientation of the therapist, and will in fact vary from therapist to therapist.

It is this variability that leads to divergent treatment options, suggesting that the treatment offered may be therapist-dependent. Nevertheless, there is some reliability in those perspectives that have a common language. An example of this is the DSM-IV in psychiatry that attempts to describe disorders and gives specific criteria for diagnosis (APA, 1994). This does not ensure a high reliability coefficient but it attempts to move assessment in that direction. This data will then be used to construct a hypothesis or formulation of the case.

The multiperspective grid offers the therapist a variety of perspectives from which to assess. Those perspectives chosen are well known to mental health professionals. Therapists from the different areas may be exposed to some of these perspectives more than to others. In psychiatry, a resident will be exposed to the biological perspective, and more than likely the psychodynamic perspective. The resident may or may not be exposed to the behavioral and cognitive perspectives since these areas have only recently been introduced into psychiatry. Many residency programs may not have individuals to teach these areas. This approach may be more available to the clinical psychology graduate student who may not be exposed to the biological perspective. The clinical psychology graduate student may or may not learn couple and family therapy, and is more likely to learn to assess from a cognitive and behavioral perspective. A social work student will be the most likely candidate to be trained in couple and family assessment but may not be exposed to the biological assessment. Consequently, different training programs will emphasize different aspects of the assessment. The multiperspective grid will enable one to assess across several perspectives and systems.

Following a discussion on how to assess within each perspective, every chapter will discuss the four Ps, the coping-response style, and treatment. Each chapter is written to introduce the reader to the particular perspective. Once a basic understanding of the perspective is obtained, additional readings are suggested in the annotated reference section at the end of the chapter. The reader is encouraged to pursue these sources to obtain a more thorough understanding and greater knowledge base. It may be useful to apply the principles learned in these chapters to a current clinical case seen by the reader. After reading a chapter the grid can be filled out for each perspective, which will test the reader's understanding of the basic principles discussed in the chapter. After a chapter is read and the grid is completed, the reader is encouraged to attempt a written formulation from that perspective. Once the entire grid is completed, an integrated formulation can be attempted. This approach can be followed in a case-rounds or seminar format, where clinical cases are presented. Each case can be viewed through the various perspectives and then understood through an integrated formulation. The formulation, along with the coping-response style, should suggest a variety of treatment options. This approach has been used with psychiatry residents at McMaster University, and it has been found clinically useful and stimulating in that it provides a comprehensive evaluation of any case, and it suggests therapeutic options that may not have otherwise been considered.

To provide more assistance with this process, a clinical illustration is presented in the book that should offer some guidance in completing this task (see chapter 14). The chapter From Formulation to Treatment Integration should assist the reader in considering treatment alternatives and treatment integration. It will take numerous trials before the grid can be completed with minimal effort. The purpose of this book is to provide a manual to carry out this process.

REFERENCES

American Psychiatric Association. (1994). Diagnostic and Statistical Manual of Mental Disorders (4th ed.) Washington, DC: American Psychiatric Association: Author.

INDIVIDUAL FACTORS

CHAPTER 5

THE BIOLOGICAL PERSPECTIVE

THE PERSPECTIVE

The first column on the grid contains the biological perspective, more commonly referred to as the biological model of human behavior. This model is represented by many disciplines that can be considered under the general heading of Neuroscience and Behavioral genetics. According to this model all human behavior is biologically based. The determinants of human behavior are understood in terms of brain function and neurophysiological mechanisms. Understanding the complex operations of the brain is one of the major areas of study within this model. Other systems that influence brain function are also considered, such as the endocrine and immune systems. Thoughts, feelings, and behaviors are all considered to be manifestations of complicated biochemical processes; it is these processes that determine behavior.

If all behavior is understood with respect to some biological mechanism, then dysfunctional behavior is seen as resulting from some alteration in the biological system. This alteration can result from a disturbance in structure, function or both. Behavioral disorders then are considered to originate from within the organism, as a consequence of some disruption or dysregulation in the biological mechanism responsible for that particular behavior. Disturbances in affect, cognition, and behavior are viewed as resulting from changes in the centres of the brain that control these experiences. Therefore mood disorders, anxiety disorders, and psychotic illnesses, are explained in terms of neurochemical changes that produce behavioral symptoms. Not all behavioral manifestations are localized to changes in the brain; changes in other systems can also have an effect on the brain, the common pathway being some metabolic process that ultimately has an effect on the brain. In many cases the mechanisms are not clearly understood. The biological perspective is not represented by one unifying theory or one discipline, but involves numerous disciplines that include the neurosciences, neuropsychiatry, neuropsychology, neurology, physiological psychology, and neurophysiology. In the mental health field most of this work falls under the general headings of brain and behavior, neuroscience, and neuropsychiatry.

Individuals belonging to any one of these disciplines will adhere to the basic premise of the biological model of human behavior, although some variability may exist with respect to the degree of adherence to this model. Within the general mental health field there are diverging opinions regarding this model of human behavior. Some professionals reduce all psychological experiences to biological mechanisms, disregarding the use for any psychological models of human behavior, such as those represented on the multiperspective grid. Others may completely disregard the biological model, seeing it as too "reductionistic" and inadequate in its ability to explain more complicated human psychological experiences; while others may see the importance of both biological and psychological models and integrate concepts from both perspectives, an approach supported in this book.

Because the focus of this book is on formulating personality and psychopathology, the contributions of the biological model in helping us understand these phenomena will be presented. Since it is not the purpose of this book to present a comprehensive discussion of each model, but rather an introductory "scan," the reader is encouraged to pursue additional references provided for a more elaborate discussion of each area. The purpose of this chapter is to encourage readers to consider the exciting contributions made by this model so that it becomes part of their "working schema" when faced with clinical problems. Psychiatry residents will gain sufficient exposure to this model because it is the major model taught in residency in the understanding and treatment of psychiatric disorders. A greater variability may be found among clinical psychology graduate students depending on their exposure to neuropsychology, abnormal psychology, and general psychiatry. Social work trainees, unless exposed to a psychiatric or other medical setting, may receive less exposure to this model. All specialties can benefit from learning more about this area, regardless of their adherence to a particular theoretical model. For the psychiatry resident it is essential, as this model is very relevant to the understanding and treatment of the psychiatric disorders.

BRIEF HISTORY

The origins of this perspective can be traced to the early Greek philosophers Alcmaeon, Empedocles, Plato, and Aristotle. Hippocrates (450–355 B.C.) was one of the first physicians to attend to biological mechanisms underlying mood disturbances (Mora, 1970). Hippocrates attributed diseases and changes in mood to imbalances of body fluids that he called "humors." The four humors, namely blood, phlegm, yellow bile and black bile, were thought to be responsible for specific conditions. Melancholia, a severe depressive condition, was considered to result from an excess of black bile.

Galen (130–200 A.D.) is credited with having been the first to identify the brain as the core structure responsible for all mental processes and human behavior. In thirteenth-century France, Bartholomaeus Anglicus was one of the first to ascribe functions to certain areas of the brain, later identifying these areas as being responsible for mental diseases. In the 1500s chemicals were being advocated for the treatment of mental illnesses, implying that these diseases resulted from chemical imbalances in the brain (Kolb & Whishaw, 1990).

The search for a connection between brain and behavior continued over the next few centuries, leading to the development of the related disciplines of neuropsychiatry, neuropsychology, and neuroscience. Neuropsychiatry was founded by Wilhelm Greisinger in the mid-1800s in Germany. He is also credited with establishing psychiatry as a subspecialty of medicine. Neuropsychology developed somewhat later as a result of a merging between neurology and physiological psychology. The term "neuropsychology" was first used by William Osler and was expanded later by Hebb (Kolb & Whishaw, 1990).

The development of neuropsychology has been influenced by two hypotheses: the brain hypothesis and the neuron hypothesis. The first identifies the brain as the source of all behavior, and the second identifies the neuron as the basic unit of brain structure and function. The first hypothesis can be traced to the early "phrenologists" of the nineteenth century, Gall and Spurzheim, who studied the relationship between skull surfaces and various individual faculties. This idea marked the beginning of the "localization of function" movement. Gall assigned various emotional and intellectual functions to 35 areas in the brain that were demarcated according to various "bumps" on the skull. Some of these centers were identified as carrying out important cognitive functions such as language and calculation. Others were assigned the responsibility of carrying human traits such as benevolence, firmness, combativeness, and many others (Kolb & Whishaw, 1990). Gall's assignment of function to structure began a controversy that has continued to this day—the localization/antilocalization debate. The first opponent of the localization movement was Pierre Flourens (1794–1867), a French neurologist who argued that the brain operated as a whole, and could not be understood by the simple assignment of function to structure. Various brain functions were thought to be carried out by the entire cortex, and injury to any area was considered to affect all functions, a position later referred to as the "aggregate field view" (Kandel, 1985a).

This debate, pioneered by Carl Wernicke and Paul Broca, continued into the mid-1800s. Wernicke argued against the localization of function, stating that there were several areas involved in any specific function, particularly in the area of language. He also claimed that there were specific connections between neurons and specific pathways between different regions of the brain that determined behavior. This theory became known as "cellular connectionism," considered to be in opposition to the aggregate field view. Broca argued the opposite, stating that functions could be localized to specific regions of the brain. Support for his theory came from studies on aphasia. Broca correlated aphasia (a disturbance in the ability to use languages) with lesions in the frontal area of the brain (later referred to as Broca's area). Further evidence for the localization of function was also provided by corticostimulation studies; however, this was once again contested by the antilocalizationists (Kolb & Whishaw, 1990; Kandel, 1985a).

The debate between the localizationists and antilocalizationists continued during the late 1800s and early 1900s. Current knowledge in neuroscience suggests that although functions can be localized to certain structures, the brain is much more complex, having many parallel processes ongoing in several locations that carry out similar functions. The complicated interconnections between several areas of the brain make it difficult to identify one location as solely responsible for a particular function. The complex nature of many human functions such as language, are likely carried out through the interconnection of many sites, each responsible for a particular component of that function (Kolb & Whishaw, 1990; Kandel, 1985a).

The second hypothesis (the neuron hypothesis) was advanced by two men: Camillo Golgi and Santiago Ramon y Cajal. Golgi developed a staining technique which permitted the first clear microscopic visualization of the nerve cell, the neuron. Cajal taking advantage of this new "view" argued that the nervous system was made up of several of these discrete cells, rather than being a conglomerate of cells that had somehow blended together (Kandel, 1985b; Kolb & Whishaw 1990).

Considerable development in modern neuropsychology and neuroscience has taken place due to improved technology in the study of the brain (Fischbach, 1992). Recent technological advances permit one to study dynamic brain function as opposed to structure, thereby influencing the types of questions being asked. At the neuronal level, technology has also provided a greater understanding of the intricate mechanisms of neurophysiology. Both these areas continue to advance and represent one of the fastest growing and exciting fields of human behavior.

BASIC PRINCIPLES

In order to discuss the biological perspective of human behavior it is necessary to have a rudimentary understanding of brain and behavior, and behavioral genetics. Under the first heading we examine the human brain in terms of structure and function, and its basic building block, the neuron. How other systems within the body affect brain and behavior will also be discussed as this has important clinical implications for mental health problems. Most of the discussion will focus on how alterations in brain structure and function affect human behavior, and contribute to psychological disturbances and psychiatric illness.

The second section entitled behavioral genetics will discuss the role of inheritance in personality and psychopathology.

BRAIN AND BEHAVIOR

The Brain

The brain weighs about three pounds and contains at least 100 billion neurons or nerve cells that decrease in number with increasing age. It is considered the most complex structure in the universe (Fischbach, 1992). It carries out numerous functions involving the interpretation of sensory data, learning, abstract thought, regulation of affect and various biological processes such as sleep, sex, hunger, aggression, and many others. These are complicated human behaviors that have all been independently studied in a variety of species including humans. Some of these behaviors have been linked to specific structures in the brain, although as mentioned above, the localization of function is much more complicated. For our purposes the more basic structural model will be presented that is still valid and sufficient for gaining an understanding of brain and behavior mechanisms.

The brain is grossly divided into three areas: the hindbrain, the midbrain and the forebrain, referring simply to the back or bottom, the middle, and the front. The hindbrain begins where the spinal cord enters the brain and contains two structures known as the medulla and the pons. This area is also known as the brain stem. These structures are responsible for carrying out the vital functions of the body such as respiration and circulation. Two other important structures in this area are the reticular formation and the cerebellum. The first is responsible for conscious experience and maintains attention and induces sleep. The latter is identified as the motor coordinator as it organizes the complex motor movements involved in everyday activity. This structure is responsible for helping us maintain an erect stable posture, a structure that is considered to have undergone significant evolutionary change as we moved from a quadrupedal to a bipedal organism, requiring much more effort to maintain balance and gait (Guyton, 1987).

The midbrain is the relay center for the auditory and visual system and contains sensory and motor nerve cells. This area has the least involvement in the regulation of emotional aspects of behavior, but is an important site for the sensorimotor system.

The forebrain contains the two large cerebral hemispheres and various structures buried in the central region of the brain. Two of these structures are called the thalamus and the hypothalamus. The thalamus is often referred to as the sensory relay station, as it directs incoming messages to various other structures in the brain. The hypothalamus located below the thalamus is one of the important structures involved in regulating human behavior. This structure is involved in controlling sexual behavior, aggression, eating, sleeping, and temperature regulation. The hypothalamus plays a central role in regulating hormone secretion throughout the body through the pituitary gland, a small gland about 1 cm in diameter located at the base of the brain. The pituitary releases substances that have an effect on various endocrine organs in the body, the organs that secrete hormones. Hormones in turn act on the brain and other organs and are involved in regulating many behaviors in the body (see section below) (Guyton, 1987; Kandel, 1985a). This hypothalamic-pituitary axis and its regulation of the release of the hormone cortisol have been implicated in the development of depression (Checkley, 1992). These "neuroendocrinological" studies have also been extended to disorders such as schizophrenia, where some have argued for a disturbance in other hormone-releasing substances emanating from the pituitary, although the evidence for this is controversial (Guyton, 1987).

Some additional structures located deep within the cerebral hemispheres are collectively called the limbic system and contain the hippocampus and the amygdala. The former is involved in learning and memory while the latter is involved in aggression, reward, punishment, and motivation. This subject has been of significant interest to schizophrenia researchers, who have found abnormalities in this area in patients diagnosed with this disorder. Breier, Buchanan, Elkashef, Munson, Patrick & Gellad (1992) found a decrease in the size of the structures in the hippocampal region in patients identified with a schizophrenic disorder. The region has also been of interest to researchers studying anxiety disorders. In panic disorder some investigators have found an increase in cerebral blood flow in the hippocampal area (Reiman, Raichele, & Robins, 1986).

The cerebral hemispheres are each divided into four lobes: frontal, parietal, occipital, and temporal. The frontal lobe is involved in abstract reasoning and social judgment; it is the area that inhibits various socially inappropriate behaviors. It is also involved in movement, and with planning (Kandel, 1985a).

Along with the limbic system, the frontal lobe has also been implicated as an important site in the development of schizophrenia. Given the complex functions of this lobe and the many extensions it receives, especially from the limbic system, it is not surprising that this area would be of interest to those studying schizophrenia, a disorder that is characterized by gross disturbances in thought, affect, and behavior. One finding has been the decreased blood flow observed in this region when these patients are asked to perform certain tasks that involve this area (Weinberger & Bergman, 1988; Berman & Weinberger, 1991). A recent review suggests that "hypofrontality" may be related to the negative symptoms of schizophrenia, characterized by apathy, social isolation, decreased drive, and restricted affect (Andreasen, Rezai, Alliger, Swayze, Flaum, Kirchner, et al, 1992).

Injuries to the frontal lobe have been associated with changes in behavior, specifically a disinhibited pattern of behavior is evident in these individuals. Any insult to this region either through a space-occupying lesion or stroke can produce a syndrome called organic personality disorder that is characterized by sexual disinhibition, decreased concern for hygiene, affective lability, impulsivity, and others, all in the presence of normal intellectual functioning (Lischman, 1987).

The parietal lobe coordinates complicated motor functions, and is the somatosensory area, meaning it receives the complex sensations from all over the body. The occipital lobe contains the visual cortex that receives the neural input from the eye and interprets this incoming sensory information (Guyton, 1987).

The temporal lobe is involved in language, memory, emotion, and audition. Abnormalities in this lobe have been connected to many neurological and psychiatric disorders. For example, temporal lobe epilepsy involves a wide range of behavioral manifestations, including aggressivity, impulsivity and others (Lischman, 1987; Guyton, 1987).

In addition to these structures the brain houses four ventricles—large fluid filled cavities that contain the cerebrospinal fluid, the substance that bathes both the brain and spinal cord. This fluid is crucial for maintaining structural integrity and regulating various functions. Two of these ventricles, known as the lateral ventricles, lie in the middle of each cerebral hemisphere extending from the frontal lobe to the occipital lobe. The third ventricle lies between the two lateral halves of the thalamus and the hypothalamus. The fourth ventricle is located in the lower brain stem. These ventricles, especially the lateral ventricles, have been the focus of study in certain psychiatric disorders (Guyton, 1987). In schizophrenia enlarged lateral ventricles have been reported in a variety of studies, suggesting the possibility of loss of cellular structure or "atrophy" in the cerebral cortex (Weinberger, Fuller, Neophytides, & Wyatt, 1979). A recent meta-analysis of studies in this area has questioned the practical significance of these findings based on the small differences found between schizophrenics and controls in ventricular size (Van Horn & McManus, 1992).

The Neuron

The preceding discussion of the brain described the structure and function; the next section focuses on the brain's basic building block, the neuron. The basic cellular unit in the nervous system is the neuron. There are at least 100 billion neurons that make up the nervous system (central and peripheral). The neuron is the nerve cell, and like all cells, it carries out a variety of functions to maintain internal equilibrium. The neuron like all other cells is encased in a membrane that selectively allows the passage of different substances in and out of the cell. It also contains receptors, special sites on the membrane that receive receptor-specific substances that lead to significant biochemical and electrical changes in the cell. Chemical substances known as neurotransmitters permit communication to occur between adjacent neurons by binding to these receptor sites and triggering a chain of events. How these neurotransmitters are stored, released, and affect other neurons is of great interest to those studying the neurochemical bases of psychiatric disorders.

There have been at least 40 neurotransmitters identified, with different neurons responding to different neurotransmitters (Reichert, 1992). These chemical messengers either excite or moderate the adjacent neuron to initiate a certain activity or inhibit the neuron to decrease its activity. The activity is usually increasing or decreasing the release of its own neurotransmitter. The neurotransmitter is released into a space between the nerve cells known as the synaptic cleft. Various neurotransmitters have been identified as being important in the experience of emotional and mental conditions. For example, pharmacological evidence suggests that the neurotransmitter known as dopamine has an important role in the etiology of schizophrenia and Parkinson's disease (Javitch & Kaufman, 1991). Other neurotransmitters known as serotonin and norepinephrine have been implicated in the mood disorders (Green, Mooney & Schildkraut, 1990). A variety of neurochemical mechanisms have also been implicated in panic disorder (Nutt & Lawson, 1992). Acetylcholine has been implicated in disorders involving memory difficulties such as in Alzheimer's disease (Kandel, 1985b). In addition to specific neurotransmitters that have been identified with certain disorders, the continuous release of large quantities of a variety of neurotransmitters has been described in seizure disorders.

Neurophysiology has been the focus of study of several disciplines including neurobiology, neuropsychiatry, and the general area of neuroscience. It is a rapidly growing area that has provided us with an illuminating picture of the chemical underpinnings of human behavior. This area is continuing to develop and has not only provided us with a greater understanding of the biological bases of human behavior, but also has influenced the treatment of many serious psychiatric disorders.

Other Systems

Other important systems interact with the brain to produce behavioral symptoms. Two important systems include the endocrine system and the autoimmune system. The endocrine system involves numerous glands throughout the body that secrete substances called hormones that have an effect on the brain, and, therefore, on behavior. These glands include the pituitary, parathyroid, thyroid, adrenals, testes, ovaries and pancreas. The anterior portion of the pituitary, after receiving chemical messages from the hypothalamus, stimulates these glands to secrete hormones. Feedback mechanisms operate between the glands and the hypothalamic-pituitary axis to regulate the secretion of these hormones into the blood stream. When there is a failure in the system, there is an over or under secretion of the hormones and emotional and behavioral symptoms develop. For example, the over or under production of thyroid hormone (secreted by the thyroid gland) has been known to produce depressive symptoms. Hyperthyroidism can also produce symptoms of anxiety. Adrenal tumors can secrete large quantities of adrenalin that can produce symptoms of panic disorder in the affected individual (Jubiz, 1985; Guyton, 1987).

More recently the association between stress and the neuroendocrine system has been further delineated with specific neurochemical events being described at the hormonal and receptor level (Post, 1992). One of the events in this "cascade of neurobiological events" (Post, 1992, p. 1002) includes the alteration of various hormone-releasing substances from the hypothalamus. The focus on the hypothalamic-pituitary adrenal axis and its role in depression and other psychiatric disorders continues to be an important area of study (Dubrovsky, 1993; DeJong and Roy, 1990; Checkley, 1992).

Connections also exist between the endocrine system and the immune system. The immune system defends the body against infection and other potential threats to survival. Recently there has been considerable interest in the relationship between stress, immunity and health with extensive research on the effects of stress on immune responsivity at a cellular level (Hickie, Hickie, Lloyd, Silove & Wakefield, 1993). The main finding has been that stress has a negative effect on the immune system. Individuals undergoing separation or divorce, bereavement, unemployment, and other significant stressors have been shown to have a decrease in lymphocytic response, the white cells that are involved in fighting infection (Dunn, 1988). A recent study with primates has shown that affiliative behaviors which result in stable social interactions enhance immunologic activity, suggesting the interaction between psychological or social support and immunity (Cohen, Kaplan, Cunnick, Manuck & Rabin, 1992).

BEHAVIORAL GENETICS

The biological model of personality infers that temperament, dispositions, and styles of personality are inherited. "Temperament" has been defined by Allport as "a person's emotional nature, including his susceptibility to emotional stimulation, his customary strength and speed of response, the quality of his prevailing mood, and all the peculiarities of fluctuation and intensity in mood" (Allport, 1961, p. 34). Temperament was initially defined globally to describe the general features of an individual's emotional life, but was later divided into three personality dispositions: activity level, sociability, and emotionality (Carver & Scheier, 1992; Hall & Lindzey, 1985). Activity level refers to the general energy level expended by the individual. The seeking of others and enjoyment of social activities is referred to as sociability. Emotionality refers to the individual's general arousability and the ease with which one becomes distressed in any given situation. The three emotions this pertains to are emotional distress, anger, and fear. There is some genetic evidence for the heritability of temperament, with a greater concordance observed between monozygotic than dizygotic twins, and adoptive children showing a temperament more like their biological sibs than their adoptive sibs (Carver & Scheier, 1992; Hall & Lindzey, 1985; Tellegen, Lyken, Bouchard, Wilcox, Segal, & Rich, 1988).

Eysenk described two personality traits that he attributed to differences in nervous system functioning: (1) neuroticism, and (2) extroversion/introversion (Carver & Scheier, 1992; Hall & Lindzey, 1985). Eysenk argued for a biological basis for neuroticism, stating that neurotics were emotionally unstable as a result of an "easy arousability" in the emotion centers of the brain. He applied this arousability theory to the extroversion/introversion dimension. Extroverts were described as dominant, uninhibited, outgoing, social seeking individuals, while introverts were seen as more inhibited and passive with a preference for being alone. These trait differences were attributed to baseline arousal levels in the reticular activating system, the structure in the brain that regulates attention and arousal. Eysenk postulated that introverts had higher resting arousal levels, and therefore their decrease in activity and preference for low social stimulation is a compensatory behavior to deal with this high level of arousal. Extroverts on the other hand were described as having a lower resting arousal level and therefore sought out stimulation to compensate for this baseline rate.

According to this view, personality traits are "reactions" to inherited arousal patterns that determine the degree to which an individual is stimulus seeking versus stimulus retreating. Based on this distinction it was predicted that introverts and extroverts would perform differently in two different situations—overstimulation and understimulation—with introverts performing poorly in the overstimulation condition. Initial results showed a differential performance between these two groups, but later research findings failed to replicate this differential response (Smith, 1993).

Others have also described similar personality profiles and have linked these to specific biological mechanisms. Zuckerman (1987; 1990) described the "sensation seeking" individual who is always in search of new experiences that are exciting and stimulating. What differentiated these individuals from others was their weak behavioral defense mechanisms against strong physiological responsiveness. Gray (1987) described three brain systems that regulated approach and avoidance behaviors that dealt with two fundamental dispositions, anxiety and impulsivity. Individuals with difficulties in impulsivity are viewed as being highly physiologically reactive to reward, whereas those with "trait anxiety" are highly reactive to cues of punishment.

All three biologically oriented personality theorists seem to focus on some form of physiological reactivity, whether this is described as extroversion, sensation seeking, or impulsivity. It is this arousal component or arousal seeking versus arousal avoiding that is described as an inherited disposition that predetermines how the individual will react in situations when this is activated.

Most of the research on the inheritance of personality has involved twin and adoption studies. In twin studies monozygotic (MZ) twins have shown a higher concordance than dizygotic (DZ) twins on measures of personality. These results have been reported for similar pairs raised apart (Tellegen et al., 1988). The investigators argue that genetic influences account for 50% of the variance, and after excluding the role of peers and the socialization process, the ultimate contribution of the family component is negligible. Their conclusion is in stark contrast to many psychological models of personality, such as the psychodynamic model, which will be discussed later.

In a meta-analysis of 103 articles on twin data McCartney and associates (McCartney, Harris & Bernieri, 1990) concluded that over time the genetic influence on personality wanes, and as twins grow older they tend to grow apart. This does not discount the genetic model of personality but it may illustrate that personality is dynamic and constantly developing or changing and although influenced by certain inherited factors, can be altered through development as a result of the interaction between predisposition and environment.

The influence of genetics is probably more evident in the major psychiatric disorders (Hyman & Nestler, 1983; Baron & Rainer, 1988; McGuffin & Thapar, 1990). In schizophrenia, twin studies have shown a higher concordance among MZ twins than DZ twins if one twin is identified to have the disorder (Schulz, 1991). First degree relatives are also at higher risk for the disorder; both pieces of evidence suggest an inherited vulnerability toward the disorder. Recent research has also focused on localizing specific genetic abnormalities in schizophrenia (Gorwood, Leboyer, d'Amato, Campion, Hillaire, Mallet & Feingold, 1992; Grove, Clementz, Iacono, & Katsanis, 1992; Schulz, 1991). The search for a genetic marker in bipolar disorder has also been investigated with mixed results. (Hebebrand, 1992; Edwards & Watt, 1989). Others have also questioned the genetic evidence for schizophrenia, bipolar disorder, and other behavioral conditions (Pam, 1990; Horgan, 1993).

In summary the biological model suggests that personality and vulnerability to certain psychological conditions or disturbances are predetermined, at least to some extent, and are based on an inherited predisposition towards a particular interactional style with the world.

The predetermined genetics gives an initial blueprint. Development, starting from in utero and thereafter, will affect how this blueprint is eventually shaped. Internal biological factors and external environmental factors will interact to produce a certain personality, and will determine whether or not a specific disorder will be expressed. Most see the importance of both genetics and environment. Some, however, pay attention only to the biological aspects, supporting their argument with the extensive research that has been carried out in this area. The scientific status of the biological model has been recently criticized by Pam (1990), who seriously questions the evidence that has been used to support this model, especially in biological psychiatry. It is possible, however, to appreciate the biological contributions to understanding human behavior without becoming overly reductionistic and impervious to the psychological models. Both contribute, and both are esssential.

ASSESSMENT

The idea that a thorough assessment should precede any form of treatment is not universal across all mental health disciplines, or even within disciplines. Psychologists, psychiatrists, and social workers will more than likely attend to different data in an initial interview. Even within groups there will be wide differences across the utilization of various assessment techniques and methods, and this difference usually depends on the clinician's orientation.

Assessment according to the biological perspective is usually carried out by psychiatrists, because this is the perspective that is taught in medical school and is well known to the psychiatry resident entering residency. This biological assessment is part of the standard medical assessment that involves taking a history, conducting a physical examination, and ordering various medical tests. First, a history of the presenting problem is obtained in order to get a clear description of the problem. Information regarding the onset and course of the presenting problem is essential for arriving at a diagnosis. While gathering this information, attention is focused on collecting a group of symptoms that conform to a particular syndrome. For example, disturbances in sleep, appetite, energy, concentration, and others, when occurring together are referred to a major depressive episode (DSM-IV; APA, 1994).

In addition to collecting data on the presenting problem, past medical and psychiatric history is also explored. Included in the past medical history are any medical or physical conditions from bith to the present that may have been responsible for the onset or progression of the presenting problem. Therefore any information about prenatal or antenatal complications, developmental milestones, and any major physical illness or injury that occurred in the early years, are all important areas to assess. Family history with respect to the presence of medical and psychiatric conditions is also noted. A family history of mood, anxiety, or psychotic disorders makes an individual more vulnerable to these conditions and may also suggest a specific medical treatment based on a family member's response to a specific treatment for the same disorder. Obtaining the history is the first and most important step in the assessment, since the information collected will direct the physical examination and determine which investigations will be ordered.

The next step is to determine whether or not there are specific biological factors responsible for the presenting problem. A physical examination is conducted to look for physical signs of a disease or illness. Although more commonly found in other areas of medicine, in psychiatry there are very few, if any, gross physical signs associated with any psychiatric conditions. Some findings include subtle movement disorders found in premedicated patients diagnosed with schizophrenia (Owens, Cunningham & Frith, 1982). At the present time there are no specific physical signs associated with the major psychiatric disorders, unless they are conditions that have an identifiable organic etiology. In most cases physical signs may be found if a medical condition is responsible for the presenting psychological condition. For example, if a stroke (or cerebral vascular incident) is responsible for the presentation of a depressive syndrome, then other neurological signs or symptoms such as weakness and aphasia may be present. If hypothyroidism is responsible for causing a depressive syndrome, then dry skin, weight gain, fatigue, and goiter, are physical signs that may be present.

Physical signs are usually more evident when there are specific medical illnesses responsible for the presenting symptoms. In psychiatry, the first step is to rule out any obvious organic pathology that may account for the symptoms. Certain illnesses are known to have affective, cognitive, and behavioral concomitants. Examples include seizure disorders (temporal lobe epilepsy), metabolic disorders (hyper/hypothyroidism), vascular events (strokes, transient ischemic attacks), infectious diseases (encephalitis), toxic disturbances (drugs-amphetamine, cocaine), and many others. Many medical conditions produce psychological symptoms, therefore this possibility needs to be assessed before embarking on a specific therapy.

After the history and physical examination are completed, the next step involves undertaking appropriate investigations. For example, blood tests that measure hormones (e.g., thyroid hormone), street drugs (amphetamines, PCPs), white cell counts to determine infection, are but a few of the investigations one can use to determine the presence of a specific disease or illness.

In psychiatry there are few if any definitive tests that confirm or disconfirm a diagnosis. Although once having held some promise, the dexamethasone suppression test, a test that was found to show a specific pattern in depression (nonsuppression of cortisol), was found to be low in specificity, and therefore lost its position as a possible biological marker for depression (APA, 1987b).

In addition to "blood tests" other investigations that assess a structural or functional change in any system can also help in determining a biological etiology. Examples include an electroencephalogram (EEG) and computed tomography (CT) scan of the brain. An EEG assesses abnormal electrical activity in the brain. A CT scan provides information regarding any structural changes in the brain, such as space occupying lesions (tumors), and vascular events (strokes). Most of these investigations are used to diagnose conditions that have a known biological etiology. Recent reports indicate that about 5% of patients discharged with a psychiatric diagnosis receive a CT scan of the head, and an even lower figure has been reported for EEGs (2.8%) (Olfson, 1992).

New technology such as the PET (Positron Emission Tomography) scan and MRI (Magnetic Resonance Imaging) scan have given us a clearer picture of the brain. The PET scan provides a picture of brain activity based on which areas are utilizing a glucose-like radioactive substance. Glucose utilization is associated with increased brain activity. The MRI scan also provides a picture of the brain with greater resolution, based on how the individual atoms within the brain tissue respond to a magnetic pulse. This gives a very sharp picture of brain in comparison to a CT scan (Kandel, 1985a; Smith, 1993). These techniques, especially the PET scan, are used primarily for research rather than diagnostic purposes.

Other investigations that assess brain function or intellectual function include cognitive and neuropsychiatric testing. Certain conditions such as dementia show a specific pattern on neuropsychological testing such as disturbance in short-term memory, visual-spatial difficulties, and various disturbances with language (Lischman, 1987). Other conditions such as schizophrenia, have also been found to have various neurocognitive deficits especially in the attention and information processing area. Neuropsychological testing is essential in diagnosing dementia, and assessing cognitive impairment in head injuries and other related conditions.

A biologically oriented or general psychiatrist may be more likely to consider medical conditions prior to considering treatment. Nonphysician clinicians may receive referrals after this assessment process has been completed.

FOUR PS

Having completed a biological assessment by obtaining the history, conducting a physical examination, and ordering the relevant investigations, it is now possible to complete the first column of the grid along the four Ps. Table 5.1 illustrates how to fill out the various columns on the grid, and for now the focus is on the biological column. Under this column ***predisposing*** biological factors include ones that contribute to an individual's biological vulnerability towards a particular disorder. Among these factors are family history for a specific disorder, or genetic abnormalities, prenatal, postnatal and early developmental insults that result in a structural or functional deficit in the brain or other system. A common biological predisposing factor is a positive family psychiatric history for a particular disorder that renders an individual more vulnerable towards that disorder. For example, a 35-year-old woman presenting with symptoms of depression and a positive family history for a mood disorder is considered to be biologically vulnerable toward this condition. A genetically transmitted disorder that can present with psychiatric symptoms is Huntington's chorea.

Any complication arising in the prenatal or postnatal period may render an individual vulnerable to a particular disorder. Some researchers have suggested various prenatal complications such as maternal viral infection to be responsible for the development of schizophrenia (Sham, O'Callaghan, Takei, Murray, Hane, & Murray, 1992) but this has been challenged by others (Crow & Dore, 1992). Certain birth complications such as prematurity, respiratory distress, and hyperbilirubinemia, have been implicated in a causal role in the development of certain psychiatric conditions in children and adults; however, the research is fraught with methodological problems and has not been successfully replicated. For the most part these birth complications have been implicated in a number of medical, psychiatric, and psychological conditions, and are therefore nonspecific findings in many disorders.

Predisposing biological factors then are those factors that make an individual biologically vulnerable to a particular disorder. As discussed above there are no definitive markers that can accurately and reliably predict the occurrence of a psychiatric or psychological condition, ex-

Table 5.1
Biological Perspective

Predisposing	* family history for specific disorder (e.g., bipolar disorder) * prenatal, postnatal complications (maternal infection, malnutrition, etc.) * developmental conditions (e.g., autism, learning disability) * inherited temperament * genetic disorders (e.g., Huntington's chorea)
Precipitating	* change in biological system: - infections (e.g., encephalitis) - toxic (e.g., drug intoxication) - neoplastic (e.g., brain tumor) - metabolic (e.g., hyperthyroidism) - vascular (e.g., stroke) - traumatic (e.g., head injury)
Perpetuating	* chronic illness - e.g., multiple sclerosis, lupus - e.g., untreated hyperthyroidism * chronic ingestion of substances - e.g., illicit drugs - e.g., alcohol - e.g., caffeine - e.g., medications
Protective	* negative family history for psychiatric disorder * negative family history for medical illnesses * good physical health/diet * intelligence * prophylactic medication (e.g., lithium) * regular physical exercise

cept in specific conditions where the genetic transmission of a disorder is known and can be relatively reliably predicted. Future research may help identify the genes responsible for specific psychiatric disorders such as bipolar disorder and schizophrenia. For now biological predisposing factors are assumed, given present research findings that suggests that vulnerability to psychiatric disorders seems to run in families.

Precipitating biological factors are physical events that trigger the onset of a disorder. Some of these include infectious (encephalitis), traumatic (head injury), toxic (drugs), metabolic (hyperthyroid), neoplastic (brain tumor), and vascular events (stroke), to name a few. A variety of biological precipitants are known to produce psychological and psychiatric symptoms. Some of these include: antidepressants precipitating mania in a vulnerable individual, panic attacks precipitated by cocaine abuse, strokes that may produce depressive or cognitive symptoms, post-viral depressions, and psychosis in amphetamine intoxication. A precipitating factor may go on to be a perpetuating factor if it becomes chronic. For example, alcohol ingested in large quantities can produce depressive symptoms in some individuals. If the individual continues to maintain a consistent level of alcohol intake, a persistent mood disturbance may ensue. Therefore when a precipitant takes on a chronic form, it is considered a perpetuating factor because it is maintaining the condition or disorder.

Perpetuating factors are those biological factors that chronically influence the brain to produce psychiatric symptoms. These include chronic substance abuse, use of prescribed medications, or chronic illnesses that produce a variety of psychiatric and physical symptoms. A good example involving alcohol abuse was described above. The use of various medications can also perpetuate a psychiatric disorder, a condition commonly seen in many elderly patients who take several medications simultaneously. Examples include depression secondary to various antihypertensive agents, confusion or psychosis in patients who are on steroidal medications, and persistent confusion and disorientation in the elderly patient taking even small doses of sedating medications such as the benzodiazapines. A more common example is chronic high caffeine intake in an individual with persistent symptoms of anxiety. All these examples involve the chronic ingestion of specific substances.

Chronic physical conditions can also perpetuate psychological symptoms. Examples include depressive-like symptoms (decreased energy, fatigue, etc.) evident in chronic anemia and persistent hypo- or hyperthyroidism, and generalized anxiety in hyperadrenalism. These are but a few examples of perpetuating biological factors that maintain chronic symptoms.

Protective biological factors are those that act as buffers to protect the individual from various psychiatric and psychological conditions, thereby making the individual less vulnerable to a specific disorder. These factors include a negative family psychiatric history (or absence of a risk factor), good physical health, above average intelligence, and even prophylactic medication, such as lithium, that protects against future illness episodes in bipolar disorder (Baldessarini, 1985). Other factors could include the daily practice of relaxation exercises, as well as regular physical exercise, that through various physical mechanisms help alleviate certain disturbing emotional symptoms such as anxiety and depression. The maintenance of a good nutritious diet as well as regular exercise may physically protect the individual by maintaining a good immune response in the presence of psychological stress.

COPING-RESPONSE STYLE

An individual with a biological coping-response style interprets signs and symptoms of psychological distress as indicative of medical illness. They may be more likely to seek a family physician for medical attention, and less likely to consider referral to a mental health professional. They may use medications more frequently to cope with distressing symptoms, or other medical or surgical interventions may be sought to obtain symptomatic relief. This persistent search for medical answers to explain psychological or physical symptoms can be viewed as a biological coping-response style in that the individual's method of coping is physically, rather than psychologically oriented. Individuals who are preoccupied with physical symptoms are sometimes referred to as somatizers or hypochondriacs, the former being preoccupied with multiple physical symptoms, while the latter believe they have a serious medical illness. Although referred to as a biological coping-response style, these methods of coping can also be seen as defenses that involve the "displacement" of psychological distress onto the body. Because the focus is on the body, it will be considered a biological coping-response style. Individuals with this type of coping response style may be more compliant with a biological rather than a psychological treatment, at least in the early phase of treatment.

Whether individuals can actually be described as having a biological coping-response style is an open empirical question. Clinical experience does suggest that some individuals are more bodily focused than others and may be more comfortable entertaining the possibility of a physical rather than a mental illness, given the stigma associated with the latter. Therefore, this may be an important coping-response style to consider when one is recommending and planning treatment.

If the assessment yields sufficient evidence for a strong biological formulation, and the coping-response style suggests an individual with a biological coping orientation, then a biological treatment is indicated if such a treatment has been demonstrated to be effective given the individual's presenting condition. If the evidence for a biological formulation is moderate then the coping-response style and current treatment practice should dictate the treatment. If however the biological formulation is weak, alternate formulation models should be explored in making treatment decisions. It may be difficult to implement psychological treatments in an individual who has a rigid biological coping-response style; however, a good therapeutic alliance should create a collaborative relationship necessary for a good outcome.

TREATMENT

Treatment according to this perspective is aimed at altering the biological structure or function implicated in the etiology of the disorder. Biological treatments are of two varieties, medical or surgical. Medical treatments include administering medications to correct chemical imbalances or other substances (e.g., radiation) to produce a desired effect. These medications are used to relieve distressing symptoms or to prevent them from occurring. Surgical techniques are those invasive procedures that attempt to remove or alter physical structures, and although used for many medical conditions, are rarely used in psychiatry except in severe intractable cases. The four biological treatments that have been discussed in the mental health field include: pharmacotherapy, electroconvulsive therapy, light therapy, and psychosurgery. In this section the first three will be discussed in more detail, as they are more frequently practiced than the last. Most of the discussion will focus on the use of medication as this is the most common biological treatment in psychiatry and medicine.

PHARMACOTHERAPY

The most common form of biological treatment for psychological disorders involves the prescribing of psychotropic medications. Although nonpsychiatric physicians use a variety of medications to alter psychological symptoms, psychiatrists are usually seen as the experts in the medical management of psychiatric disorders. The major pharmacological agents used in psychiatry are the psychotropic or psychoactive medications. In psychiatry they are more traditionally known as: antipsychotics, antidepressants, antimanics and antianxiety or anxiolytics. This is the traditional classification that has been used in most textbooks of psychiatry and psychopharmacology until recently (Kaplan and Sadock, 1991; 1993). This classification system is considered less valid today due to the variety of disorders that are treated by each of these agents. For example, antidepressants, although originally used for treating depression, are also used for treating many other disorders such as panic disorder, chronic pain syndromes, and cocaine withdrawal. For the trainee however, this classification system is practical and provides an organizational framework for learning the major pharmacotherapeutic agents used in psychiatry.

Historically these classes of medications have been relatively new, all being developed after the 1950s. Most of these drugs were discovered accidentally, in that they were originally designed for other purposes and were coincidentally found to be effective in relieving certain psychological conditions. The biological theories of the major psychiatric disorders were therefore developed retrospectively; once a medication was found to be effective, the mechanism of action of the specific agent was then said to be responsible for the disorder.

Antipsychotics

The first class of pharmacological agents to be discovered was the antipsychotics. This was the more traditional name given to a class of medications found helpful in treating severe agitation and psychosis. They are now more commonly referred to as the neuroleptics. The first antipsychotic that was discovered was chlorpromazine (thorazine). As mentioned above this medication was discovered rather serendipitously, when Charpentier in 1950, synthesized this drug to be used as an adjunct in anaesthesia (Baldessarini, 1985). In the same year Delay and Deniker used this medication to treat severe agitation and psychotic symptoms (Carlson, 1988). Toward the end of the 1950s Janssen discovered another antipsychotic, Haloperidol. Over the next few decades numerous other antipsychotics were developed that significantly changed the milieu in psychiatric hospitals. Patients with chronic psychotic disorders such as schizophrenia, now required much less restraint and supervision, and were able to leave the hospital. The psychiatric hospital became a much quieter, more controlled environment, and these medications brought dramatic relief to many patients who had suffered for years with these distressing symptoms. Prior to the use of antipsychotics, treatment such as insulin coma and frontal lobotomies were carried out in such patients.

Psychopharmacological research produced additional antipsychotic drugs. Efficacy across the various antipsychotics remains equal, in that all antipsychotics seem to be equally effective, and differ with respect to their potency and side effect profile (Bernstein, 1988). Haloperidol is considered to have the highest potency in that a small amount of the drug is needed to produce the desired effect. Chlorpromazine is the least potent requiring larger dosages to produce the same effect as a small dose of Haldol. In between these two antipsychotics are several others that differ in their potency and side effect profile.

Although antipsychotics revolutionized the treatment of psychosis and schizophrenia, their side effects made it difficult to obtain compliance. Side effects can be described as acute or chronic. Acute side effects include various movement disorders such as dystonic crises (sudden muscles spasms), parkinsonism and akathesia referred to as extrapyramidal side effects (Cassey & Keepes, 1988). The underlying pathophysiology of these side effects involves the blockade of dopamine receptors. Because the antipsychotics were found to block dopamine, it was hypothesized that the etiology of schizophrenia must be due to an excess of dopamine. Antipsychotics were found to block dopamine receptors, thereby preventing it from acting on the post synaptic cell. This creates a hypodopaminergic state similar to that seen in Parkinson's disease.

A worrisome side effect known as tardive dyskinesia was noted in patients who received long term administration of these medications (Yassa, Nair, Iskandar & Schwartz, 1990; Bernstein, 1988). Involuntary lip smacking movements which were not always irreversible once medication was discontinued were observed. Stopping the medication can sometimes reverse the situation, but can also for a brief period worsen the symptoms. A relatively new neuroleptic known as Clozapine has been developed that blocks dopamine in the cortical and limbic areas, thereby decreasing the risk of these side effects (Gerlack & Hansen, 1992). However, clozapine has its own serious side effects that require careful monitoring (agranulocytosis—dramatic decrease in white cell count). Despite this, it has been shown to be an effective antipsychotic agent, particularly in treatment resistant schizophrenia (Kane, Honigfeld, Singer & Mal, 1988; Krupp & Barnes, 1992).

Neuroleptic malignant syndrome, a potentially life threatening condition has been observed in a small percentage of patients taking these medications (Rosebush & Stewart, 1989). Symptoms such as fever, tachycardia, tachypnea, and other symptoms of autonomic hyperarousal are present. Mortality is high. There is no specific treatment for this condition except for the maintenance of fluids and electrolytes, although the use of some specific agents has been discussed.

Antipsychotics can be given in a variety of forms, orally in pills or liquid or through intramuscular injection. Long-acting forms are also available that can be given every 2–3 weeks or once a month. This is ideal for the noncompliant patient, and although highly effective it has a higher risk of producing the side effects described above (Bernstein, 1988).

Antipsychotics are indicated in the treatment of severe agitation and psychosis. They are therefore used in the treatment of schizophrenia and other psychotic disorders such as mania and psychotic depression. In small doses they can be effective in treating the agitation associated with dementia, as well as certain movement disorders such as Tourette's syndrome and Huntington's chorea.

Antidepressants

The next group of medications discovered were the antidepressants. Although referred to as antidepressant, these medications have come to be used in the treatment of other disorders such as panic disorder, obsessive-compulsive disorder, eating disorders, chronic pain, attention deficit disorder, enuresis, migraine headaches, and others. Their discovery significantly changed the course of depressive illness by alleviating the depressive symptoms over a few weeks and preventing relapse. Prior to the discovery of antidepressants, a depressive episode could go on for up to a year untreated. The first antidepressant, imipramine (a tricyclic antidepressant) was discovered in the 1950s, again rather accidentally. Given its structural similarity to chlorpromazine, Thomas Khune first used it as an antipsychotic and found that it was not successful in relieving agitation. He later found that it seemed to improve depressive symptoms in some patients. In the late 1950s another antidepressant was discovered belonging to the group now known as the monoamine oxidase inhibitors (MAOI). Iproniazid, an antituberculous agent, was found to improve depressive symptoms in these patients. The first report on the effectiveness of this MAOI in depressed patients was published in 1958 by Nathan Kline (Baldessarini, 1985).

Today numerous antidepressants exist; again all equally effective in treating depressive symptoms (APA, 1993). The first group was called the tricyclics due to the three-ring nucleus these compounds contained. They included imipramine, amytriptyline, and others. Later newer antidepressants similar to the tricyclics but containing additional rings were discovered, and the new name heterocyclics was given to include both groups. The MAOIs were also used and two compounds were isolated, phenelzine and tranylcypromine. MAOIs were initially unpopular given the dietary restriction necessary when administering this medication. Tyramine-containing foods such as some red wines, beers, pickled products, cheese, and others were prohibited while on this medication due to the hypertensive crisis that could occur. Other adverse reactions were also discovered when these drugs were used in conjunction with medications such as antihistamines and demerol. As a result, psychiatrists were initially hesitant to use these medications. Nevertheless, the positive results obtained with these drugs, especially in patients that presented with a more agitated, anxious, atypical depression increased their use (Baldessarini, 1985; Bernstein, 1988).

Most of these medications cause side effects making compliance difficult. The heterocyclics produce side effects such as dry mouth, blurred vision, constipation, urinary hesitancy, weight gain, tremor, and agitation. Dizziness, weight gain, agitation, and insomnia are commonly experienced with the MAOIs.

Following the heterocyclic and MAOIs were the atypical antidepressants: Trazodone, Alprazolam, Buproprion, and Nomifensine, now referred to as the second generation antidepressants. (Baldessarini, 1985; Bernstein, 1988). These were all found to be effective with their own side effect profiles. Still newer antidepressants were discovered and became available in the late 1980s (APA, 1993). These included the newer serotonergic agents such as fluoxetine (Prozac), fluvoxamine (Luvox), paroxetine (Paxil) and sertaline (Zoloft). Moclobemide, a new MAOI, has also been developed that does not demand the dietary restriction of the earlier forms (Versiani, Nardi, Figueria & Stable, 1990). All these medications are effective antidepressants without having the side effect profile of the older medications. They do, however, have their own side effects which include nausea, headaches, restlessness, and insomnia. Their effectiveness continues to be evaluated and future research will confirm their wide applicability.

Although not strictly considered an antidepressant, lithium has been used as an adjunct in treating refractory depression, and is effective in many cases (Baldessarini, 1985; Bernstein, 1988). The thyroid hormone triiodothyrorine (T3) has also been used as an adjunct in treatment resistant cases.

Antimanics

In addition to the use of lithium as an adjunct in the treatment of depression, it is commonly used in the treatment of mania and in the prophylactic treatment of bipolar disorder. Lithium is a salt, which was discovered in 1950 by an Australian psychiatrist, John Cade, who found that when administered to monkeys they became lethargic (Kaplan & Sadock, 1988). This finding led him to administer lithium to agitated psychiatric patients. Later the drug was used in treating individuals with bipolar disorder, some cases of schizophrenia, and impulse disorders.

The mechanism of action of lithium is not yet clearly understood but is speculated to occur at the intracellular level affecting certain enzymes responsible for determining the cells' response to neurotransmitters. Prior to the administration of lithium, a work-up to assess hydration status, as well as thyroid and renal function, should be carried out. Side effects include gastric symptoms such as diarrhea, frequent urination, tremor, acne, weight gain, and fatigue. Side effects can lead to poor compliance in patients. Blood levels can be drawn to monitor compliance and should determine the proper dosage as lithium has a narrow margin of safety. Toxic levels of lithium can be hazardous and result in permanent brain damage, especially to the cerebellum.

Unfortunately, not all patients are responsive to lithium, and a small group known as rapid cyclers (four illness episodes for two weeks or more/year) required additional medications to achieve good results (Baldessarini, 1985). Alternate medications include the anticonvulsants carbamezapine (tegretol) and valproic acid (valproate) (Calabrese & Delucchi, 1990). These medications can be used by themselves or as an adjunct to lithium.

Antianxiety

The final group of psychoactive drugs discovered were the antianxiety or anxiolytics. These medications have also been used as muscle relaxants, anticonvulsants, hypnotic-sedatives, and in managing aggression. The benzodiazepines, a new class of drugs, were discovered by Sternback at the Roche laboratories in the late 1950s (Greenblatt & Shader, 1974). The more commonly known medications in this group include Valium, Ativan, and the long acting Clonazepam. These medications were initially used extensively by family physicians to treat anxiety and insomnia, with Valium being the most common drug prescribed in the 1960s. Since then there has been a decrease in prescribing Valium for these conditions, and newer benzodiazepines and other classes of drugs have been used. The most common use of benzodiazepines has been in the treatment of anxiety disorders; however, these drugs have also been used in conjunction with neuroleptics in the treatment of agitation associated with psychosis and mania. Benzodiazepines have also been combined with antidepressants to treat the "agitated-anxious" depressed individual. However, newer antidepressants have been developed to alleviate these symptoms, decreasing the need for an anxiolytic agent.

The major difficulty with the benzodiazepines was their potential for abuse. Patients on these medications for an extended period of time had difficulty terminating these drugs due to withdrawal symptoms. The sedating side effects of most benzodiazepines led to the discovery of another antianxiety drug known as buspirone. This medication has been found to have less addictive potential, a longer onset (1–3 wks) and does not have the sedative/hypnotic effects of the benzodiazepines that contribute to excessive sedation and drowsiness. Its efficacy, however, is questionable (Baldessarini, 1985; Bernstein, 1988).

Despite the potential for abuse, the benzodiazepines are one of the safest medications when taken in an overdose, and their effectiveness in the treatment of a variety of conditions has made them a very useful pharmacological agent.

ELECTROCONVULSIVE THERAPY

All the medications discussed above have significantly reduced the very distressing symptoms present in patients suffering from major psychiatric disorders. Another medical treatment that has been found very effective in the treatment of severe depression is electroconvulsive therapy (ECT). ECT was discovered by Ugo Cerletti and Lucio Bini in the late 1930s in Rome (Endler & Persad, 1988). Since that time, this procedure has been altered from bilateral to unilateral placement of the electrodes, although controversy exists as to which is more effective. Recommendations regarding the energy required to produce a seizure has also changed from a larger to a smaller dose. The most common regimen practiced today is nondominant unilateral, brief pulse ECT (APA, 1993). This method produces a low energy bilateral seizure of at least 30 seconds duration and is associated with less cognitive impairment. This form of therapy has been highly controversial and has been criticized by many ex-patients and their families. A task force was assembled to address the concerns expressed by this group, that this procedure was archaic, and produced significant cognitive impairment. Extensive research to date has not demonstrated any long-term cognitive impairment associated with ECT. Short-term memory loss for events just prior to the procedure has been reported (APA, 1990). However, an 80–90% improvement rate was noted in severe depression associated with extensive psychomotor retardation and delusional symptoms. ECT has also been recommended for those severely ill patients who need more rapid improvement, since antidepressants require several weeks before positive effects are observed. Examples include the severely depressed elderly who refuse to eat or drink, and are a high suicidal and medical risk. This therapy has also been used in the treatment of mania, catatonia, and refractory schizophrenia.

The specific mechanism of action responsible for the effectiveness of ECT has not been defined, although neurochemical theories have been suggested. This procedure is not undertaken in any individual who has a space occupying lesion, or increased intracranial pressure secondary to any etiology. Nevertheless, according to the APA Task Force (1990), there is no absolute contraindication for ECT. The major risk in administering ECT is due to the anaesthetic given prior to producing the seizure. Although at one time categorized as psychosurgery, ECT is considered a medical treatment in that the process affects neurochemistry rather than neural structure.

LIGHT THERAPIES

In addition to ECT another form of non-pharmacological medical treatment is the use of light therapy in the treatment of seasonal affective disorders (Rosenthal, Sekis, Carpenter, Tary, Mendelson & Whert, 1985). A particular seasonal pattern was discovered in some individuals who reported depressive symptoms that coincided with the onset of a particular season. There has been speculation that this disorder results from an interaction between light and the hormone melatonin. If these individuals are given light therapy that consists of 2,500 lux (200 times indoor light) for a specific period of time, there is an improvement noticed in the amelioration of their depressive symptoms. These symptoms, in addition to the classic symptoms of depression, included hyperinsomnia, carbohydrate craving, and lethargy, all of which improved after light therapy. The diagnosis and treatment are still controversial but have been included in the DSM-IV under the category Mood Disorders (APA, 1994).

PSYCHOSURGERY

The last form of biological therapy to be discussed is psychosurgery. Psychosurgery which alters the structure of the brain is rarely practiced today. The first investigators to use these techniques were two U.S. scientists, Jacobsen and Fulton, who in 1935 performed frontal lobotomies in monkeys and found that this had a calming effect. Two Portuguese psychiatrists Moniz and Lima found a similar effect when severing white matter in the frontal lobe in 20 psychotic patients. Moniz won a Nobel Prize for this work in 1949. Freeman and Watts refined this procedure and called it transorbital frontal leucotomy. They performed the procedure by inserting an instrument through the orbit into the frontal lobe. By 1940 the rate of this surgical procedure rose to 5,000 a year. As research accumulated, this process was discontinued due to postsurgical cognitive deficits, the high risk and invasiveness of the procedure, and the discovery of antipsychotic medications. Today psychosurgery is seldom practiced and is used only in very rare, intractable cases of some disorders such as a severe form of obsessive compulsive disorder (Kaplan & Sadock, 1988).

SUMMARY

The biological treatments described above are very effective in the treatment of the major psychiatric disorders. Most of these treatments are prescribed by psychiatrists or family physicians. Psychiatry residents are expected to learn all these treatments, and they receive three or four years of training in how to administer these medications successfully. Most psychiatrists prescribe psychotropics, but differ according to the type of patients seen in their practice. A psychiatrist who practices psychoanalysis or other forms of psychodynamic psychotherapy may be less likely to prescribe these medications than one who works in a chronic psychiatric institution or in a general hospital psychiatric unit. Psychiatric nurses, social workers, and psychologists who work in these settings will have some exposure to these therapies. Other non-M.D. mental health professionals who do not have adequate exposure to these therapies should keep in mind that in some cases, a medication or alternate medical therapy may be the first treatment of choice. Having some knowledge of this literature and this perspective will prevent the administration of nonpharmacologic therapies that may be ineffective as a first line treatment.

Prescribing medications does not mean that psychotherapy is contraindicated. In fact this is rarely the case. The treatment of the major psychiatric disorders requires the careful combination of medication and psychotherapy to produce the best outcome. It is the timing and the specific psychotherapy chosen that are important. For example, in the treatment of obsessive compulsive disorders it has been found that the serotonergic antidepressant clomipramine and the behavioral intervention of exposure and response prevention are the treatments of choice for these disorders, which have generally been shown to be unresponsive to the more traditional psychoanalytic therapies. Knowledge of this information will prevent the therapist from using other less effective therapies. Non-M.D. professionals can refer these patients to a psychiatrist or work collaboratively to provide the best possible combination of therapies. In this situation, the psychiatrists could prescribe and monitor the medication, while the psychologists can carry out the behavior therapy, an area that is better known and more commonly practiced by this group of professionals.

Therefore, knowledge of this perspective gives another dimension to the understanding and treatment of psychiatric and psychological disorders.

REFERENCES

Allport, G. W. (1961). *Pattern and Growth in Personality.* New York: Holt, Rinehart & Winston.

American Psychiatric Association. (1994). *The Diagnostic and Statistical Manual of Mental Disorders* (4th ed.). Washington, DC: Author.

American Psychiatric Association Task Force on Laboratory Tests in Psychiatry. The Dexamethasone Test: An Overview of its Current Status in Psychiatry. (1987b). *American Journal of Psychiatry, 44,* 1253–1262.

American Psychiatric Association. (1990). *American Psychiatric Association Task Force on Electroconvulsive Therapy: The Practice of Electroconvulsive Therapy.* Washington, DC: Author.

American Psychiatric Association. (1993). Practical Guidelines for Major Depressive Disorder in Adults. *American Journal of Psychiatry, 150,* (4 suppl).

Andreasen, N., Rezai, K., Alliger, R., Swayze, V. W., Flaum, M., Kirchner, P., Cohen, G., & O'Leary, D.S. (1992). Hypofrontality in Neuroleptic Naive Patients and in Patients with Chronic Schizophrenia. *Archives of General Psychiatry, 49,* 943–958.

Baldessarini, R. J. (1985). *Chemotherapy in Psychiatry: Principles and Practice.* Cambridge, MA: Harvard University Press.

Baron, M., & Rainer, J. D. (1988). Molecular Genetics and Human Diseases: Implications for Modern Psychiatric Research and Practice. *British Journal of Psychiatry, 152,* 741–753.

Berman, K. F., & Weinberger, D. R. (1991). Functional Localization in the Brain in Schizophrenia. In A. Tasman, & S. M. Goldfinger (Eds.), *Review of Psychiatry.* Washington, DC: American Psychiatric Press.

Bernstein, G. G. (1988). *Handbook of Drug Therapy in Psychiatry* (2nd ed.). Littleton, MA: PSG Publishing.

Breier, A., Buchanan, R., Elkashef, A., Munson, R., Patrick, B., & Gellad, F.

(1992). Brain Morphology and Schizophrenia. *Archives of General Psychiatry, 49,* 921–926.

Calabrese, J. R., & Delucchi, A. (1990). Spectrum of Efficacy of Valproate in 55 Patients with Rapid Cycling Bioplar Disorder. *American Journal of Psychiatry, 147,* 431–434.

Carlson, A. (1988). Reflections on the History in Psychopharmacology: Current Trends. In D. E. Cassey, & A. Vibeke Christensen (Eds.), *Psychopharmacology Series: Number 5.* Berlin, Germany: Springer-Verlag.

Carver, C. S., & Scheier, M. F. (1992). *Perspectives on Personality* (2nd ed.). Needham Heights, MA: Allyn and Bacon.

Cassey, D. E., & Keepes, G. A. (1988). Neuroleptic Side Effects: Acute Extra Pyramidal Syndromes and Tardive Dyskinesia in Psychopharmacology: Current Trends. In D. Cassey, & A. V. Christensen, (Eds.), *Psychopharmacology Series #5.* Berlin, Germany: Springer-Verlag.

Checkley, S. (1992). Neuroendocrine Mechanisms and the Precipitation of Depression by Life Events. *British Journal of Psychiatry, 160* (suppl 15), 7–17.

Cohen, S., Kaplan, J. R., Cunnick, J. E., Manuck, S. B., & Rabin, B. S. (1992). Chronic Social Stress, Affiliation, and the Cellular Immune Response in Non Human Primates. *Psychological Science, 3,* 301–304.

Crow, T. J., & Dore, D. J. (1992). Prenatal Exposure to Influenza Does Not Cause Schizophrenia. *British Journal of Psychiatry, 161,* 390–393.

DeJong, J. A., & Roy, A. (1990). Relationship of Cognitive Factors to CSF Corticotropin-Releasing Hormone in Depression. *American Journal of Psychiatry, 147,* 350–352.

Dubrovsky, B. (1993). Effects of Adrenal Cortex Hormones on Limbic Structures: Some Experimental and Clinical Correlations Related to Depression. *Journal of Psychiatry and Neuroscience, 18*(1), 4–16.

Dunn, A. J. (1988). Nervous System Immune System Interaction: An Overview. *Journal of Receptor Research, 8,* 589–607.

Edwards, J. H., & Watt, D. C. (1989). Caution in Locating the Gene for Affective Disorder. *Psychological Medicine, 19,* 273–275.

Endler, N. S., & Persad, E. (1988). *ECT: The Myths and the Realities.* Toronto, Ontario: Hans Hober.

Fischbach, G. D. (1992). Mind and Brain. *Science, 267*(3), 48–57.

Gerlack, J., & Hansen, L. (1992). Clonazepam and D1/D2 Antagonism in Extrapyramidal factors. *British Journal of Psychiatry, 160* (suppl 17), 34–37.

Gorwood, P., Leboyer, M., d'Amato, T., Campion, J. M., Hillaire, D., Mallet, I., & Feingold, J. (1992). Evidence for a Pseudo Autosomal Focus for Therapy: I: A Replication study Using Phenotype Analysis. *British Journal of Psychiatry, 161,* 55–58.

Gray, J. A. (1987). Perspectives on Anxiety and Impulsivity: A Commentary. *Journal of Research in Personality, 21,* 495–509.

Green, L. A., Mooney, J., & Schildkraut, J. J. (1990). The Biochemistry of Affective Disorders: An Overview. In A. M. Nicholi Jr. (Ed.), *The New*

Harvard Guide to Modern Psychiatry. Cambridge, MA: Belknap Press of Harvard University Press.

Greenblatt, D. J., & Shader, R. I. (1974). *Benzodiazepines and Clinical Practice*. New York: Raven Press.

Grove, W. M., Clementz, B. A., Iacono, W. G., & Katsanis, J. (1992). Smooth Pursuit, Ocular Motor Dysfunction in Schizophrenia. Evidence for a Major Gene. *American Journal of Psychiatry, 49,* 1362–1368.

Guyton, A. C. (1987). *Basic Neuroscience: Anatomy and Physiology*. Philadelphia: W. B. Saunders.

Hall, C. S., & Lindzey, G. (1985). *Introduction to Theories of Personality*. New York: John Wiley and Sons.

Hebebrand, J. (1992). A Critical Appraisal of X-linked Bipolar Illness: Evidence for the Assumed Mode of Inheritance is Lacking. *British Journal of Psychiatry, 161,* 1–11.

Hickie, I., Hickie, C., Lloyd, A., Silove, D., & Wakefield, D. (1993). Impaired In-vivo Immune Response in Patients with Melancholia. *British Journal of Psychiatry, 162,* 651–657.

Horgan, J. (1993). Eugenics Revisited. *Scientific American, 263,* 121–131.

Hyman, S. E., & Nestler, E. J. (1983). *The Molecular Foundation of Psychiatry*. Washington, DC: American Psychiatric Press.

Javitch, J. A., & Kaufman, C. A. (1991). Schizophrenia and the Dopamine D-2 Receptor. In A. Tasman, & S. Goldfinger (Eds.), *Review of Psychiatry*. Washington, DC: American Psychiatric Press.

Jubiz, W. (1985). *Endocrinology: A Logical Approach for Clinicians* (2nd ed.). New York: McGraw-Hill.

Kandel, E. R. (1985a). Brain and Behavior. In E. R. Kandel, & J. H. Schwartz, (Eds.), *Principles of Neuroscience* (2nd ed.). New York: Elsevier.

Kandel, E. R. (1985b). Nerve Cells and Behavior. In E. R. Kandel, J. H. Schwartz (Eds.), *Principles of Neuroscience* (2nd ed.). New York: Elsevier.

Kane, J., Honigfeld, Singer, J., & Mal, H. (1988). Clonazapine for the Treatment Resistant Schizophrenic. *Archives of General Psychiatry, 45,* 789–796.

Kaplan, H. I., & Sadock, B. J. (1988). *Synopsis of Psychiatry: Behavioral Sciences. Clinical Psychiatry* (5th ed.). Baltimore, MD: Williams and Wilkins.

Kaplan, H. I. & Sadock, B. J. (1991). *Synopsis of Psychiatry: Behavioral Sciences. Clinical Psychiatry* (6th ed.). Baltimore, MD: Williams and Wilkins.

Kaplan, H. I., & Sadock, B. J. (1993). *Pocket Handbook of Psychiatric Drug Treatment*. Baltimore, MD: Williams and Wilkins.

Kolb, B., & Whishaw, I.Q. (1990). *Fundamentals of Human Neuropsychology*. New York: W. H. Freeman.

Krupp, P., & Barnes, P. (1992). Clozapine-Associated Agranulocytosis: Risk and Aetiology. *British Journal of Psychiatry, 160* (supp 17), 38–40.

Lischman, W. A. (1987). *Organic Psychiatry, the Psychological Consequences of Cerebral Disorders* (2nd ed.). London, England: Blackwell Scientific Publications.

McCartney, K., Harris, M. J., & Bernieri, F. (1990). Growing up and Growing

Apart: A Developmental Meta-analysis of Twin Studies. *Psychological Bulletin, 107,* 226–237.
McGuffin, P., & Thapar, A. (1990). The Genetics of Personality Disorder. *British Journal of Psychiatry, 160,* 12–23.
Mora, G. (1970). The History of Psychiatry: It's Relevance for the Psychiatrist. *American Journal of Psychiatry, 126,* 957–967.
Nutt, D., & Lawson, C. (1992). Panic Attacks: A Neurochemical Overview of Models and Mechanisms. *British Journal of Psychiatry, 160,* 165–178.
Olfson, M. (1992). Utilization of Neuropsychiatric Diagnostic Tests for General Hospital Patients with Mental Disorders. *American Journal of Psychiatry, 149,* 1711–1717.
Owens, D. G., Cunningham, J. C., & Frith, C. D. (1982). Spontaneous Involuntaary Disorders of Movement. *Archives of General Psychiatry, 39,* 452–461.
Pam, A. (1990). A Critique of the Scientific Status of Biological Psychiatry. *Acta Psychiatria Scandanavica, 82* (suppl 362), 1–35.
Post, R. M. (1992). Transduction of Psychosocial Stress into the Neurobiology of Recurrent Affective Disorder. *American Journal of Psychiatry, 149,* 999–1010.
Reichert, H. (1992). *Introduction to Neurobiology.* New York: Oxford University Press.
Reiman, E. M., Raichele, M. E., & Robins, E. (1986). Application of Positron Tomography to the Study of Panic Disorder. *American Journal of Psychiatry, 143,* 469–479.
Rosebush, P., & Stewart, T. (1989). A Prospective Analysis of 24 episodes of Neuroleptic Malignant Syndrome. *American Journal of Psychiatry, 146,* 717–725.
Rosenthal, M. E., Sekis, D. A., Carpenter, C. J., Tary, B. L., Mendelson, U. B., & Whert, A. (1985). Antidepressant Effects of Light in Seasonal Affective Disorder. *American Journal of Psychiatry, 142,* 163–170.
Schulz, S. C. (1991). Genetics of Schizophrenia: A Status Report. In A. Tasman, & S. M. Goldfinger (Eds.), *Review of Psychiatry.* Washington, DC: American Psychiatric Press.
Sham, P. C., O'Callaghan, E. O., Takei, N. Y., Murray, G. R., Hane, E. H., & Murray, R. M. (1992). Schizophrenia Following Prenatal Exposure to Influenza Epidemic between 1939 and 1960. *British Journal of Psychiatry, 160,* 461–466.
Smith, R. E. (1993). *Psychology.* St. Paul, MN: West Publishing.
Tellegen, A., Lyken, D. T., Bouchard, T. J., Wilcox, K. J., Segal, N. L., & Rich, S. (1988). Personality Similarities in Twins Reared Apart and Together. *Journal of Personality and Social Psychology, 54*(6), 1031–1039.
Van Horn, J. D., & McManus, I. C. (1992). Ventricular Enlargement in Therapy: A Meta-analysis of Studies of the Ventricle: Brain Ratio, (VBR). *British Journal of Psychiatry, 160,* 687–697.
Versiani, M., Nardi, A. E., Figueria, I. L. V., & Stable, M. (1990). Tolerability of Moclobemide and New Reversible Inhibitors of Monoamineoxidase-A com-

pared with other antidepressants and placebos. *Acta Psychiatria Scandanavica, 360* (suppl), 240–328.

Weinberger, D. R., Fuller, T. E. Neophytides, A. N., & Wyatt, J. R. (1979). Structural Abnormalities in the Cerebral Cortex of Chronic Schizophrenic patients. *Archives of General Psychiatry, 36,* 735–739.

Weinberger, D. R., & Bergman, K. F. (1988). Speculation of the Meaning of Metabolic Hypofrontality in Schizophrenia. *Schizophrenia Bulletin, 14,* 157–168.

Yassa, R., Nair, N., Iskandar, H., & Schwartz, G. (1990). Factors in the Development of Severe Forms of Tardive Dyskinesia. *American Journal of Psychiatry, 147,* 1156–1163.

Zuckerman, M. A. (1987). Critical Look at Three Arousal Constructs in Personality Theories. In J. Strelau, & H. J. Eysenk, (Eds.), *Personality Dimensions and Arousal.* New York: Plenum Press.

Zuckerman, M. A. (1990). The Psychophysiology of Sensation Seeking. *Journal of Personality, 58,* 313–345.

CHAPTER 6

THE BEHAVIORAL PERSPECTIVE

THE PERSPECTIVE

The first psychological perspective presented on the grid is the behavioral perspective. This view of human behavior differs from more traditional models, in that it focuses on the circumstances under which certain behaviors occur. Various personality and psychological constructs defined by personality theorists were rejected by behaviorists, who recommended an empirical approach to the study of human behavior that identified observable behaviors as the only valid data for the scientific study of psychology. Since thoughts, feelings, and other inner experiences could only be inferred, they were called intervening variables, and were unavailable for study. Behaviors on the other hand, were observable and measurable, making them the only legitimate data in any scientific study of human behavior (Kimble, 1961; Schwartz, 1989).

This empirical approach to studying human behavior was initially developed with nonhuman subjects in animal learning laboratories in experimental psychology departments. The application of this animal research to human problems led to the development of the behavioral model and behavior therapy. Even today this perspective is more widely shared by psychologists than psychiatrists or social workers; however, its introduction into psychiatry over the last two decades has provided a major form of treatment for a variety of psychiatric disorders.

Since its birth almost a century ago, behavior theory and therapy have evolved over the years and continue to be very influential in many experimental and clinical settings. The initial preferential status given to this approach has been affected by recent attention given to cognitive and affective processes. Some of these intervening variables have been incorporated into the behavioral model as is evident in cognitive-behavioral therapy (CBT). The introduction of these new variables split the original group into two factions: (1) one that still adheres to the rule that behavior is the only unit of analysis and, (2) a cognitive-behavioral school that gives importance to both intervening variables and observable behaviors (Carver & Scheier, 1992). Although the majority of clinicians likely adhere to this latter group, this chapter will focus on the "pure" behavioral approach (not CBT), in order to emphasize its theoretical distinctiveness and divergence from the other perspectives. Additional reasons for maintaining this distinction are to facilitate the learning of each theory so that a more sophisticated theoretical and technical integration can be undertaken later, and to encourage the practice of behavioral formulations that may be sufficient in understanding some cases. Therefore, it may be important to understand behavioral principles first, before considering the cognitive-behavioral model. In clinical practice it is probably the latter that is more frequently used.

BRIEF HISTORY

Behavior therapy grew out of animal learning theory and can be traced to the late 1890s when Russian physiologist, Ivan Pavlov, discovered that physiological responses could be triggered by novel stimuli after learning experiences, later referred to as classical conditioning (Mackintosh, 1974). Around the same time an American psychologist, E. L. Thorndike, described "instrumental conditioning," a form of learning that emphasized the role of response outcome (reinforcement and punishment) in determining human behavior. The first to use these principles to establish a psychology of human behavior was American psychologist, John B. Watson. Watson, credited with coining the term "behaviorism," applied principles of classical conditioning to human behavior. He took an extreme view stating that subjective views of psychology were invalid and only a psychology that can objectify and empirically study behavior could be seen as a valid model for psychology.

The most well-known individual to have developed a complete theory of human behavior is B. F. Skinner. Skinner, considered one of the most distinguished psychologists of this century, had a significant impact on shaping the field of psychology and has been considered as influential as Freud in shifting its direction and developing a new approach to the study of human behavior (Schwartz, 1989; Hall & Lindzey, 1985). Skinner published extensively in experimental psychology (animal learning) and in the applied behavioral field. Skinner coined the term "operant" conditioning and substituted this word for "instrumental," stating that most behavior operated on the environment in that it often brought about a specific environmental response—reinforcement or punishment. He pioneered a major area of animal learning research and applied the principles discovered in the laboratory to human behavior

(Ferster & Skinner, 1957). He published numerous articles and books in this field and was well known for his controversial novel *Walden Two* (Skinner, 1948), the description of a utopian community designed by rules of behavior theory. Principles such as shaping, schedules of reinforcement, primary and secondary reinforcers, stimulus generalization, and discriminative stimulus (all discussed below), were originally described by Skinner. This work probably more than any other was responsible for the development of a strong animal learning group in experimental psychology departments.

As behaviorism was gaining strength and popularity in America similar developments were occurring in other countries (Wilson, 1989). In the late 1950s a South African psychiatrist, Joseph Wolpe, continued to apply learning theory principles to human behavior. Wolpe adamantly contested that psychoanalysis was ineffective in changing behavior and offered behavior therapy as an alternative which he considered superior and more efficient. Wolpe has been credited by some for having been the first to develop a formal behavior therapy, applying principles of classical conditioning to develop systematic desensitization—a specific behavior therapy developed for phobic disorders. Followers of Wolpe include Lazarus and Rachman who continued to pioneer this new behavior therapy. In England, Hans J. Eysenk established the first journal of behavior therapy: *Behavior Research and Therapy*. He also developed the Institute of Psychiatry in London, which continues to be a major center for behavior therapy. More recently, Isaac Marks has maintained this focus and has published extensively on the application of behavioral principles to anxiety disorders (Marks, 1986). Behavior therapy continued to flourish in the United Kingdom and extended to Western Europe and Scandinavia.

In the United States behavior therapy began to challenge other therapies, particularly psychoanalysis and psychodynamic psychotherapy. Dollard and Miller, while at Yale University in the 1950s, attempted to integrate principles of psychoanalysis and behavior theory (Carver & Scheier, 1992). Having received psychoanalytic training, they tried to explain drives, conflicts, and needs via learning theory principles—an early attempt at theoretical integration. Although well respected for their emphasis on motivation and other important intervening variables, they were criticized for not presenting a novel theory but rather interpreting an old theory from a new perspective. Miller and Banuazi, (1968) went on to demonstrate that contrary to earlier beliefs autonomic responses could be instrumentally conditioned, leading to the development of biofeedback.

Behavior therapy has had a significant impact on the mental health field, and its influence is evident by the numerous journals devoted solely to this topic. Some of these include: *Behavior Therapy and Research, Behavior Modification,* and the *Journal of Applied Behavioral Analysis*. This therapy has been applied to a variety of psychological and medical conditions with favourable results. As mentioned earlier this area continues to be dominated by psychologists; however, psychiatrists and social workers in increasing numbers are being trained in the use of behavioral methods for the treatment of psychiatric disorders.

BASIC PRINCIPLES

There are three models that are represented within the behavioral perspective. They are (1) classical conditioning, (2) operant conditioning, and (3) modeling (Schwartz, 1989). Each of these models has been extensively studied through animal and clinical research and will be discussed separately below.

Classical Conditioning

Classical conditioning as mentioned above was first discussed by Pavlov, who showed that a neutral stimulus such as a bell, when repeatedly associated with a stimulus such as food, could by itself produce salivation in a dog (Mackintosh, 1974; Schwartz, 1989; Kimble, 1961). Therefore, a situation or stimulus previously unable to produce a specific response by itself, now becomes able to elicit the response. In this paradigm food is considered the unconditioned stimulus (US), because on its own it produces the unconditioned response (UR) of salivation. After repeated pairings of the food (US) and the bell, the bell by itself acquires the capacity to elicit the salivation response. The bell then becomes conditioned, and is therefore called the conditioned stimulus (CS), while the salivation now elicited by the bell is called the conditioned response (CR).

As research in classical conditioning advanced, other phenomena were observed in the laboratory, eventually comprising the laws of classical conditioning: extinction, generalization, and discrimination. Extinction is observed when repeated presentations of the bell without the food results in a decreased and eventual disappearance of the salivation response. That is, if the bell is presented numerous times without the food, the bell no longer elicits the salivation response, and the response is said to be extinguished.

Also discovered was that other stimuli similar to the CS, could become CSs for a CR. Any stimulus that was present at the time the US occurred could potentially become conditioned. For example, the experimenter carrying the bell or the surroundings where the experiment occurred, all seemed to elicit the salivation response, although at different intensities, a process called generalization.

Discrimination is considered complementary to generalization. In generalization the same response occurs to physically similar stimuli; in discrimination a different response occurs to different stimuli. For example, in conditioned discrimination two CSs are presented, such as two different tones. The first tone (CS-1) would be assoicated with food, whereas a second tone (CS-2), would not be associated with food. Initially salivation would occur to both tones with equal intensity, but over time the response to CS-1 would increase and the response to CS-2 would decrease, and eventually disappear. In this situation conditioned discrimination learning is said to have taken place.

Although Pavlov and others focused on physiological responses such as salivation and heart rate, other investigators found that affective responses could also be classically conditioned (Mackintosh, 1974). Therefore emotions such as fear and anxiety that may have been experienced in one context could later be conditioned to certain stimuli that were present in the original context. For example if a frightening event occurred in a particular situation, the situation itself could come to elicit the fear, as a result of the association. In some cases, intense emotional responses only require one trial of learning in order for conditioning to take place.

Therefore, the classical conditioning model can be applied to a variety of emotional and psychological difficulties (Barlow, 1981; Hawton, Salkovskis, Kirk & Clark, 1989; Marks, 1986). The most popular condition this model has been applied to is phobias. In a phobia, a neutral stimulus that did not previously produce an intense emotional response, becomes associated with intense fear or anxiety as a result of classical conditioning. For example, an individual with a fear of flying may have had a frightening experience on a plane or suffered anxiety about an unrelated issue while sitting on a plane. The person experiences anxiety *on the plane,* regardless of whether an alarming event actually occurred; the plane now acts as a conditioned stimulus. Subsequent exposure to any plane will by itself elicit the anxious response via association. Other stimuli may come to be assoicated with this anxious response, such as getting on the plane, waiting at the departure gate, entering the airport, and even thinking about traveling. Through generalization other modes of transportation such as driving a car may initially produce the conditioned response. Nevertheless, with repeated episodes the anxious response to the car will diminish and eventually disappear due to discriminative conditioning.

Another example is agoraphobia. Individuals who have this condition are unable to leave their homes unless accompanied by a family member or friend. If they attempt to go outside the house by themselves, they become anxious and eventually housebound. A classical conditioning model would explain this behavior in a similar fashion to the flying phobia. In this situation it is likely that a frightening event occurred when the individual was out of the house that caused anxiety. There could have been a specific event that triggered the anxiety or the individual may have been anxious for other reasons and hence "out of the house when alone" was paired with anxiety, leading to the CS ("out of the house when alone") now producing the CR (anxiety). However, if the individual leaves the house with a family member, this new stimulus (out of house but not alone) is sufficiently different from the CS, so as not to produce the CR (anxiety).

The application of this model to anxiety disorders has enhanced the treatment of these very distressing and often disabling conditions. This model has also been applied to other disorders, some of which include sexual, eating, and somatic disorders (Barlow, 1981; Barlow & Cerny 1988; Hawton et al., 1989). For example, in sexual disorders it is possible that a negative, anxiety-arousing sexual experience would make future sexual encounters difficult because the sexual behaviors and associated stimuli would become conditioned to produce an anxiety response in the next sexual situation. The classical conditioning model explains the development of this anxiety and suggests a method of treatment. The focus of the treatment is to weaken the association between the CS and the CR.

In eating disorders food has become a noxious stimulus through its association with weight gain. Weight gain produces anxiety, and food is related to weight gain. Therefore, food becomes a conditioned stimulus for anxiety and is avoided. This explains the development of the disorder, and therapy focuses on pairing food with alternative more favorable stimuli.

All these terms, conditioning, extinction, generalization, and discrimination have come to play important roles in the understanding and treatment of psychological and physical disorders. The mechanism of classical conditioning provides a behavioral explanation for the development of various disorders. Various noxious events, once paired with a neutral stimulus can create a powerful association, explaining how fears, anxieties, and other negative emotions develop. To be complete, however, most behavioral explanations of psychological disorders require the integration of two learning mechanisms: classical conditioning and operant conditioning.

Operant Conditioning

Perhaps even more applicable to the understanding of what maintains psychological problems is the operant conditioning paradigm which stipulates that behavior that is reinforced increases in frequency, and behavior that is not reinforced or punished decreases in frequency (Schwartz, 1989). Reinforcers are thought to be powerful in governing our behavior. A reinforcer is defined as a stimulus that increases the behavior that precedes it. There are two types of reinforcers: positive and negative. Positive reinforcers can be specific rewards such as food, activities, money, or they can be social rewards such as attention and affection by a significant other. Social reinforcement can sometimes be more powerful than nonsocial reinforcement in determining the frequency of certain behaviors. Numerous examples from everyday life include punching a clock to receive a pay check, exercising to obtain a thinner, fitter body, and working hard to receive approval from employers. In the example presented earlier, an individual with agoraphobia who remains at home may be taken care of by their spouse and family, who are seen as reinforcing the avoidance behavior. This model of reinforcement has been applied extensively in behavioral medicine, a specialty that uses behavioral techniques, especially positive reinforcement, for increasing "well" behaviors, and decreasing "illness behaviors."

In negative reinforcement an anticipated aversive stimulus is removed if a particular behavior occurs (Schwartz, 1989). Examples include someone pressing a bell to prevent the occurrence of a shock, a child completing homework to avoid punishment, and an individual afraid of heights avoiding tall buildings to prevent the experience of anxiety. In the first two examples, "pressing the bell" and "doing the homework" prevent the occurrence of negative events such as a shock, and other forms of punishment. Some everyday examples include arriving on time at work to avoid punishment, exercising to prevent weight gain (can be viewed as both a positive and negative reinforcer), and driving carefully to avoid an accident. In some cases, such as in phobias, the individual avoids a particular stimulus to prevent the occurrence of a distressing affect, in this case anxiety. Avoidance behaviors are common in many anxiety disorders. Although classical conditioning explains the development of anxiety, operant conditioning explains how avoidance behaviors are maintained; the avoidance behavior is reinforced by anxiety reduction, explaining how in phobias these avoidance behaviors are difficult to treat.

Additional principles of operant conditioning that have important clinical implications are shaping, extinction, discrimination, generalization, and schedules of reinforcement (Schwartz, 1989; Smith, 1993; Mackintosh, 1974). Some of these principles were discussed in the classical conditioning section, but have different meanings when discussed within the operant conditioning paradigm. In shaping, successive approximations to the desired behavior are reinforced in order to reach a target behavior. For example, in order to get a child to do his or her homework, a parent may initially provide a small reinforcement if the child first spends time in his or her room for 10 minutes in the evening doing anything that he or she likes. Later he or she may be required to read a favorite story for 15–20 minutes. This will eventually be substituted by having the child do his or her homework a little at a time, with each segment of behavior being reinforced, until eventually he or she is able to spend 45 minutes to an hour doing the homework. Instead of requesting that the homework be completed right away, the child is asked to engage in behaviors that approach the ultimate task, but each approximation is reinforced, increasing the likelihood that they will continue to occur. This technique of shaping has been applied to many situations where a desired response is required that has been hard to obtain.

Extinction, discrimination, and generalization are phenomena of operant conditioning. Extinction refers to the gradual decrease in responding when reinforcement is no longer delivered. If in the example above, the child is no longer reinforced for homework behavior, this behavior will eventually decrease. In this situation, however, other reinforcers such as success at school may also act as additional reinforcement if parental reinforcement decreases. If there are no reinforcers, however, the behavior will decrease. In discrimination learning selective reinforcement leads to a differential response rate of the same behavior in two separate conditions. For example, a child may be reinforced for "good" behavior in the classroom, but not at home. This would lead to an increase in "good" behaviors in only the classroom situation. The classroom has become a discriminative stimulus for reinforcement and home is a discriminative stimulus for no reinforcement for the same behavior, explaining why the child may behave quite differently in the two situations. In generalization, responses that have been reinforced in one situation may increase in other, similar situations: the behavior is said to generalize to these situations. Using the same example, the child who has been reinforced for "good" behaviors in the classroom may also generalize these behaviors to other situations in the school such as the auditorium, playground, gymnasium, and other school areas.

Operant behaviors are learned as a result of reinforcement that is contingent upon a specific behavior. Reinforcement, however, can be delivered in many different ways to produce a variety of frequencies in responding. There are a variety of reinforcement schedules that can predict various behavior patterns specific to a particular schedule (Smith, 1993; Schwartz, 1989; Ferster & Skinner, 1957). The rate of reinforcement determines the frequency of behavior. Reinforcement schedules differ with respect to (1) the number of responses that are required before reinforcement is received, and (2) the time interval between availability of reinforcement. In the first case reinforcement can occur after a fixed number of responses, or after an unpredictable number of responses. In the second case, reinforcement will occur after a fixed period of time, or a variable period of time since the previous reinforcer. In situations where the reinforcement is unpredictable (with respect to number of responses, or time interval), a more persistent rate of responding is observed. In this case the individual is unsure when reinforcement will occur and engages in a higher and more regular rate of responding, increasing the likelihood of eventually receiving reinforcement. This form of reinforcement is also known as intermittent reinforcement.

Variable reinforcement schedules are seen in situations such as gambling, fishing, and most sporting or recreational activities such as golf, tennis, and others. The rate of reinforcement in these situations is unpredictable and variable. This keeps the individual responding over and over again until reinforcement is received. Variable reinforcement is considered more potent in increasing the frequency of behavior than a fixed rate of reinforcement. In a fixed ratio reinforcement schedule, reinforcers are available after a constant number of responses. This results in an increase in behavior just prior to the expected reinforcer, followed by a rapid decrease in behavior until just before the next reinforcer, when the behavior once again increases. This pattern of behavior has been observed in experiments with animals and humans and can be applied to various human conditions. One example is studying behavior that increases just prior to an exam, and then decreases rapidly until the next exam.

Operant conditioning principles have been helpful in understanding why certain behaviors occur, and they have been used to develop a variety of effective treatment programs for such problems as anxiety (Barlow & Cerny, 1988), depression (Hawton et al., 1989), marital problems (Jacobson & Margolin, 1979), family dysfunction (Falloon, 1988), and child behavioral problems (Hersen & Van Hasselt, 1987).

Another clinically important observation within the operant conditioning paradigm is the apathetic behavior observed when people are exposed to situations where there is no relationship between behavior and reinforcement. This was initially described by Seligman (1975) and referred to as "learned helplessness." Seligman's research was conducted in animal learning laboratories with dogs in a learning task involving avoiding electric shock. For example, a dog would be given a shock that was preceded by a tone at varying intervals. If the dog made a specific response such as jumping over a barrier and going to one side of the cage, the shock would not be given. With repeated trials the dog would learn to avoid the shock by going to the other side of the cage when the tone was heard. Avoiding shock was *contingent* on the dog's response at the presentation of the tone. If the dog was exposed to a separate situation in which he was given unavoidable and inescapable shocks when he was presented with the avoidance learning task, he could not learn. He did not make any operant responses and acted as if he was "helpless," and unable to learn.

This concept of learned helplessness in animals was compared to the syndrome of depression in humans, as similar symptoms were noted in both conditions, for example, lack of initiative in learning situations, low energy, poor appetite, weight loss, and social withdrawal. The depressive like behaviors were attributed to the lack of contingency experienced between behavior and outcome. In other words one learns helplessness as a function of experiencing no connection between action and either positive or negative reinforcement. This model has been used to describe the general apathy noticed in institutionalized individuals, who experience very little or no relationship between their behaviors and reinforcers. Such apathy has been especially noticed in geriatric institutions, where individuals remain inactive and develop a helplessness regarding the influence they have on receiving reinforcement (Seligman, 1975).

The learned helplessness model illustrates the important relationship between behavior and reinforcement. Although "motivation" was not a construct used by the original behaviorists, the learned helplessness model suggests that this learned connection between reinforcement and behavior is important in maintaining a variety of behaviors. If reinforcement or punishment occurs independent of behavior, the result is a dramatic decrease in behavior.

Modeling

In addition to classical and operant conditioning, a third form of learning often cited is observational learning or modeling (Carver &

Scheier, 1992). From birth, infants observe their environment, and the first evidence of observational learning is seen in imitation. The first models are the parents and sibs, with peers, teachers, and popular social figures becoming more important for older children and adolescents. Observational learning involves "observing" someone else or others engaging in a particular behavior that has a specific outcome. If the model is reinforced for the behaviors that are being observed, then these behaviors are more likely to be modeled or imitated. Therefore, observed behaviors that are reinforced tend to be imitated, whereas those that are punished or not reinforced are not imitated. This is an efficient form of learning in that the individual does not have to engage in the behavior and learn through trial and error, but can learn the consequences of certain behaviors simply by observing others. For example, in school, when a child observes a teacher praising another child for a particular behavior, the observing child may be more likely to imitate the observed behavior, given its positive outcome.

Other examples include observing social norms and behaviors in certain situations, such as refraining from using obscenities in church, school, or at home with parents, where punishment is likely to follow. Of recent interest is the effect of observing violence on television on children's subsequent behavior. A well-known experiment conducted by Albert Bandura (1965) showed that children who observed aggression that was reinforced were more likely to engage in aggressive behaviors themselves, compared to those children who viewed the same aggressive behaviors being punished. This area is of current interest given the increase in violence seen in many television programs and motion pictures. Many individuals have concerns that the modeling of violent behavior by "hero" figures desensitizes children to aggressive behaviors and increases the likelihood that they will engage in these behaviors themselves (Bandura, 1986; Eron, 1987).

Therefore, does observing a particular behavior automatically result in imitation or modeling? One important finding in Bandura's original research was that all children learned the aggressive behaviors, but not all children *performed* these behaviors (Bandura, 1965). The outcome in the observational learning experiment was dependent on whether the behavior was reinforced or punished. Therefore, imitating a behavior is more likely if a positive outcome is associated with it. In addition, modeling is more likely to occur if the model is perceived to be similar to the observer with respect to gender, race, age, and other physical and social characteristics (Perry & Bussey, 1984).

Other important behaviors that children learn from their parents through modeling include respect for authority figures, management of anger, expression of affect, assertiveness, resolution of conflicts, physical and sexual abuse, and many others. Social roles are also modeled by parents, and this is how children first learn about gender specific behaviors, how mothers and fathers are different, and how marital partners and families function, all important observations for future development and later adult functioning (Perry & Bussey, 1984; Carver & Scheier, 1992). Modeling and imitation are not restricted to childhood and adolescence, but continue to play an important role in adult learning in later life. Mentors, supervisors, and employers all have the potential to be powerful role models in early and even late adulthood.

All these learning concepts are very useful to mental health professionals and although there are subtle aspects to them that the interested reader can pursue, a basic understanding of what has been presented is sufficient to attempt a behavioral assessment and formulation.

ASSESSMENT

Behavior therapists are probably by far the most meticulous assessors. A thorough behavioral assessment includes collecting historical data, present data, and ongoing data as therapy progresses. The assessment therefore involves obtaining (1) the reinforcement and punishment history prior to the disorder, (2) the classical conditioning history predating the disorder, (3) the reinforcers and punishers in the present environment, (4) the individual's ability to access reinforcers, and finally (5) data regarding a baseline of the frequency of the problematic behavior and other associated activities are often collected over a two-week period prior to treatment. Usually the behavior in question is problematic because there is either too much of it (as seen in compulsive rituals), or "not enough of it" (such as remaining in feared situations, e.g., a plane in aviaphobia).

Reinforcement and Punishment History

The assessment begins at the first session and treatment is not initiated until the assessment is completed. First, the reinforcement and punishment history is obtained. The history of the frequency and variety of reinforcers prior to the onset of the behavioral disorder is evaluated. This information is obtained to determine if there has been a significant change in either the frequency or quality of reinforcers, or an increase in punishers prior to the development of the behavioral disorder. Identifying previous reinforcers will also help in developing a list of the variety of reinforcers that have been effective in the past; this information will be useful in planning treatment. For example, a patient who is mildly to moderately depressed whose reinforcers are primarily social may have lost a significant relationship with a friend or family member prior to the onset of their symptoms. A person who is normally active and is reinforced by behaviors that lead to productive ends might have had a recent decrease in the opportunity to engage in such behaviors, as is seen in the elderly or disabled, leading to symptoms of depression. Individuals who receive reinforcement through recreation or hobbies may have had a recent decline in these. Simple as it may sound, it is important not to ignore how powerful one's reinforcers can be in maintaining certain behaviors.

Classical Conditioning History Predating the Disorder

After the reinforcement and punishment history, the classical conditioning history is obtained to understand the development of the disorder, that is important in determining how a particular stimulus became associated with fear or anxiety. This history can certainly be applied to phobic disorders but can also be applied to more subtle interpersonal conditions. An individual may be able to perform quite well in most situations, but may perform poorly in a specific situation, especially if the specific situation has been associated with an anxious or feared response. For example, a student may do very well in school, yet perform poorly at home. Home could have been classically conditioned with fear, especially if home is associated with a punitive, critical father who elicits fear and interferes with good performance. Therefore, the feared stimulus is father, and father has been associated with being at home so that the home by itself elicits the now conditioned feared response. This is the common behavioral explanation given for the development of phobias and other anxiety disorders. It is important to note, however, that the patient may not be aware of the link between a specific situation in the past and the feared response.

In addition to anxiety disorders, physical symptoms as first shown by Pavlov can also be classically conditioned. In this area various physical symptoms such as palpitations, hyperventilation, headaches, etc., have been paired with various stressful conditions at work (with an employer), or at home (marital distress). These situations would then become CSs for the headache or other responses. Therefore it is important to obtain a good assessment of the various situations that have become classically conditioned to a certain maladaptive behavioral response. Treatment often involves pairing the CS with an incompatible response, such as relaxation. This will be discussed below.

Consistent with the classical-conditioning model it is important to assess the degree of generalization of the targeted response to other stimuli. This will also indicate the severity of the condition. For example, are the headaches occurring elsewhere, such as in different offices in the building where the individual works, to the entire building, to any situation close to the building, and to any social interactions with colleagues from work. Assessing the extent of generalization is important in order to develop a hierarchy of situations for treatment.

Present Reinforcers and Punishers

After establishing the classical conditioning history one obtains the frequency of reinforcers and punishers in the present environment to understand what is maintaining the behavior. This information is often acquired by asking the patient to keep records of the frequency of behaviors, reinforcers, and punishers. Information regarding the function of these behaviors in the patient's environment is collected by asking the patient to note antecedents and consequences to the target behaviors, the so-called ABCs (Barlow, 1981; Marks, 1986). The antecedents are those situational factors that precede the onset of the behavior, and the consequence is the reinforcement or punishment that follows the behavior in question. Due to the recent joining of cognitive and behavior therapy (cognitive-behavioral therapy), beliefs have been added, resulting in antecedent-behavior—beliefs, and consequences (O'Leary & Wilson, 1989). As mentioned above, for the purposes of learning, these two areas will be kept separate, but the reader is reminded that in practice these two therapies are usually integrated.

A behavioral assessment would then examine the frequency of certain negative behaviors such as avoidance (in anxiety disorders), rituals (in obsessive-compulsive disorders), tantrums or acting out (in conduct disorders), self-injurious behaviors (in borderline personality disorder), and others (Hawton et al., 1989). It also requires assessing low frequency behaviors such as social interaction (in depressive disorders and social phobias).

Accessing Reinforcers

In addition to present reinforcers and punishers, it is important to assess the individual's ability to access certain reinforcers in the environment. This requires the assessment of behavioral skills that are necessary to obtain and maintain reinforcers. Interpersonal skills such as communication and assertiveness are important to assess in order to predict future ability to access reinforcers. Also the wider the behavioral repertoire, the greater the number of behaviors to access available reinforcement, and accordingly, the greater the chance of reinforcement. For example, a shy individual may have a very low frequency of "social approach" behaviors. As a result, there is a very poor chance that he or she will receive reinforcement for social behaviors. Social behaviors then decrease in frequency and the individual will maintain a social avoidance pattern. In contrast, individuals who have a wide repertoire of social behaviors such as good communication and listening skills and an ability to be empathic as well as assertive, increase the chance that their social behaviors will be reinforced, thereby increasing the frequency of these behaviors. According to behavior theory this can also lead to the appearance of new behaviors, which will also be reinforced. This cycle of reinforcement—increase behavior—more reinforcement, will be repeated over and over again and will result in the development of a wide range of skilled behaviors that will likely be reinforced. The shy individual with a limited social behavioral repertoire, will continue to maintain a low frequency of social behaviors and will not have the opportunity to widen this area unless specific skills are acquired. The teaching of various skills such as assertiveness and good communication is a very popular technique used in behavioral therapy.

Baseline of Problematic Behavior

Once the behavioral history is obtained, the patient is instructed to keep a daily record of behaviors, reinforcers, and punishers so that a baseline is collected that will determine the appropriate specific behavioral intervention. Obtaining a baseline is crucial to the therapy because it will give objective data that does not rely completely on recall and self-report. Once the data is collected, a treatment plan is agreed upon by patient and therapist together. Behavior continues to be recorded throughout treatment in order to monitor progress. This assessment process not only provides more objective data, but also enables the patient to become more aware of his or her behaviors.

Clinical behavior therapists have developed a wide variety of assessment instruments that can be used for a range of conditions. These instruments are available in most behavior therapy texts but a good selection has been provided by Isaac Marks (1986) and David Barlow (1981). In these texts one will find numerous assessment instruments for a variety of disorders that can be utilized by patients and therapists. Familiarizing yourself with a few of these instruments will help in understanding how a behavioral assessment is completed. In order to use a behavioral intervention successfully it is imperative that a thorough behavioral assessment be completed, which requires the collection of a certain amount of objective data.

THE FOUR PS

Having presented a discussion on behavior theory and behavioral assessment, we can now turn to the behavioral heading on the grid (see Table 6.1). ***Predisposing*** behavioral factors are defined as those past behavioral events that increase the likelihood of the development of a particular disorder. The main areas considered in this section of the grid are the classical conditioning, operant conditioning, and modeling history. With classical conditioning, the various situations that have been associated with a particular response are recorded in this box, such as the original conditioning environment, and later, discrimination and generalization history. With the operant conditioning, the specific reinforcement history that may predispose an individual to a particular condition is recorded. This history includes the frequency, variety, and availability of past reinforcers. For example, individuals who are currently experiencing a depressive episode may have been behaviorally vulnerable to depression as a result of a low frequency and limited variety of reinforcers. If the individuals relied on only a few reinforcers, then they would be vulnerable if they were to lose these few reinforcers in their lives. An individual who is inactive and partially paralyzed at home after a physical injury, may be less likely to improve if his or her behavioral repertoire, prior to the injury, was limited to physically active events. This individual would then be more vulnerable to depression or other maladaptive responses as a result of their limited behavioral repertoire, thus predisposing him or her to a particular condition.

Individuals with social phobias or other disorders where there is a fear of social punishment may have had social approach behaviors punished in the past by embarrassment or some other form of social disapproval. Such experience would make these individuals fearful of any social perfor-

Table 6.1
Behavioral Perspective

Predisposing	* classical conditioning history –stimulus-response –discrimination –generalization * reinforcement (R*) history –frequency –quality –variety –accessibility –availability * punishment history (e.g. social rejection, physical abuse) * modeling history (e.g. aggressive behavior) * learned helplessness
Precipitating	* loss of reinforcement (e.g. relationship, money, job) * change in frequency of R* * punishment (rejection, humiliation, failure, divorce)
Perpetuating	* specific reinforcement schedule—variable *R * lack of reinforcement for desirable behavior * persistent low rate of reinforcement for positive behavior * ↓ variety of R* * inability to access R*—limited behavioral repertoire * noncontingent reinforcement * learned helplessness
Protective	* good rate of reinforcement * ↑ variety of R* * ↑ accessibility to R*—wide behavioral repertoire * ↓ punishment

mance situations, increasing the chance that similar situations would be avoided later. The modeling history is also important to consider. Children who observed aggressive behavior modeled by their parents may be at risk of displaying these behaviors as adults. Therefore predisposing behavioral factors such as specific paired-associations, reinforcement, punishment and modeling histories make an individual more vulnerable to a particular behavioral disorder.

Precipitating behavioral events trigger or bring on a condition in a vulnerable individual. These events are usually loss of reinforcement or punishment. Loss of a significant reinforcer such as an important relationship, or sudden unemployment, are seen as behavioral precipitants in that their occurrence triggers the onset of a particular disorder. Loss of secondary reinforcers such as money may make it difficult to access primary reinforcers such as food, drink, and recreational activities. Punishment such as social disapproval, verbal, physical or emotional abuse may all trigger the onset of a particular behavioral disorder. Precipitating events are seen as precursors to the development of a classically or operantly conditioned behavioral disorder. Additional examples include separation or divorce that precipitates depressive symptoms, a physical illness that increases illness behavior that is immediately reinforced by family, and a humiliating experience at school that leads to school refusal and social withdrawal in a child. Precipitants then increase the chance of a particular disorder or condition developing in an individual with a vulnerable behavioral history.

Perpetuating behavioral factors are those factors that continue to maintain a specific response or behavior. These factors are viewed in terms of their ability to perpetuate a behavioral disorder. One common factor is a specific reinforcement schedule such as variable reinforcement that is known to maintain a continuous, high rate of response. An example of this is seen when a spouse or family member gives consistent yet unpredictable attention to a "sick" individual in the family. Various avoidance and illness behaviors are maintained as a result of this rate of social reinforcement, especially if this rate was previously low. Negative reinforcement such as removal and escape from work also reinforces illness behaviors. Another type of reinforcement schedule that can perpetuate a specific behavioral condition is a low rate of reinforcement. Apathy and withdrawal could be maintained in individuals living in institutional settings, if there is no reinforcement for positive interactive social behaviors. The lack of adequate reinforcement of more socially appropriate behaviors will prevent these behaviors from developing and being maintained.

In addition, the lack of skills an individual has to obtain alternate reinforcers in the face of significant reinforcement loss, will also determine whether a problematic behavior is perpetuated. For example, if following the loss of a significant relationship, an individual possesses the social skills to create new relationships, this will produce new opportunities to engage in behaviors that will ultimately be reinforced. If, however, these skills are not possessed, the loss may perpetuate depressive and withdrawal behaviors for a greater period of time. Perpetuating behavioral factors then are those behavioral events that continue to maintain maladaptive behaviors, and decrease the chance of alternate more adaptive responses from occurring, and being reinforced.

Protective behavioral factors maintain adaptive responses and thereby protect the individual from the development of behavioral disorders. Individuals in environments that offer sufficient reinforcement would be protected from reinforcement deterioration, unlike individuals in low-rate environments (geriatric institutions). Therefore, adequate quantity and quality of reinforcement is a protective behavioral factor. Individuals who have a wide behavioral repertoire that can be reinforced are also protected from significant reinforcement loss. Learning various skills to increase access to reinforcers and avoid punishers are also viewed as protective behavioral factors.

In addition to adequately reinforcing environments, it is important to have a variety of reinforcers for protection against behavioral disorders. If there is a greater variety of reinforcers available to the individual, then there is less reliance on one or a few reinforcers, so that the individual is less affected by the loss of any particular reinforcer. For example, if an individual's major source of reinforcement is from work, and very little reinforcement is received from other areas (such as social, interpersonal, and recreational areas), then loss of work will be more of a problem for this individual than for persons who have a variety of reinforcers available to buffer them from depression and other behavioral problems. Individuals with infrequent and limited reinforcers would then be more likely to experience these conditions.

A behavioral formulation integrates the four Ps to provide a hypothesis as to why an individual is presenting with a specific behavioral disturbance at this point in time. The emphasis in the formulation is on behavior and on how this behavior is maintained through either classical or operant conditioning, or in most cases a combination of both. Treatment then will focus on altering this maladaptive behavioral pattern.

COPING-RESPONSE STYLE

Individuals with a behaviorally oriented coping-response style can be described as "action oriented." These individuals may already engage in various activities to deal with stress. They may prefer "to do" something about their difficulties as opposed to talking about them or taking medications. In a sense they may already be their own behavior therapist, and may only need additional "coaching" to help them deal more effectively with their difficulties. Some common examples include individuals who participate in exercise and recreational activities when they are experiencing uncomfortable emotions such as anxiety, anger, or sadness, and those who avoid distressing situations. In order to assess coping-response style, one needs to obtain information regarding past and present coping responses to situations involving the identified problem. This information will give you some idea of the particular coping style of the individual.

In addition to obtaining a history of coping methods used, specific instruments (as discussed in chapter 3) may be used to obtain information regarding a behavioral coping-response style. For example, Billings and Moos (1981) described an "active-behavioral" coping-response style which included participation in activities such as exercise, and "talking" with significant others in a personal or professional capacity. Although exercise is certainly a behavioral coping-response style, in this book, "talking" to obtain advice or support will be considered a social coping-response style (see chapter 3).

Folkman and Lazarus (1988) developed a self-report escape-avoidance coping scale that assesses the "behavioral effort" used by the individual to escape or avoid a particular stressful situation. For example, one item states "tried to make myself feel better by eating, drinking, smoking, using drugs or medication." In this book, such responses will not be considered behavioral but rather biological coping responses in that substances are ingested in an attempt to alter bodily sensations.

In contrast to the escape-avoidance scale, others have focused on behavioral methods used to deal with intrapsychic issues. For example, defense mechanisms inventories (Gleser & Ihilevich, 1969) assess "sublimation," which refers to the channeling of anxiety to a more acceptable form of behavior, such as exercise. An individual who uses this defense mechanism more than others could be seen as using a behaviorally oriented method of coping since an action is used to decrease anxiety created by an intrapsychic conflict. Although behavioral therapists do not use concepts involving "intrapsychic conflicts," sublimation can be viewed as a behavioral defensive style, because it is the redirection of an emotional response to a physical activity.

As noted earlier, it is unlikely that individuals can be easily slotted into one coping-response style over another. Nevertheless, it is possible to ascertain a particular preference for a style of coping that may be more prevalent at the time the patient is being assessed. Individuals who use a behavioral coping style may be more responsive to this approach especially at the beginning of treatment, when it is important to obtain compliance and build a good therapeutic alliance. Since "doing" things to deal with distress is consistent with their method of coping, it is possible that they may be more amenable to a behavioral approach that emphasizes more action-oriented components in therapy, giving patients and therapists a place to begin. This does not mean that the treatment plan include *only* behavioral approaches, but rather that this approach be considered first. One may find that a behaviorally oriented individual as a result of behavior therapy may become more available to other therapies that focus on thoughts (cognitive) and inner experiences (dynamic, humanistic). Alternative therapies may be sequentially planned or simultaneously integrated (as seen in CBT) at different times as the therapy progresses and the patient becomes more available to these different approaches.

TREATMENT

Behavioral psychotherapy differs significantly from most traditional therapies such as psychoanalysis and psychodynamic psychotherapy. It also differs from client-centered and other humanistic therapies. In behavior therapy the therapist is seen as the expert, the teacher, or the coach. Although the therapeutic relationship is considered important, in that a warm, empathic, supportive therapist is regarded as necessary to engage a patient into therapy, it is not considered the active ingredient of change. The active component is the specific behavioral technique that is used with the patient such as relaxation training or systematic desensitization. Although a good supportive therapeutic relationship is necessary, it is not considered sufficient to obtain a good outcome.

Behavior therapy also differs from other therapies in its emphasis on collecting data prior to, during, and after treatment. Behavior therapy is time limited, and usually involves 10 to 20 sessions, with some variability in duration based on the severity of the disorder. This therapy is goal focused, present oriented, and directive, with treatment and outcome being clearly specified. This does not mean that behavior therapists simply "throw techniques" at patients to "control" their behavior, as is sometimes implied. The therapeutic approach encourages a collaborative interaction between therapist and patient; treatment planning is done together and the desired goals are set by the patient with the help of the therapist. The ultimate goal in therapy is not just to change the maladaptive behavioral pattern, but to teach the patient skills that can help him or her exert control over their own behavior.

Behavioral therapy focuses on two areas: (1) decreasing maladaptive behaviors such as avoidance, disruptive (conduct), or dysfunctional behaviors (e.g., anxiety, depression, illness, rituals), and (2) increasing adaptive behaviors (e.g., relaxation, acquisition of skills in communication, assertion, social functioning, parenting, etc.). In treating behavioral disorders identifying both types of behaviors is essential. For example, a behavioral analysis will usually reveal that avoidance and disruptive behaviors need to be decreased while skills deficits and relaxation behaviors need to be increased.

Therefore, the basic principles of behavior therapy include (1) identifying target behaviors that have to be increased or decreased, and (2) the specific application of learning principles (e.g., reinforcement, punishment, extinction, etc.) in designing treatment programs. A variety of behavioral techniques have been applied to increase and decrease various behaviors. These include systematic desensitization and relaxation training, exposure, behavioral training through reinforcement and punishment, and specific skills training.

Systematic Desensitization and Relaxation Training

Avoidance behaviors are usually evident in conditions associated with anxiety. This is seen in all the phobic disorders such as the simple phobias, agoraphobia, social phobia, school phobias; in sexual disorders such as erectile dysfunctions and arousal/desire problems; and in personality disorders where social situations and social interactions are avoided as is seen in schizoid disorders (Hawton et al., 1989). The behavior exhibited is maladaptive in that the avoidance behavior prevents the possibility of learning new more adaptive behaviors. Avoidance behaviors are maintained because they are reinforced by anxiety reduction. With repeated trials the avoidance behavior becomes well established and is resistant to extinction, since there is no opportunity to pair the feared situation with an alternative more adaptive response. Treatment of anxiety symptoms and avoidance behaviors includes systematic desensitization and relaxation training, and exposure and response prevention. In behavior therapy the individual is gradually exposed to the feared situation and an alternate more adaptive response is learned.

In systematic desensitization (Goldfried & Davison, 1976; Wilson, 1989) the patient is asked to first develop a hierarchy of items from the least anxiety provoking to the most anxiety provoking item. Next, the patient is taught progressive muscle relaxation, a technique originally described by Jacobson (1929) and later developed by Wolpe (1958) that involves progressive sequential relaxation of the various muscle groups in the body, either from head to toe, or in the other direction. The initial phase involves the patient learning these relaxation exercises so that a successful state of relaxation can be reached. Following this training, the patient is asked to imagine the first item on the list (lowest on the hierarchy in anxiety) and then practice relaxation. Because relaxation is incompatible with anxiety, pairing it with the feared stimulus reduces the intensity of the experienced anxiety until eventually it disappears. This procedure is repeated with each item, and only after successful relaxation is attained is the patient asked to move up to the next item. If the phobia involves airplanes, the lowest item ranked could be looking at or imagining a suitcase, while the highest ranked item could be imagining being on an airplane. Desensitization begins with the lowest ranked item. The patient is asked to imagine a suitcase and rate from 0–10 (0-no anxiety to 10-worst anxiety) the level of anxiety experienced. When successful relaxation is achieved with the first item, the patient is allowed to move to the next item and so on, until eventually the first item is reached.

Exposure Training

The above describes how systematic desensitization was originally conducted. Initial results showed dramatic improvements in treating phobias (Emmelkamp, 1986). As the therapy became more widely used new findings showed that actual graduated exposure to the feared stimulus rather than imaginal exposure produced better and faster results. Therefore instead of imagining a suitcase the individual would be instructed to actually look at a suitcase for a certain period of time. They would then practice relaxation and progress up the hierarchy as described above, except in this case actual *exposure* to each situation would occur until the patient was finally able to fly on an airplane relatively free of anxiety.

As clinical research advanced it became apparent that the key ingredient responsible for a good outcome was the actual exposure to the feared stimulus. It was also discovered that pairing relaxation with the feared stimuli was not essential, and that exposure by itself with response prevention, (in this case leaving the plane) was the active ingredient necessary to produce change. This behavioral technique now known as exposure and response prevention has been used to treat a variety of phobias, agoraphobia with panic disorder, compulsive rituals, and sexual disorders (Hawton et al., 1989; Barlow, 1981; 1988).

However, in some cases as in treating certain sexual dysfunctions (e.g., anorgasmia) relaxation is still very much part of the therapy (Hawton et al., 1989). In order to weaken the association between sexual stimuli and anxiety, an alternate response such as relaxation is paired with the sexual stimuli. Repeated pairings of this new response (relaxation) that is opposite in direction to the conditioned response (anxiety), with the sexual stimuli, weaken the previous association and form a new association between relaxation and sexual stimuli. The sexual stimuli no longer produce anxiety, and an alternate relaxation response is now associated with sexual stimuli, thereby alleviating the problem.

In panic disorder, patients are taught various relaxation and breathing techniques, to help them substitute a more adaptive and incompatible response to anxiety (Barlow, 1981; Marks, 1986).

Behavioral Training

In addition to avoidance behaviors behavioral therapists have focused on disruptive or dysfunctional behaviors that need to be decreased to promote adaptive functioning. Examples include conduct problems in children, habit disorders, illness behaviors, and depressive behaviors (Hawton et al., 1989). In some of these cases there is "too much" of a disruptive behavior, and the goal is to decrease these behaviors and learn alternate more adaptive ones. A good example is the application of behavioral principles to decrease disruptive behavior in children (Mash & Terdal, 1988). During treatment a child who throws temper tantrums and becomes destructive will be given either punishment for the tantrum or positive reinforcement for the absence of tantrums, or both, to control the behavior. In negative punishment a positive stimulus will be removed if the undesirable behavior occurs. For example, an eight-year-old boy who destroys his toys in anger will not be able to play with his favorite toy for the rest of the week. This is negative punishment since a positive stimulus (favorite toy) is removed ("negative" operation) contingent on the occurrence of an undesirable behavior. Another method of dealing with this is to reinforce more positive behaviors while ignoring the more disruptive ones, a combination of positive reinforcement and extinction. In this case for example, at the end of the day both parents will assess whether the toys have been put away in the proper place. If this has occurred, the boy will receive a reinforcer. If it has not occurred, a reinforcer will not be presented. Any tantrum or destructive behavior will be ignored.

In some cases secondary reinforcers can be used to obtain primary reinforcers at a later point in time. For example, in the case described above, the young boy can earn a star for each day he takes care of his toys and does not destroy any family property. These daily stars can be accumulated over a week to earn a special gift such as going to a movie with a parent, or some other reinforcing activity. Parental attention is a strong reinforcer for children. These techniques have been used extensively with children with behavioral disorders and have been found very effective in not only reducing the disruptive behavior, but in increasing more appropriate less disruptive ones (Hersen & Van Hasselt, 1987). These techniques have also been used to deal with disruptive behaviors in the classroom, and have been found to be very effective (Kerr & Nelson, 1989). In most of these situations with children the focus has been on positive reinforcement of desirable behaviors rather than punishment of undesirable ones. Punishment is not advocated except in special circumstances, and if necessary negative reinforcement is preferred to punishment.

These techniques have also been used with great success in developmentally handicapped children and adolescents. Certain disruptive, physically damaging behaviors such as head banging, self-biting, and other self-mutilating behaviors have been well controlled with behavior therapy (Gardner, 1988). Adolescents and young adults with eating disorders have also benefitted from this therapy (Hawton et al., 1989). In anorexia nervosa, weight gain is reinforced while weight loss is associated with the loss of a reinforcer such as certain privileges. In obesity, certain eating behaviors and weight loss have been reinforced to reach the desired weight.

One of the first applications of behavioral principles was the token economy established in psychiatric institutions (Ayllon & Azarin, 1968). In this situation patients' self-care behaviors such as washing, dressing, and cleaning were reinforced with tokens that could be exchanged for cigarettes or other goods that were valued by the patients at that time. This approach significantly changed the behavior of institutionalized patients, who went from being chronically dependent on nursing care to more independent management of their own daily hygiene. This was surprising to the mental health professionals who worked with these patients who considered these behaviors to be secondary to the patients' psychiatric condition, treatable only through medication. The practice of behavior therapy in these settings has helped patients and staff deal with very disruptive and sometimes dangerous behaviors.

Behavioral principles have also been applied to other psychological disorders. In depression, symptomatic behaviors such as inactivity and social withdrawal have been targeted for change and alternate behaviors such as a gradual increase in activity and social contact have been reinforced (Becker, Heinberg & Bellack, 1987; Fennell, 1989). In such cases a structured daily program encourages daily hygiene, physical activity, and social interaction as part of a behavioral attempt to decrease depressive behaviors and increase more healthy nondepressive ones.

In addition to psychiatric and educational settings, behavior therapy has also been applied to patients in other areas of medicine. The now well established area of behavioral medicine applies behavioral principles to deal with physical symptoms such as chest pain, temporomandibular joint pain, headaches (Blanchard, 1992), chronic pain (Tunks, Bellissimo, & Roy, 1990; Keefe, Dunsmore & Burnett, 1992), and any other illnesses that have a behavioral component to their maintenance. The underlying hypothesis here is that any physical symptom can be influenced by the laws of reinforcement and punishment. Therefore, certain illness behaviors such as verbal complaining and seeking support develop and are maintained by reinforcement over time in the form of increased attention received from a spouse, family member or friend, decreased responsibility at home and at work, or even dismissal from work due to "disability."

Chronic pain provides a well researched example (Tunks et al., 1990). A significant number of individuals experience a great deal of frustration attempting to seek relief from chronic pain. Many attempts to obtain relief are futile, creating frustration for both patient and physician. Behavioral medicine has been useful in not only helping these individuals with their pain, but in also helping them lead better lives. As with all behavior therapy the basic principle is to increase more adaptive productive behaviors by reinforcing them, while decreasing reinforcement given to illness behaviors. This process can be implemented by instructing family members not to attend to the individual when they are exhibiting helpless behaviors, but to increase their attention when the individual shows more adaptive, "well" behaviors. Other "well" behaviors that are reinforced are independent self-care, increased activity or exercise, increased social interaction, and increased attention given to occupational or other productive areas. Controlled evaluations of these types of programs have been provided by Fordyce (1976).

The behavioral medicine field has grown rapidly over the last 10 years, and continues to provide a unique approach to some very complex conditions (Blanchard, 1992). Some have mistakenly accused this approach of blaming patients for their difficulties and manipulating their environment in order to "control" behavior. Therapists in behavioral medicine do not blame their patients for their symptoms because they do not view behaviors as being consciously motivated, but rather as learned due to reinforcement, which is considered an automatic process.

Skills Training

A final, very popular application that will be discussed involves increasing adaptive behaviors in the area of social skills and assertiveness training (Becker et al., 1987; Bower & Bower, 1991). Both these areas have effectively utilized behavioral principles and have been helpful to individuals with social skills deficits and assertiveness problems that contribute to poor social, occupational, and interpersonal relationships. The basic learning principles that have been developed for this area involve modeling, role playing, corrective feedback, and generalization. More simply these terms refer to the main components of teaching: show, try or practice, get feedback, and try elsewhere. These training programs usually involve groups to facilitate practice among individuals with similar concerns. An instructor or group leader will demonstrate certain skills and members of the group will be asked to role play and practice these skills in the group situation. Feedback will be given to correct unskilled behaviors and shape more complex skills, reinforcement is given for behaviors that approximate the desired response. The instructor and other members also encourage individuals to practice with reinforcement. Once these skills are learned and practiced successfully within the confines of the group, they are then encouraged to practice these in real life situations (generalization). These programs are very helpful in increasing more socially adaptive behaviors in individuals who show a deficit in this area.

SUMMARY

Behavior therapy has been demonstrated to be effective in treating many of the conditions described above and is the first choice of treatment in conditions such as phobias and certain behavioral disorders in children. The major treatments in behavior therapy involve relaxation exercises for anxiety, systematic desensitization for phobias, exposure and response prevention for OCD and agoraphobia with panic disorder, reinforcing alternative more desirable behaviors in childhood behavioral problems, and increasing adaptive behavior through skills training and reinforcement.

All these therapies are very effective in producing behavior change and the reader is referred to the references for practical treatment guides. Supervision with an individual who is trained in this field is encouraged. In most psychiatric programs this is difficult to obtain due to the restricted training of most available supervisors; however psychologists and psychiatric supervisors who have discovered the effectiveness of these therapies may be able to offer good supervision in these areas. Anxiety disorders and behavioral medicine clinics, as well as parent-child training programs, and other child treatment clinics are usually good places to learn these techniques.

Behavior therapy has changed over the last four decades. There has been a shift in focus from classical and operant conditioning principles in the 1950s and 1960s, to the integration of concepts from cognitive and social psychology in the 1980s. Affective variables have also been integrated and this emphasis will continue to be an important part of behavior therapy in the 1990s (Wilson & Agras, 1992).

REFERENCES

Ayllon, T., & Azrin, N. H. (1968). *The Token Economy.* New York: Appleton-Century-Crofts Inc.

Bandura, T. (1965). Influence of Models' Reinforcement Contingencies in the Acquisition of Imitated Responses. *Journal of Personality and Social Psychology, 1,* 589–595.

Bandura, A. (1986). Social Foundations of Thought and Action. *A Social Cognitive Theory.* Englewood Cliffs, NJ: Prentice Hall.

Barlow, D. H. (1981). *Behavioral Assessment of Adult Disorders.* New York: Guilford Press.

Barlow, D. H., & Cerny, J. A. (1988). *Psychological Treatment of Panic.* New York: Guilford Press.

Becker, R. E., Heinberg, R. G., & Bellack, A. S. (1987). *Social Skills Training Treatment for Depression.* New York: Pergamon Press.

Billings, A. G., & Moos, R. (1981). The Role of Coping Responses and Social Resources in Attenuating the Stress of Life Events. *Journal of Behavioral Medicine, 4,* 139–157.

Blanchard, E. B. (1992). Introduction to the Special Issue in Behavioral Medicine: An Update on the 1990's. *Journal of Consulting and Clinical Psychology, 60*(4), 491–492.

Bower, S. A., & Bower G. H. (1991). *Asserting Yourself: A Practical Guide for Positive Change.* Reading, MA: Addison-Wesley.

Carver, C. S., & Scheier, M. F. (1992). *Perspectives on Personality* (2nd ed.). Needham Heights, MA: Allyn & Bacon.

Emmelkamp, P. M. J. (1986). Behavior Therapy with Adults. In S. L. Garfield, & A. E. Bergin, (Eds.), *Handbook of Psychotherapy and Behavior Change* (3rd ed.). New York: John Wiley and Sons.

Eron, L. D. (1987). A Development of Aggressive Behavior from the Perspective of a Developing Behaviorism. *American Psychologist, 42,* 435–442.

Falloon, I. R. H. (1988). *Handbook of Behavioral Family Therapy.* New York: Guilford Press.

Fennell, M. (1989). *Cognitive Behavior Therapy for Psychiatric Problems. A Critical Guide.* New York: Oxford University Press.

Ferster, C. B., & Skinner, B. F. (1957). *Schedules of Reinforcement.* New York: Appleton-Century-Crofts Inc.

Folkman, S., & Lazarus, R. S. (1988). *Manual for the Ways of Coping Questionnaire*. Palo Alto, CA: Consulting Psychologists.

Fordyce, W. (1976). *Behavioral Methods for Chronic Pain and Illness*. St. Louis: Mosby.

Gardner, W. I. (1988). Behavior Therapies, Past, Present and Future. In J. A. Stark, F. J. Menolseino, M. H. Albarelli, & V. C. Gray, (Eds.), *Mental Retardation and Mental Health: Classification, Diagnosis, Treatment, Services*. New York: Springer-Verlag.

Gleser, G. C., & Ihilevich, D. (1969). An Objective Instrument for Measuring Defense Mechanisms. *Journal of Consulting and Clinical Psychology, 33*, 251–260.

Goldfried, M. R., & Davison, G. C. (1976). *Critical Behavior Therapy*. New York: Holt, Rinehart & Winston.

Hall, C. S., & Lindzey, G. (1985). *Introduction to Theories of Personality*. New York: John Wiley and Sons.

Hawton, K., Salkovskis, M., Kirk, J, & Clark, D. M. (1989). *Cognitive Behavior Therapy for Psychiatric Problems: A Practical Guide*. Oxford: Oxford Medical Publications.

Hersen, M., & Van Hasselt, V. B. (Eds.). (1987). *Behavior Therapy With Children and Adolescents: A Clinical Approach*. New York: John Wiley and Sons.

Jacobson, N. S., & Margolin, G. (1979). *Marital Therapy*. New York: Brunner/Mazel.

Jacobson, E. (1929). *Progressive Relaxation*. Chicago: Chicago University Press.

Keefe, F. J., Dunsmore, J., & Burnett, R. (1992). Behavioral and Cognitive Approaches to Chronic Pain: Recent Advances and Future Direction. *Journal of Consulting and Clinical Psychology, 60*(4), 528–536.

Kerr, M. M., & Nelson, C. M. (1989). *Strategies for Managing Behavior Problems in the Classroom* (2nd ed.). Columbus, OH: Merrill Publishing.

Kimble, G. A. (1961). *Hilgard and Marquis's Conditioning and Learning* (2nd ed.). New York: Appleton Century Crofts Inc.

Mackintosh, N. J. (1974). *The Psychology of Animal Learning*. London: Academic Press.

Marks, I. M. (1986). *Behavioral Psychotherapy*. Bristol, England: Wright Publishers.

Mash, E. J., & Terdal, L. (1988). *Behavioral Assessment of Childhood Disorders:* Selected Core Problems. (2nd ed.) New York: Guilford Press.

Miller, N. E., & Banuazi, C. (1968). Instrumental Learning by Curarized Rats of a Specific Visceral Response: Intestinal or Cardiac. *Journal of Comparative and Physiological Psychology, 65*, 1–7.

O'Leary, K. D., & Wilson, G. T. (1989). Behavior Therapy: Application and Outcome. In K. Hawton, P. M. Salkovski, J. Kirk, J. & D. Clark, (Eds.), *Cognitive Behavior Therapy for Psychiatric Problems*. Oxford: Oxford Medical Publications.

Perry D. G., & Bussey, K. (1984). *Social Development*. Englewood Cliffs, NJ: Prentice Hall.

Schwartz, B. (1989). *Psychology of Learning and Behavior* (3rd ed.). New York: Norton.

Seligman, M. E. P. (1975). *Helplessness*. San Francisco: W. H. Freeman.

Skinner, B. F. (1948). *Walden Two*. New York: Macmillan Press.

Smith, R. E. (1993). *Psychology*. St. Paul, MN: West Publishing.

Tunks, E., Bellissimo, A., & Roy, R. (1990). *Chronic Pain and Social Factors in Rehabilitation* (2nd ed.). Melbourne, FL: Krieger Publishing.

Wilson, G. T. (1989). Behavior Therapy. In R. J. Corsini, & D. Wedding, (Eds.), *Current Psychotherapies* (4th ed.). Itasca, IL: F. E. Peacock.

Wilson, G. T., & Agras, W. S. (1992). The Future of Behavior Therapy. *Psychotherapy, 29,* 39–43.

Wolpe, J. (1958). *Psychotherapy by Reciprocal Inhibitions*. Stanford: Stanford University Press.

CHAPTER 7

THE COGNITIVE PERSPECTIVE

THE PERSPECTIVE

The cognitive perspective of personality and psychopathology identifies cognition as the key variable that determines human behavior. This perspective views the human organism as an information processing machine not unlike a computer. Although this is a useful analogy, the human processing system is far more complex than a computer. Unlike a computer, an individual must filter all the daily incoming stimuli and selectively attend, encode, and process only that which has some relevance or importance to the individual, an essential task for survival.

This information processing model was developed in cognitive psychology, a discipline within experimental psychology. Cognitive scientists who study the acquisition of knowledge, human memory, and various other cognitive functions challenged the behaviorally oriented animal learning group, who at that time discounted the study of internal intervening variables between stimulus and response. Cognitive psychologists developed empirical methods that could be applied to the inner experiences of the individual, and began to find intriguing results that led to very sophisticated theories of human cognition. This group, however, did not develop a cognitive theory of personality; its influence, however, was important. Cognitive theories of personality developed from three areas: the phenomenological perspective, social learning theory, and cognitive therapy.

The main focus of the cognitive model of human behavior is on how individuals interpret or construe the events they experience around them. It is the meaning assigned to an event that is important, rather than the event itself. The same external stimuli presented to a variety of individuals will not be experienced the same. Each individual will *interpret* the stimulus quite differently. These differences reflect the unique interpretations given to the stimulus and explain why when two individuals see the same movie, read the same book, or share a common event, they can leave these situations with very different experiences. These differences are a result of the complex internal factors that influence human information processing.

According to the cognitive perspective, thinking affects feeling and behavior. Therefore, any disturbance in affect or behavior is attributed to a disturbance in thinking. Certain dysfunctional thinking styles are considered etiologically significant in emotional and personal difficulties. Identifying these maladaptive thoughts, beliefs, or assumptions is the first step towards correcting them. Cognitive therapy is aimed at altering these thought processes in order to return the individual to a more adaptive level of functioning.

As mentioned in the behavioral chapter, there has been a recent integration of cognitive and behavioral techniques (Fishman & Franks, 1992); however the focus of this chapter will be on the cognitive model, and not cognitive-behavioral therapy. More recently, interpersonal processes (Safran & Segal, 1990), and object-relations theory (Ryle, 1990) have also been incorporated into cognitive therapy once again reflecting the general trend towards integration in psychotherapy.

Cognitive therapists are usually psychologists who receive training in this form of therapy in graduate school. Psychiatrists have traditionally not received this training until recently, and many still refer patients needing this form of psychotherapy to clinical psychologists. Social workers are the least likely to obtain this training and may not be exposed to this area until they work on a multidisciplinary team that includes psychologists and psychiatrists.

The cognitive perspective has made a significant impact in the mental health field, especially in the treatment of certain psychological and psychiatric disorders (Hawton, Salkovskis, Kirk, & Clark, 1989), and it is an important model to learn in training.

BRIEF HISTORY

Although the development of the cognitive perspective of human behavior is relatively new, the idea that thoughts can determine affect and behavior has been traced to the fourth century B.C. (Beck, Rush, Shaw, & Emery, 1979). Ancient eastern philosophies such as Buddhism also emphasized the relationship between thoughts and human suffering. Although Freud focused on the unconscious, thought processes were considered important in the generation of affect. Freud's followers, the neo-Freudians, gave more attention to conscious perceptions and developed a phenomenological perspective of human behavior that gave precedence to the individual's experience of the self, the other and the world. However it was the social psychologists who first developed a formal, cognitively oriented theory of personality.

Frita Heider (1944; 1958) was one of the first social psychologists to emphasize how individuals perceive and interpret the events around them. According to Heider an individual's experience of the world is not always consistent with reality; it is an interpretation of the perceived reality. Therefore, individuals can attribute several different causes to the same event.

Another influential figure who had a significant impact on the development of the cognitive perspective, particularly in developmental psychology, was Jean Piaget. Piaget made meticulous observations of children at different ages and found that cognitive capabilities followed a developmental course, with older children showing a greater capacity for abstract thought than younger children who are more concrete in their thinking (Ginsburg & Opper, 1979). Although Piaget did not develop a cognitive theory of personality, his work stimulated a great deal of research in cognitive psychology. His theory on the development of *schemas* has been borrowed by cognitive personality theorists.

The individual credited with having been the first to develop a cognitive theory of personality is George Kelly (Carver & Scheier, 1992). While working with children with behavioral problems, Kelly concluded that it was not always the behavior per se that disrupted the classroom but the teacher's interpretation of the situation. Like Heider, Kelly focused on the interpretation given to events rather than their objective reality. According to Kelly (1963) individuals use a variety of constructs or mental representations to organize incoming information. These personal constructs develop over time, and enable the individual to predict events and make decisions about what actions need to be taken. Personality, according to Kelly, is an organization of mental structures that helps the individual interpret reality. Therefore, each individual's view of reality is different because individuals will use personal constructs that are unique to them. Kelly referred to this as "constructive alternativism" meaning that individuals will use constructs that are or have been useful to them. Whether a construct works depends on its ability to predict events. A construct that has a high predictive ability will survive; one that does not, will not survive. This became known as Kelly's Personal Construct Theory.

Kelly went on to develop a grid to measure an individual's personal constructs, later known as the Rep Test (Hall & Lindzey, 1985). According to the model underlying this test, problems arose when there was a difficulty in interpretation or in prediction. New situations were considered problematic because no constructs were available to interpret or predict events. Therefore, any novel event will generate anxiety because existing constructs will be inadequate in being able to interpret them. In addition, existing constructs can become unable to interpret and predict events, necessitating a change in the construct system. Thus, Kelly believed that constructs were changeable, and he developed a therapy he called Fixed Role Therapy, which focused on modifying any inadequate personal construct. His ideas could probably be considered the first cognitive therapy.

Although Kelly's Personal Construct theory can be viewed as the first cognitive theory of personality, Mischel (1983), a student of Kelly's, has been credited with having had the greatest influence on the development of a cognitive theory of personality. Mischel argued that any adequate theory of personality had to account for five classes of "cognitive-social-learning-person variables": a person's competence, personal constructs, expectancies, subjective values, and goal orientation. These variables determined the interpretation given to events and the behavior that would follow. Mischel described the human organism as a self-regulatory system that is able to make plans and direct these toward a specific goal.

One of the first to develop a cognitive therapy based on a cognitive model of personality was Albert Ellis. Ellis (1962) developed Rational-Emotive therapy, a confrontational approach that challenged irrational beliefs, the major cause of psychological problems. Despite Ellis's unique contribution to cognitive therapy this area did not become established until Aaron Beck's cognitive model of depression and now well-known cognitive therapy for depression (Beck, 1963; 1964; 1967; 1976).

Having received psychoanalytic training, Beck's interest was in confirming Freud's hypothesis that depression resulted from anger turned inward. While conducting analysis he became aware of his depressed patients' negative view of themselves and the world around them. He proposed that certain "depressogenic" cognitions were responsible for depressed affect. Beck's cognitive therapy was later applied to anxiety (Beck, Emery, & Greenberg, 1985), marital discord (Baucom & Epstein, 1990), and personality disorders (Beck, Freeman, et al., 1990). Beck's therapeutic approach differed from Ellis's in that he emphasized the development of a collaborative rather than confrontational relationship with the patient. Beck also discarded the notion of a patient's thoughts as being "irrational," and described them as "dysfunctional," emphasizing their effect on the patient's adaptation to the world.

Along with Beck, many others expanded this cognitive model of human behavior and applied it to a variety of psychological conditions. Arnold Lazarus and Susan Folkman (1984) are well known for their model of Stress and Coping and have emphasized the cognitive function "appraisal," as an important intervening variable that determines an individual's response to stress. Once again, the emphasis is on how individuals interpret various life events; it is the final appraisal of these events that determines whether or not they are experienced as stressful. Lazarus combined behavioral and cognitive theory to explain the experience of stress as a method of coping. Other influential behaviorists who contributed to cognitive therapy include Bandura (1977), Mahoney (1974) and Meichenbaum (1976; 1977). Bandura is well known for his social-cognitive learning theories of human behavior. Mahoney also emphasized cognitive aspects as being helpful in the control of behavior. Donald Meichenbaum (1977), described cognitive-behavior modification, a true integration of cognitive and behavioral techniques and has provided many clinical applications in his work.

More recently attention has focused on personal schemas and how they contribute to personality disorders and other psychological difficulties (Beck et al., 1990; Young, 1990). The origin of the concept schema has been traced to Bartlett (1932), a cognitive psychologist who borrowed this term from a neurologist who originally used it to explain the body's awareness of all parts. Bartlett later used this term to explain how information was organized in memory. Since then this concept has been widely used in a variety of disciplines including cognitive psychology and cognitive personality theory.

Cognitive psychology and cognitive therapy developed in parallel; a movement that continues today. Cognitive psychologists did not apply their empirically derived research to theories of personality, psychopathology, or cognitive therapy. However, cognitive psychology influenced cognitive theories of personality, even though both theories developed relatively independently. Therefore, the historical development of this perspective is not as straightforward as the behavioral perspective, which clearly grew out of animal learning psychology. Several independent yet related fields of developmental psychology, cognitive psychology, cognitive science, cognitive personality theory and cognitive therapy, contributed to a model of human behavior that has become very useful, not only in understanding, but in treating a variety of mental health conditions.

BASIC PRINCIPLES

The basic principles of the cognitive perspective can be divided into two areas: dysfunctional thinking and early maladaptive schemas. The three dysfunctional thought processes include negative automatic thoughts, cognitive distortions and core irrational beliefs. All three reflect certain maladaptive cognitive processes that contribute to psychological distress. The latter form, core irrational beliefs, are similar to early maladaptive schemas, in that they both reflect stable, enduring beliefs about self and other that have developed over time, and significantly determine reactions and behavior in various situations. However, since the concept of a schema is more complicated and has been a recent focus in long-term cognitive therapy, this will be discussed separately.

Dysfunctional Thinking

Negative automatic thoughts

While listening to his patients in analysis Beck became aware that they experienced ongoing thoughts that were not readily apparent to them (Beck, 1976). He later suggested that these unreported streams of thoughts were important in the etiology of emotional problems and could be accessed by enhancing the patient's introspective capabilities. Because of their rapid onset and spontaneous nature they were called automatic thoughts. These automatic thoughts were found to precede affective responses and were therefore important in actually determining the type of affect that would be experienced. These thoughts were at times dysfunctional, in that they could lead to distressing emotions and problematic behaviors. The greater the disturbance, the greater the likelihood of having numerous negative automatic thoughts.

Beck (1976) assigned certain characteristics to these negative automatic thoughts. They are discrete, specific, and follow a telegraphic style. They are involuntary in that they come on reflexively without any effort exerted by the individual. They are disturbing because they are difficult to control and generate negative affective experiences. In the dysfunctional cases, the patient regards these thoughts as valid and possessing a high degree of accuracy. Even if these negative automatic thoughts are invalidated in the external world, they often are not discounted, indicating their persistence and resistance to extinction. Part of this persistence is attributed to the individual developing cognitive habits through sheer repetition and practice, like the development of an automatic motor skill.

Further analyses of these negative automatic thoughts revealed that individuals with the same difficulties shared similar themes in the content of their automatic thoughts. For example, individuals with social

Table 7.1
Cognitive Distortions

Cognitive Distortions
arbitrary inference selective abstraction maximizing/minimizing dichotomous thinking labeling mislabeling personalizing

from Beck (1976)

phobias had similar automatic thoughts such as "they're looking at me critically," "they can see I'm anxious," "they won't like me," and "I'll embarrass myself." Individuals with depression were found to have similar thoughts that suggest a theme of hopelessness about the self and the future such as "I will never be happy" or "things will never improve for me." Several other automatic thoughts were described in depressed patients (Beck, 1976).

Cognitive distortions

Once these negative automatic thoughts were analyzed it became apparent that they contained certain identifiable logical errors. These errors, although present in the thinking patterns of many individuals, appeared much more frequently in those experiencing psychological problems. Beck (1976) referred to these errors as cognitive distortions, and he identified six distortions that were originally described in the depressed patient and others that were described later (see Table 7.1). These include arbitrary inference, selective abstraction, generalization, maximizing/minimizing, dichotomous thinking, labeling, mislabeling, and personalization. These distortions, also described as errors in reasoning, lead to misinterpretations of the environment and subsequent distress.

In arbitrary inference, conclusions are drawn in the absence of sufficient evidence or in the presence of evidence that appears contradictory to the inference. For example, a very competent man involved in successful activities may incorrectly assume that he is incompetent despite all the evidence to the contrary. Selective abstraction involves attending to a small detail, while ignoring the context, such as when an individual giving a presentation focuses on one person in the audience who may appear disinterested, while ignoring the rest of the audience that is displaying significant interest. By focusing on the one disinterested individual, a conclusion is made that the presentation is being received in a negative manner. Generalization, as the name suggests, involves the application of a belief to a broad group of situations when its validity applies only to a single instance. Generalization occurs when an individual having received critical feedback in one situation about a specific task, applies it to all situations that involve some performance. For example, a student may have received an unexpectedly low grade in one subject and consequently may conclude that he is inadequate and will fail all subjects. In this example, the individual generalizes a single instance of negative feedback to all aspects of performance.

Other distortions include magnification/minimization, labeling, mislabeling, personalizing, and dichotomous or black and white thinking. As the name suggests, magnification involves perceiving a situation as more negative or positive than it really is; minimization is the opposite. An individual receives a minor critical comment, blows it out of proportion, and interprets it as defamation of his or her character. This is an example of magnification. Minimization is seen when an individual after receiving a positive comment, dismisses it as insignificant. Personalization is a common cognitive error that occurs when an individual attaches personal meaning to another's action. For instance, an individual receiving a cold reception from an acquaintance who has otherwise been friendly, may interpret this response as "he is angry with me," rather than "he seems upset, or preoccupied," an interpretation that does not personalize the other's action. Dichotomous thinking, also referred to as black and white thinking, is a form of cognitive error that involves extremes in thinking. For example, situations are considered as either all good or all bad, as in an employer who perceives an employee as always being negative with no positive attributes. Other individuals and situations may also be interpreted in this manner. All these cognitive distortions, although evident to some extent in most people's thinking, are more prevalent in individuals suffering emotional disorders such as depression and anxiety. Like negative automatic thoughts, cognitive distortions are maintained through practice and repetition.

These errors in thinking are usually regarded as the product of other deeply held beliefs about the self and the world. Such beliefs are referred to as core beliefs, in Beck's system.

Core irrational beliefs/underlying assumptions

Albert Ellis (1962) was the first to describe ten irrational ideas that contributed to psychological distress. These were referred to as core beliefs or underlying assumptions. Examples of these core beliefs are always needing love and approval from everyone, having to be perfect at everything, and never failing at anything. Other irrational ideas were suggested by Ellis that were considered to be part of the individual's core belief system. This idea of a "core belief" led to the concept of the early maladaptive schema that was originally described by Beck (et al., 1979) and later expanded by Jeffrey Young (1990). This concept of personal or self-schemas has broadened the applicability of the cognitive model to include chronic conditions such as personality disorders, where more pervasive dysfunctionality is often evident.

Early Maladaptive Schemas

The idea that information is processed and stored according to various classes or categories has been developed and researched by cognitive psychologists (Smith, 1993). Piaget (Ginsburg & Opper, 1979), was one of the first to advocate the concept of a schema as a model for understanding the acquisition of knowledge in the early developmental years. Schemas offer a method to organize the vast array of information available to us on a daily basis. Schemas determine what will be selectively attended to and what will be ignored. Incoming information is always attended to, encoded, and processed in a specific manner that is determined by the operating schema. Storage of information is also determined by the schema, and it is this schema that is then accessed to aid in recall. Schemas develop through the years and become more complicated with increasing experience.

A schema is necessary to interpret a stimulus and carry out an action, a process that occurs quite rapidly and outside the level of awareness. This process is evident when a new experience needs to be attended to for which there is no schema, or for which the existing schema is insufficient. For example, the schema that allows one to drive a car has developed after years of experience. All the activities associated with driving have become so well practiced that little attention is needed to carry out any of these activities. However, if one is now to drive in another country where the rules are different, the situation dramatically changes. Initially, increased attention is paid to every aspect of driving. This increased attention is necessary to process new rules associated with an old schema. The old schema dictated that one drive on the right side of the street, while sitting in the left side of the car. The new rule is the opposite; driving on the left side of the street while sitting on the right side of the car. This creates some confusion and anxiety because the old schema is inadequate in this new situation. However, with experience, driving in this new situation becomes easier as one's old car schema accommodates to this new information—a simple yet sufficient example to illustrate the importance of schemas in real life situations.

Similarly, one develops self-schemas, which are organized bits of information about one's self that gives individuals a sense of who they are, providing them with a self-concept. Self-schemas are much more complicated in that there are more affective elements attached to them than to other cognitive schemas, such as the schemas for animals, plants, and food.

The self-schema contains a social schema that guides behavior. Research indicates (Carver & Scheier, 1992) that individuals develop schemas about a vast array of social stimuli. Schemas can be developed for social behavior, gender roles, prejudices, emotional experiences, and an endless variety of social situations. These schemas help us attend to our environment and provide us with a framework to interpret many different social stimuli. These schemas are much more complicated but can be appreciated by anyone who has traveled to a foreign country and experienced a different culture. Initially some anxiety is experienced for the existing social schema is inadequate in this situation and a new, broader schema needs to be developed to help interpret and guide behavior.

The social schema influences the self-schema by providing norms for behavior and a context for self-comparison. The self-schema contains the person's organization of selected information about one's experiences of the self. A self-schema becomes more and more complex with increasing introspection (Nasby, 1985; Carver & Scheier, 1992). That is, the more one thinks about one's self, the more likely that the self-schema will change. Self-schemas develop early in life and are maintained and at times modified by life experiences. Certain self-schemas can be dysfunctional in that they lead to maladaptive affective and behavioral responses. Therefore dysfunctional schemas lead to dysfunctional thinking, which leads to distressing emotions and maladaptive behaviors. By examining an individual's cognitive distortions one can begin to develop hypotheses about dysfunctional self-schemas. According to Beck and others (Beck et al., 1990) self-schemas can be inferred by observing behavior and monitoring thoughts, and according to Burns (1989), by a technique called vertical questioning.

In chronic conditions such as personality disorders the cognitive therapist focuses on gaining access to maladaptive schemas so that they can be modified. These schemas reside at the deepest level of cognition and contain various themes that influence the individuals' experience of themselves and their environment. According to Young (1990), as a result of certain early experiences, some individuals develop schemas so maladaptive that they create personal and interpersonal difficulties for them throughout their lives. These maladaptive schemas such as "I am unloveable," "I can never succeed at anything," or "I cannot survive alone," influence how the individual deals with various life experiences. These early maladaptive schemas are very rigid in comparison to the underlying assumptions described earlier. These schemas continue to be self-perpetuating in that they impose an interpretive bias, forcing the individual to selectively attend and to interpret events according to the schema. Therefore, an individual who has an "incompetent". self-schema may reinforce this sense of incompetence by attending to and interpreting only those events that confirm that the individual is incompetent, illustrating a very important property of maladaptive schemas, their self-perpetuating nature.

These early maladaptive schemas are affectively charged and influence the individual throughout their life. Young (1990) has proposed 15 maladaptive schemas that fall into four categories: Autonomy, Connectedness, Worthiness, and Limits and Standards (see Table 7.2).

Autonomy

Four maladaptive schemas have been described under the Autonomy category: dependence, subjugation/lack of individuation, vulnerability to harm and illness, and fear of losing self-control. These maladaptive schemas prevent the individual from attaining a sense of autonomy that leads to independence, individuation, and an internal sense of security that decreases fears of self-harm, or loss of control.

Connectedness

Four maladaptive schemas are identified under the Connectedness category: emotional deprivation, abandonment/loss, mistrust, and social isolation/alienation. The themes in this category center around the ability to form trusting relationships and attachments to significant others. The maladaptive schemas listed play an important role in preventing

Table 7.2
Early Maladaptive Schemas

Categories	Early Maladaptive Schemas
Autonomy	dependence subjugation/lack of individuation vulnerability to harm or illness fear of losing self-control
Connectedness	emotional deprivation abandonment/loss mistrust social isolation/alienation
Worthiness	defectiveness/unlovability social undesirability incompetence/failure guilt/punishment shame/embarrassment
Limits & Standards	unrelenting standards entitlement/insufficient limits

from Young (1990)

individuals from developing stable, intimate relationships or create difficulties in existing relationships.

Worthiness

The Worthiness category includes five schemas: defectiveness/unlovability, social undesirability, incompetence/failure, guilt/punishment and shame/embarrassment. These schemas contribute to low self-esteem, negative self-perceptions, relationship difficulties, inhibited ambition, and an inability to take risks necessary for self-growth.

Limits and standards

The final category deals with Limits and Standards, and contains two schemas: unrelenting standards and entitlement/insufficient limits. These schemas set rules or standards for behavior, and if unmet, create considerable distress for the individual.

According to Young (1990) these schemas make up the core of what we call personality. Schemas influence self-esteem and determine how we interact and relate to others. Cognitive distortions and self-defeating behavior patterns maintain these maladaptive schemas. In addition, relevant information that contradicts these rigid schemas is ignored, thereby increasing their resistance to alternate more accurate interpretations. The maladaptive schemas apparent in adulthood may have been adaptive in childhood, especially in a dysfunctional family environment.

Young (1990) discusses different effects that schemas may have. Some schemas may be avoided given the negative affect associated with their activation. This "cognitive avoidance," as he calls it, is carried out by blocking certain thoughts that arouse the schema, a process not that different from the psychodynamic defense mechanism known as suppression. *Affective avoidance* involves the activation of automatic thoughts that help block painful feelings associated with a particular schema. Situations can also be avoided that are known to trigger a distressing schema, this is known as *behavioral avoidance.* A form of avoidance called "compensation" occurs when the cognitive and behavioral style go in an opposite direction to the known schema. Compensation is observed in situations where an individual who has been emotionally deprived exhibits narcissistic traits. The tendency to move in an opposite direction may be regarded as adaptive, in that it leads to behaviors that are opposite in direction to the maladaptive schema; however since this is an extreme position it is considered dysfunctional.

These early schemas influence how we perceive ourselves and significant others in our world. Some maladaptive schemas may make one more vulnerable to certain conditions. An individual with maladaptive schemas that center around feelings of unworthiness may be more vulnerable to depression if they experience a series of circumstances that make them feel incompetent, guilty, and embarrassed. An individual with fears of abandonment and loss may be more vulnerable to anxiety disorders, specifically agoraphobia, if the environment becomes unpredictable and feelings of isolation and alienation prevail. Different self-schemas have been suggested for depression and anxiety, with depression prone individuals using a characterological self-blame schema, and anxiety prone individuals using a behavioral self-blame schema (Beck et al., 1985). The difference is that in anxiety disorders the individuals negative view of self centers on performance anxiety and not on maladaptive schemas at the characterological level.

These maladaptive schemas have also been applied to the personality disorders (Beck et al., 1990), and a long term cognitive therapy has been developed to deal with these disorders. However, before this or any form of cognitive therapy takes place, a thorough cognitive assessment is undertaken so that data can be obtained regarding automatic thoughts, cognitive distortions, core beliefs, and early maladaptive schemas.

ASSESSMENT

A full cognitive assessment precedes any form of cognitive therapy. The assessment process is structured and organized, and not that dissimilar to the behavioral assessment in behavior therapy. During the first interview the therapist obtains a clear description of the problem as it is described in the patient's own words. A collaborative relationship is developed and the therapist offers an initial hypothesis that the patient's difficulties could be a result of a dysfunctional thinking style. In order to test this idea the patient is asked to self-monitor daily thoughts, feelings and behaviors at certain times of the day and in certain situations. Self-monitoring is important in that it provides the necessary data for organizing a treatment plan, and has the additional benefit of increasing the patient's awareness of the relationship between thoughts, feelings, and behaviors. Before a patient can self-monitor, instructions are given regarding what is to be recorded. Numerous assessment instruments have been developed to collect data generated from self-monitoring (Barlow, 1981). Specific cognitive self-monitoring sheets have been developed for depression, anxiety disorders, eating disorders, conduct disorders and many others (Beck et al., 1979; Hawton et al., 1989).

Before patients can record their thoughts, feelings, and behaviors they need to be informed about what is to be recorded. This explanation involves educating the patient on what constitutes an automatic thought, and in some cases instructions will have to be given regarding recognizing certain affects and behaviors, as most of these phenomena likely go unnoticed. Therefore, some degree of training is required before a patient can successfully monitor this information. The amount of education needed will vary from patient to patient. It is not necessary for the patients to have insight into their difficulties (in the psychoanalytic sense) because they can be trained to monitor their thoughts and learn this skill with practice. Obtaining compliance at this initial phase of assessment is important since it will predict future compliance to a therapy that invovles a significant amount of homework exercises. A patient who is very resistant to providing the initial data, may not be a good candidate for this therapy because it requires a collaborative effort on the part of the patient and the therapist. In order for the patient to engage in therapy, this resistance needs to be assessed.

Once the assessment is completed, the data is examined according to a particular hypothesis. Various situations are analyzed with respect to the patient's ability to generate specific automatic thoughts. The affects associated with these thoughts are also recorded so that the patient can see this relationship. The specific behaviors that precede and follow these thoughts are also noted. In addition to automatic thoughts, the data is also examined for major cognitive distortions so that these can be challenged in therapy. It is important for the patient to collect and record the data so that it has more personal meaning and relevance than if the therapist collects it through the initial interview. Nevertheless, spouses and family members are sometimes used as co-therapists to collect additional data or to corroborate what has been obtained from the patient.

In addition to examining automatic thoughts and cognitive distortions, the patient's thoughts are examined for early maladaptive schemas. Young (1990) has developed a schema questionnaire consisting of 123 items rated on a six-point rating scale, that assesses early maladaptive schemas. Although this questionnaire has not been normed or validated, it can be used to help patients develop hypotheses about their own maladaptive self-schemas. This questionnaire once scored identifies whether or not a specific maladaptive schema is present. Once a schema is identified it can be modified in therapy through a variety of cognitive techniques.

THE FOUR PS

When examining the four P's under this perspective attention is given to the cognitive predisposing, precipitating, perpetuating, and protective factors (see Table 7.3).

Predisposing factors include early maladaptive schemas, dysfunctional automatic thoughts, and frequent cognitive distortions that reinforce maladaptive schemas. The four categories of early maladaptive schemas described by Young (1990) can be used to predict future difficulties. Individuals with maladaptive schemas that center around autonomy issues may have relationship difficulties as a result of excessive dependency needs, difficulties separating from their families and fears of being alone, and they may be vulnerable to anxiety (especially agoraphobia), hypochondriasis, and somatic disorders, as a result of fears of being

Table 7.3
Cognitive Perspective

Predisposing	* Early maladaptive schemas (EMS) related to –autonomy (dependency, individuation, hypochondriasis, etc.) –connectedness (mistrust, fear of abandonment) –worthiness, (self-esteem, fear of failure) –limits and standards (high expectations) * vulnerability to negative automatic thoughts—dependent on schema * vulnerability to specific cognitive distortions (minimization, selective abstraction, etc.)
Precipitating	* events that activate EMS and trigger negative automatic thoughts (NAT) –e.g. failure (performance, exams, etc.) –loss of relationship –loss of job –social rejection –interpersonal problems –increased demands at work
Perpetuating	* persistent NAT—maintain EMS * chronic use of specific cognitive distortions (CD) (e.g. generalization) maintain EMS * chronic conditions that maintain EMS, NAT, CD, e.g., chronic marital discord occupational stress poor school performance poor social relationship
Protective	* minimal EMS * situations that challenge EMS (supportive, self-validating relationship) * introspective (challenges NAT < CD) * series of overwhelming positive experiences –reattribution

harmed. These individuals may in extreme situations meet the criteria for dependent or histrionic personality disorder.

Individuals with early maladaptive schemas related to the connectedness category will more than likely have difficulties in interpersonal relationships as a result of fears of mistrust and abandonment, and in extreme situations be predisposed towards avoidant (defectiveness/unlovability), paranoid (mistrust), schizoid (social isolation/alienation), and narcissistic (defectiveness/unlovability) personality disorders, depending on the specific maladaptive schema.

A vulnerability towards low self-esteem, relationship difficulties, fear of failure, depression, and dysthymic disorders are probably more likely in individuals who have early maladaptive schemas associated with the worthiness category. Maladaptive schemas in this category may also render one vulnerable to avoidant or schizoid personality disorders. Individuals with a maladaptive schema that centers around limits and standards may be predisposed toward perfectionistic tendencies, obsessional or compulsive traits, and in extreme conditions, obsessive-compulsive personality disorder.

Other schemas have also been described that predispose individuals towards specific conditions. Individuals vulnerable to anxiety and depression have also been described as possessing different self-blame schemas, either at a behavioral or characterological level respectively. Certain schemas developed in childhood predispose individuals or make them more vulnerable to a particular condition or disorder. Different schemas have been discussed for the various emotional (Guidano & Liotti, 1983) and personality disorders (Beck et al., 1990). Understanding the early maladaptive schemas that predate the disorder helps the therapist comprehend how the individual views self and other and what psychological vulnerability he or she possesses. These early maladaptive schemas will determine the negative automatic thoughts and cognitive distortions that will be generated given a specific precipitating event.

As mentioned above, these predisposing vulnerabilities are activated by environmental events. For the depression-prone individual a breakup of a significant relationship, failure on an exam, death of a close relative, or other significant loss will activate the maladaptive schema of "I am unloveable" or "I am incompetent at everything," leading to a series of automatic thoughts that perpetuate the schema. It is not the events per se that activate the schema, but rather the interpretation or meaning given to the event that determines the response. As mentioned above, individuals with a particular maladaptive schema likely use certain cognitive distortions to interpret events. Therefore, the schema makes them vulnerable to specific cognitive distortions, and these distortions strengthen the schema.

Precipitating events are interpreted in accord with the self-schema and are biased toward maintaining this negative view of self. Consequently, the meaning given to these events will determine the response. One who sees a failure on an exam as another indication of overall inadequacy and incompetence will experience this event very differently from one who sees it as an unfortunate experience, that is not reflective of overall self-competence. Precipitating events by themselves are not as important as the meaning given to them, and are, therefore, unique to the individual. Other common precipitating events that trigger dysfunctional automatic thoughts or early maladaptive schemas include increased demands at work, interpersonal difficulties, loss of a job, any experience of failure, social rejection, and many others.

Perpetuating cognitive factors maintain maladaptive schemas, negative automatic thoughts, and cognitive distortions. As already explained, the cognitive system itself maintains the various schemas. Therefore, once a maladaptive schema has developed, it is self-perpetuated by the cognitive system. However, in addition to the inherent operations of the system, certain ongoing events may serve to reinforce and maintain this internal system. For example, a woman who has low self-esteem (due to an early maladaptive schema) and has been experiencing significant depressive symptoms after losing her job, may maintain these symptoms if she is in a chronically distressing marriage where she is verbally and physically abused. In this situation the predisposing vulnerability and a recent significant loss have resulted in depressive symptoms. Once these symptoms have developed, they are likely to be maintained if other environmental events continue to reinforce this negative view of herself, thereby perpetuating the depressive symptomatology. The precipitant activates the early maladaptive schema and sets off a series of negative automatic thoughts that maintain a negative self-perception. An unsupportive, destructive relationship could maintain these thoughts and perpetuate the woman's depression.

Similarly a child or adolescent with an overanxious disorder may have fears of failing at school, a likely result of parental pressures emphasizing success. This anxiety could generate a maladaptive schema such as "I have to be very successful in order to be loved." This schema will lead to certain cognitive distortions such as selective abstraction, where the child distressingly concentrates on the one B on a report card filled with As. This distortion may be perpetuated by the parent who also focuses on the B, and reprimands the child for not getting straight As. This parental response confirms the child's cognitive distortion of selective abstraction and maintains or perpetuates the maladaptive schema. Therefore, perpetuating events, according to the cognitive perspective, are those events that maintain a maladaptive schema by supporting the various cognitive distortions associated with that schema.

Protective cognitive factors buffer against psychological distress. If in the previous example the depressed woman has a supportive spouse in a time of crisis, his support is a protective cognitive factor. In this case, the spouse offers counter evidence that the event does not mean she is totally incompetent or inadequate. In other words, the spouse behaves like a cognitive therapist, challenging his wife's assumptions. The woman is forced to examine her interpretation of the situation and may arrive at a different conclusion. Protective cognitive factors act to challenge cognitive distortions and early maladaptive schemas. Positive experiences that continue to challenge a negative view of self may buffer against significant psychological distress. Other protective cognitive factors include a supportive network that challenges maladaptive schemas, introspective capabilities that facilitate more complex adaptive self-schemas, and a series of successful experiences that challenge rigid early maladaptive schemas or negative automatic thoughts. All these factors protect the individual cognitively in that they challenge maladaptive styles of thinking that lead to psychological disorders.

COPING-RESPONSE STYLE

An individual with a cognitive coping-response style may already be using various cognitive techniques to cope with stress. Informal techniques may have been learned through many years of adaptation to stress. These individuals are "problem solvers." They use self-talk methods to help them reach solutions to their problems. They are more than likely introspective individuals who reflect on their thought processes. This may allow them to effectively deal with daily hassles and significant stressful life events, even though these methods may not always be successful.

There are many techniques used by individuals to deal with stress that can be described as cognitive in style. These include "thinking through" the problem, "distracting" oneself from the problem by attending to something else, "stopping" the disturbing thoughts so that they are out of awareness, and reevaluating or reinterpreting the stressor so that it is perceived in a more positive light. All these coping methods could be described as cognitive coping techniques because the method of coping involves altering in some way the thought processes that contribute to emotional distress.

Understanding the cognitive mechanism of coping was first described by Gardner and associates (Gardner, Holzman, Klein, Linton, & Spense, 1959) who used the term "cognitive controls" to refer to processes used by individuals to maintain equilibrium. Although not referred to as a cognitive coping-response style, these cognitive controls were described as adaptive methods by which the ego maintained some form of homeostasis. Various methods were described such as leveling-sharpening (perceiving things as similar or different), focusing or scanning (referring to the attention given), and others that focused on various responses of the organism.

Folkman and Lazarus (1988) in their Ways of Coping Questionnaire discussed eight coping styles, some of which can be viewed as cognitive. The distancing coping style refers to cognitive operations such as "refused to think about it too much," "tried to forget the whole thing," and "tried to look on the brighter side." Some cognitive techniques are also seen in the self-controlling style, such as "I went over in my mind what I would do," and "I thought about how a person I would admire would handle the situation."

In the style described as planful problem solving, numerous cognitive techniques are used such as "concentrated on what I had to do," "came up with a couple of different solutions," and "I made a plan of action," to name a few. And finally, positive reappraisal involves rethinking about the problem.

All these cognitive techniques may be used by all individuals at different times and in different situations. It may be possible to use the Ways of Coping Questionnaire to evaluate a cognitive-coping style because many items reflect this method of coping. This would be helpful in identifying an individual who utilizes a predominantly cognitive coping-response style. An individual who already tends to use cognitive controls or cognitive techniques to cope, may be more likely to respond to a cognitive therapeutic approach. This approach is not necessarily the only one indicated, but rather it may be a place to begin, especially if research supports the use of this therapy for the individual's presenting problem.

TREATMENT

Cognitive therapy has flourished since it was first introduced by Albert Ellis and Aaron Beck. Today one can find texts on cognitive therapy for depression (Beck et al., 1979; Nezu, Nezu, & Perri, 1989); (Williams & Mark, 1984, Lewinsohn, Munoz, Yongeren, & Zeiss, 1986), anxiety disorders (Beck et al., 1985; Wolpe & Wolpe, 1988), personality disorders (Young, 1990; Beck et al., 1990), anger management (Ellis, 1977), child and adolescent disorders (Kendall, 1991), couple and family problems (Baucom & Epstein, 1990), sexual disorders (Hawton, 1985), and many others (Schuyler, 1991; D'Zurilla, 1986). As mentioned earlier, there has been an integration of cognitive and behavior therapy and most of the published material describes cognitive-behavioral therapies for the various disorders discussed above.

Cognitive therapy follows a similar format to behavioral therapy. It is a brief, directive, highly structured therapy that is problem focused and goal directed. The therapist is viewed as a teacher, advisor, or coach who guides the patient through learning a variety of techniques directed at changing cognitions. Beck et al. (1979) describes three fundamental concepts of cognitive therapy: collaborative empiricism, Socratic dialogue, and guided discovery. Collaborative empiricism refers to the scientific, joint line of inquiry undertaken by both the patient and the therapist in examining the evidence for a particular belief. The Socratic method is used to question and explore maladaptive thoughts so that the patient can arrive at logical conclusions based on the therapist's style of questioning. The therapist also serves as a guide creating new experiences for the patient in order to teach new skills and change perceptions. These fundamental principles are common to all forms of cognitive therapy. Although therapist factors such as warmth, genuineness, and empathic ability are important in creating a good therapeutic alliance, they are insufficient for a successful outcome. They are essential for creating a safe, collaborative environment so that cognitions can be explored and cognitive techniques can be implemented. The active ingredient of change is the technique utilized to alter dysfunctional cognitions.

Therapy is usually conducted over 16 to 25 sessions and can be divided into three stages: beginning, middle, and end. Initial sessions focus on establishing a relationship, conducting a comprehensive assessment, teaching self-monitoring, and assigning homework, with a focus on symptoms. In the middle of therapy there is greater concentration on thinking styles than on symptoms and emphasis is placed on learning effective techniques. The final sessions address predicting future problems and refining techniques so that they can be used more efficiently and across a variety of situations.

The major work of cognitive therapy is to (1) identify and challenge negative automatic thoughts, (2) correct cognitive distortions, (3) identify and challenge dysfunctional assumptions, and to (4) modify early maladaptive schemas, the latter being the major focus in treating personality disorders.

Identifying and Challenging Negative Automatic Thoughts

Through the assessment phase negative automatic thoughts are identified, and the therapeutic focus is on challenging these maladaptive thoughts. Challenging is carried out empirically, either verbally or through conducting small experiments. Recent events are used as data to identify and challenge these negative automatic thoughts. For example, if in a recent public speaking situation the patient experienced severe anxiety, this event is discussed at length to identify the automatic thoughts that preceded the anxious response. The patient may have seen one person in the audience yawning and may have immediately thought "Every one is bored with my talk." This thought is then challenged for its accuracy and validity, and alternative explanations are considered for the individual's yawn. Alternate hypotheses such as "The yawner may have been tired due to lack of sleep" are considered. By challenging the plausibility of the negative automatic thoughts the patient comes to see how their *interpretation* of an event leads to certain emotional reactions, and that an alternate interpretation will lead to a different affective response. This process is repeated with other negative automatic thoughts (Beck et al., 1979; Hawton, et al., 1989).

In addition to verbally challenging these thoughts a "behavioral experiment" is suggested to test out the belief. One common example is testing a negative thought that is associated with someone else. For example, if a friend is perceived as being "angry or upset" the patient may automatically assume that the friend is angry at him. To test this assumption the patient will be instructed to first check his interpretation by asking if the friend is in fact angry or upset, and then finding out if the friend is responsible in some way for creating these negative feelings. This process forces the patient to test his or her automatic thoughts in real situations so that they can be verified.

Correcting Cognitive Distortions

The automatic thoughts are also examined for their errors in thinking or for cognitive distortions. Once identified they are challenged by the therapist in an open nonconfrontational manner. This teaches patients to challenge their own cognitive distortions. With repeated challenges the patient comes to see the logical errors that are prevalent in his or her thinking, and can then be taught a variety of techniques to counter these maladaptive thoughts.

Identifying and Challenging Dysfunctional Assumptions

Once the automatic thoughts have been identified and challenged and cognitive distortions have been corrected, attention shifts to identifying the dysfunctional assumptions and core beliefs that underlie negative automatic thoughts. These are harder to identify since individuals are usually unaware of them. Assumptions such as "I have to succeed at everything" may underlie the negative automatic thought described above in the public speaking example. Because these dysfunctional assumptions generate the negative automatic thoughts, it is important that they be challenged and modified to reflect more realistic statements.

Cognitive Techniques

Numerous techniques have been devised to deal with negative automatic thoughts and dysfunctional assumptions (see McMullin, 1986). Most of these techniques incorporate a behavioral component. These techniques have been applied to various psychological disorders and several references illustrate how this has been done. Examples of specific techniques include countering, perceptual shifting, conditioning, paradoxical methods, logical analysis, and many others. Although these techniques have been divided into categories, in practice numerous techniques and strategies within each group may be applied to any condition. The cognitive technique known as countering is probably the most familiar to cognitive therapists and others who incorporate some of these techniques into an integrative or eclectic therapy. Countering refers to the use of an alternate, philosophically more adaptive statement that challenges an irrational or maladaptive thought. Under the broad heading "countering" are specific techniques known as disputing, challenging, reappraisal, de-catastrophizing, and others. In disputing and challenging the patient is encouraged to examine his or her negative thoughts such as "I must never get angry," and is then assisted to challenge this statement by discovering his or her own disputing counters such as "It is o.k. to be angry." Reappraisal is a very common countering technique that directs the individual to seek an alternate, more accurate, adaptive interpretation of a stimulus that is perceived as distressing.

Common examples are seen when individuals appraise ambiguous situations negatively, leading to distressful emotions. In cognitive therapy these events are reappraised and alternate meanings are explored that are not personal and do not reflect the individual.

In de-catastrophizing, countering statements are used to neutralize an exaggerated response. This technique may be used in anxiety disorders such as panic disorder, generalized anxiety disorder, and phobias, as well as in somatic disorders such as hypochondriasis. In many of these disorders individuals exaggerate or catastrophize a neutral stimulus such as an innocuous physical symptom. The catastrophizing leads to anxiety. De-catastrophizing involves challenging the meaning attributed to the symptom, so that it is interpreted more accurately. For example, a minor physical symptom may be interpreted as evidence of cancer or other serious disease. This assumption will be challenged, and other interpretations more consistent with the evidence will be offered, such as a minor ailment or hypervigilance resulting in more acute awareness of bodily symptoms. Many other cognitive techniques are used to treat a variety of conditions associated with negative automatic thoughts.

Modifying Early Maladaptive Schemas

Negative automatic thoughts and underlying assumptions are considered to follow certain themes that reflect early maladaptive schemas developed in childhood. The focus of the therapy in this case is not just to alter the negative automatic thoughts, but to modify or change the maladaptive schema (Beck et al., 1990; Young, 1990). Since the schema guides the interpretation of events and stimuli, schema restructuring attempts to shift the particular bias in the information processing system to a more neutral position. Cognitive distortions help the therapist and patient gain access to the "core" cognitions or schemas that generate the negative automatic thoughts.

This form of cognitive therapy that focuses on changing schemas is similar to psychodynamic therapy with respect to the importance given to early developmental experiences, and the therapeutic relationship. This approach has been extensively described in the treatment of personality disorders (Beck et al., 1990; Young, 1990) and is a recent development in cognitive therapy. The first task is to identify the various schemas that contribute to psychological and interpersonal distress. Schemas are identified by the therapist in the initial evaluation by the patient completing the Schema Questionnaire (Young, 1990), and by further sessions that focus on triggering schemas through inter-session homework or in-session interventions. Before triggering schemas, the patient is informed about them and the rationale for triggering them is explained. Once this explanation is complete, the schemas are triggered by various methods including imagery, current events, past memories, the therapeutic relationship, books, movies, dreams, homework, and in some cases group therapy. In imagery the patient is instructed to report any images that come to mind at the moment, and these images are examined for their schema content. Another method is to focus on any current upsetting event that may have triggered a particular schema. Because schemas are very closely tied to strong affective experiences, any event that produces a significant affective response may be reflecting a schema. Since these schemas are developed in childhood, past memories are also elicited to trigger schemas that may not always be in awareness. Interpersonal issues in the therapeutic relationship are also examined for their ability to trigger various schemas associated with perception of the self and others. For example, the patient may interpret the therapist's comments as hostile and rejecting, and this attitude may be explored to examine schemas centering around worthiness, such as social undesirability and incompetence/failure. This appears similar to the concept of transference and is an example of how cognitive therapy shares some similarity with psychodynamic therapy. Another similarity is in the value given to the examination of dreams that may produce more information about schemas.

When schemas are identified, schema driven behaviors and schema avoidance are confronted and brought into awareness so that the patient can see the relationship between early schemas and how they are maintained (Young, 1990). After this is realized, the therapist and patient arrive at a formulation regarding how these schemas contribute to personal and interpersonal difficulties. Once the formulation is agreed upon, a common goal of reconstructing the early maladaptive schemas can be undertaken. Various cognitive, behavioral, interpersonal and emotive techniques are used to (1) loosen and trigger schemas, (2) examine the situations in which they arise, and (3) change schemas so that they lead to more adaptive functioning. Similar cognitive techniques as described with negative automatic thoughts and cognitive distortions are used to do deal with early maladaptive schemas. In schema oriented-therapy it is the core beliefs that are the target of therapy. Given their fixed nature and length of survival, more time is required to produce change in this area.

These techniques have been well described in a variety of sources and the reader is referred to them in order to obtain a deeper understanding of schemas and the method of therapeutic change. In addition to schema theory, there has also been a recent interest in examining interpersonal process in cognitive therapy (Safran & Segal, 1990), once again illustrating the merging of cognitive therapy with other forms of therapy (Beck & Haaga, 1992).

SUMMARY

The cognitive perspective offers a unique model for understanding human behavior and psychological disorders. This perspective offers a coherent theory of human information processing that can be applied to understanding personality and psychopathology. Cognitive therapy is a highly effective therapy that has been subjected to empirical research, with effectiveness noted in the treatment of depression (Hollon, Shelton, & Davis, 1993), anxiety disorders (Chambless & Gillis, 1993), eating disorders (Wilson & Fairburn, 1993), and many other conditions (Beck & Haaga, 1992). This perspective continues to be open to new information and recent developments that involve the incorporation of experiential, emotional, interpersonal and unconscious processes, revealing the "adaptability" of cognitive therapy to consider other perspectives in the development of its own theory (Mahoney, 1993). This is a rapidly developing field that will no doubt continue to offer effective intervention strategies in the treatment of many mental health problems. As this therapy is applied to a broad range of clinical problems some of its limitations may also be discovered, assisting us with this difficult process of differential therapeutics.

REFERENCES

Bandura, A. (1977). *Social Learning Theory.* Englewood Cliffs, NJ: Prentice Hall.

Barlow, D. H. (1981). *Behavioral Assessment of Adult Disorders.* New York: Guilford Press.

Bartlett, F. C. (1932). *Remembering.* Cambridge: Cambridge University Press.

Baucom, D. H., & Epstein, N. (1990). *Cognitive Behavioral Marital Therapy.* New York: Brunner/Mazel.

Beck, A. T. (1963). Thinking and Depression: 1, Idiosyncratic Content and Cognitive Distortions. *Archives of General Psychiatry, 9,* 324–333.

Beck, A. T. (1964). Thinking and Depression: 2, Theory and therapy. *Archives of General Psychiatry, 10,* 561–571.

Beck, A. T. (1967). *Depression: Clinical, Experimental, and Theoretical Aspects.* New York: Harper and Row.

Beck, A. T. (1976). *Cognitive Therapy and the Emotional Disorders.* New York: New American Library.

Beck, A. T., Freeman, A. & Associates. (1990). *Cognitive Therapy of Personality Disorders*. New York: Guilford Press.

Beck, A. T., & Haaga, D. A. (1992). Future of Cognitive Therapy. *Psychotherapy, 29,* 34–38.

Beck, A. T., Rush, A. J., Shaw, B. F., & Emery, G. (1979). *Cognitive Therapy of Depression*. New York: Guilford Press.

Beck, A. T., Emery, G., & Greenberg, R. L. (1985). *Anxiety Disorders and Phobias: A Cognitive Perspective*. New York: Basic Books.

Burns, D. D. (1989). *The Feeling Good Handbook*. New York: William Morrow.

Carver, C. S., & Scheier, M. F. (1992). *Perspectives on Personality* (2nd ed.). Needham Heights, MA: Allyn & Bacon.

Chambless, D. L., & Gillis, M. M. (1993). Cognitive Therapy of Anxiety Disorders. *Journal of Consulting and Clinical Psychology, 61,* 248–260.

D'Zurilla, T. J. (1986). *Problem Solving Therapy: Social Competence Approach to Clinical Intervention*. New York: Springer Publishing.

Ellis, A. (1962). *Reason and Emotion in Psychotherapy*. Secaucus, NJ: Lyle Stewart.

Ellis, A. (1977). *Anger: How to Live with and without it*. Secauçus, NJ: Citadel Press.

Fishman, D. B., & Franks, C. M. (1992). Evolution and Differentiation within Behavior Therapy: The Theoretical and Epistemological Review. In D. K. Freedheim (Ed.), *History of Psychotherapy: A Century of Change*. Washington, DC: American Psychological Association.

Folkman, S., & Lazarus, R. S. (1988). *Manual for the Ways of Coping Questionnaire*. Palo Alto, CA: Consulting Psychologists.

Gardner, R. W., Holzman, P. S, Klein, G. S., Linton, H. B. & Spense, D. P. (1959). Cognitive Control: A Study of Individual Consistencies and Behavior. *Psychological Issues, 1*(4), 1–185.

Ginsburg, H., & Opper, S. (1979). *Piaget's Theory of Intellectual Development* (2nd ed). Englewood Cliffs, NJ: Prentice Hall.

Guidano, V. F., & Liotti, G. (1983). *Cognitive Processes and Emotional Disorders: A Structural Approach to Psychotherapy.* New York: Guilford Press.

Hall, C. S., & Lindzey, G. (1985). *Introduction to Theories of Personality.* New York: John Wiley and Sons.

Hawton, K. (1985). *Sex Therapy: A Practical Guide*. Oxford: Oxford University Press.

Hawton, K., Salkovskis, M., Kirk, J., & Clark, D. M. (1989). *Cognitive Behavior Therapy for Psychiatric Problems: A Practical Guide*. Oxford: Oxford Medical Publications.

Heider, F. (1958). *Psychology of Interpersonal Relations*. New York: Wiley.

Heider, F. (1944). Social Perception and Phenomenal Causation. *Psychological Review, 58,* 371–374.

Hollon, S. D., Shelton, R. C., & Davis, D. D. (1993). Cognitive Therapy for Depression: Conceptual Issues and Clinical Efficacy. *Journal of Consulting and Clinical Psychology, 61,* 270–275.

Kelly, G. A. (1963). *Theory of Personality. The Psychology of Personal Constructs*. New York: W. W. Norton.

Kendall, P. C. (1991). *Child and Adolescent Therapy: Cognitive Behavioral Procedures*. New York: Guilford Press.

Lazarus, A., & Folkman, S. (1984). *Stress, Appraisal, and Coping*. New York: Springer Publishing.

Lewinsohn, P. M., Munoz, R. F., Yongeren, M., & Zeiss, A. M. (1986). *Control Your Depression*. New York: Simon and Schuster.

Mahoney, M. J. (1993). Introduction to Special Section: Theoretical Development in the Cognitive Psychotherapies. *Journal of Consulting and Clinical Psychology, 61,* 187–193.

Mahoney, M.J. (1974). *Cognition and Behavioral Modification*. Cambridge, MA: Ballinger.

McMullin, Ryan E. (1986). *Handbook of Cognitive Therapy Techniques*. New York: W. W. Norton.

Meichenbaum, D. P. (1977). *Cognitive Behavioral Modification: An Integrative Approach*. New York: Plenum Press.

Meichenbaum, D. (1976). Cognitive Behavior Modification. In J. T. Spense, R. C. Carson & J. W. Thibaut, (Eds.), *Behavioral Approaches to Therapy*. Morristown, NJ: General Learning Press.

Mischel, L. (1983). Toward a Cognitive Social Learning Reconceptualization of Personality. *Psychological Review, 80,* 252–283.

Nasby, W. (1985). Private Self-Consciousness: Articulation of Self-Schema and the Recognition Memory of Trait Adjectives. *Journal of Personality and Social Psychology, 49,* 704–709.

Nezu, A. M., Nezu, C. M., & Perri, M. G. (1989). *Problem Solving Therapy for Depression: Theory, Research, and Clinical Guidelines*. New York: John Wiley and Sons.

Ryle, A. (1990). Cognitive-Analytic Therapy: Active Participation in Change. Chichester: Wiley.

Safran, J. D., & Segal, Z. (1990). *Interpersonal Process and Cognitive Therapy*. New York: Basic Books.

Schuyler, D. (1991). *A Practical Guide to Cognitive Therapy*. New York: W. W. Norton.

Smith, R. E. (1993). *Psychology*. St. Paul, MN: West Publishing.

Williams, J., & Mark, G. (1984). *The Psychological Treatment of Depression: Guide, Theory and Practice of Cognitive Behavior Therapy*. London: Croom Helm.

Wilson, G. T., & Fairburn, C. G. (1993). Cognitive Treatments for Eating Disorders. *Journal of Consulting and Clinical Psychology, 61,* 261–269.

Wolpe, J., & Wolpe, D. (1988). *Life Without Fear*. Oakland, CA: New Harbinger Publications.

Young, J. E. (1990). *Cognitive Therapy for Personality Disorders: A Schema Focused Approach*. Sarasota, FL: Professional Resource Exchange.

CHAPTER 8

THE PSYCHODYNAMIC PERSPECTIVE

THE PERSPECTIVE

The psychodynamic perspective offers a psychology of human behavior that is unique and rich in theory. This perspective is represented by a variety of theoretical models with more recent theories challenging earlier ideas. Historically, the major difference between this perspective and the others is the importance given to unconscious determinants of human behavior. According to psychodynamic theory, behavior is motivated by unconscious processes. In the earlier views, conscious experiences such as thoughts and behaviors were considered secondary phenomena, limited in providing us with a complete understanding of human behavior. There has been some modification to this original view with more contemporary theorists giving more attention to conscious experiences.

According to the psychodynamic perspective, human behavior and psychological distress are not fully explained by reinforcement contingencies or dysfunctional beliefs, but are seen as resulting from complicated intrapsychic processes that involve instinctual drives, internal conflicts, attachment patterns, and an "inner" representation of the world that begins at birth and evolves throughout development. It is this inner world experience that determines the adult's relationship with the external world.

The psychodynamic perspective offers a developmental theory of personality. The first few years of life are viewed as the critical period—when the roots of personality take shape. By adulthood, certain patterns have been ingrained and changing personality characteristics, although possible, requires considerable effort. Personality is a function of the intrapsychic forces that are constantly in motion, hence the term "dynamic." Most of these experiences are out of awareness but can be made conscious through self-reflection and introspection. Personality change occurs by making the unconscious, conscious—a process by which the individual gains insight into why certain maladaptive behaviors have developed and are continuing to be maintained. Since most of these behavior patterns result from early relationships with primary caretakers, unresolved issues surrounding these relationships are worked through in a therapeutic relationship with an analyst or therapist.

The psychodynamic perspective is represented by many theoretical models, all having developed from or in reaction to, the original psychoanalytical theory of Sigmund Freud. Three models will be discussed in this chapter: (1) Freud's drive conflict theory, (2) the British Object-Relations theory, and (3) self-psychology. The development of these theories and their contribution to our understanding of personality and psychopathology will be discussed. It is beyond the scope of this book to present a comprehensive discussion of each theory; several sources are cited in the reference section for more detailed study. The major effort here will be to try to present the essential elements of each theory that have enhanced our understanding of the psychodynamics of human behavior.

The psychodynamic view of personality has intrigued many mental health professionals who practice psychotherapy according to this perspective. They are usually referred to as analysts or psychodynamic therapists. Analysts receive formal training from analytic institutions and are required to undergo self-analysis. Therefore, there is some consistency in training analysts. Psychodynamic therapists on the other hand are a heterogeneous group who have received some form of supervised training in psychodynamic psychotherapy, through psychiatry residency, graduate school, or a fellowship experience. They are not necessarily analytically trained, so an analyst may be called a psychodynamic therapist; a psychodynamic therapist is not necessarily an analyst.

BRIEF HISTORY

Sigmund Freud is the father of psychoanalytic theory. Freud, trained as a physician, was originally interested in research in neurology, spending most of his time in the laboratory studying the neurophysiology of microorganisms. His description of the neuroanatomy of these organisms earned him great respect. Due to difficulties encountered in gaining a desired position and an increased demand for greater financial security (to support a wife and family), Freud turned away from his research interests and developed a private practice (Jones, 1953). It was the patients Freud encountered in his general medical practice that led him to develop his psychoanalytic theory. Freud became interested in patients who complained of neurological symptoms in the absence of any physical evidence of disease. Influenced by Charcot and Janet, he began to explore the area of hypnosis and catharsis in relieving these "hysterical" symptoms (Jones, 1953; Freud & Breuer, 1974).

Freud's explorations led him to develop four models of the mind. He developed his theories from the late 1800s to the 1930s. Freud's emphasis on sex and aggression as the primary instinctual drives, placed humans on the same level as other species. This was of course consistent with Darwin's theory of evolution, but it was opposed by the more "civilized" Victorian views of human behavior. It is not surprising that in this era Freud's emphasis on sexuality led to such controversy and heated debate among academic and public circles (Jones, 1953; Symington, 1986).

Freud's psychoanalytic theories and clinical practice led him to develop "psychoanalysis," a treatment aimed at helping individuals suffering from "hysterical or neurotic symptoms." It is important to note that the evidence Freud used to develop his theories was based on sexual themes presented by his patients; these were recollections of childhood sexual contact with parents. The possibility that sexual contact might have occurred between parent and child was unacceptable to Freud. As a result, he explained these recollections as representing the patient's childhood fantasies and unconscious sexual wishes (Freud, 1905). Given our current knowledge of the prevalence of childhood sexual abuse, it is possible that these recollections reflected reality more than they did fantasy, but such an interpretation could not have been considered during the Victorian era.

Freud had many followers, some of whom adhered to his original theories and others who departed from them to develop their own. Important figures include Carl Jung, Alfred Adler, Erik Erikson, Karen Horney, Erich Fromm, and Harry Stack Sullivan (Carver & Scheier, 1992; Hall & Lindzey, 1985; Guntrip, 1961). The latter three individuals became later known as the neo-Freudians. They expanded their own theories based on the psychoanalytic theory originally developed by Freud.

Psychoanalysis developed rapidly, and the Vienna Institute of Psychoanalysis became the center for psychoanalytic training. With the Nazi occupation of Austria in 1938, Freud left Vienna for London, England. He died a year later on September 23, 1939, of throat cancer (Jones, 1953).

Following the Freudian psychoanalytic movement were two separate movements: British Object-relations theory and Self-Psychology. The British Object-Relations school developed in England in the early 1930s and was pioneered by a social worker named Melanie Klein. Klein, although adhering to some of Freud's theories, focused on the inner world of the child and its experience with the primary caretaker, referred to as the object. Object-relations theory focused on the subject's experience with this relationship (Grotstein, 1991a; 1991b; 1991c; Guntrip, 1961; Greenberg & Mitchell, 1983; Ogden, 1983; Sutherland, 1980).

Others belonging to the British Object-Relations school include Michael Balint, Donald Winnicott, Ronald Fairbairn, Harry Guntrip and John Bowlby. Fairbairn developed his theories in isolation in Scotland, the others in England. Object-relations theory focused on the capacity of the individual to relate to and differentiate from the primary object. This school continued to develop in Britain, with very little movement observed in the United States.

The second movement known as Self-Psychology, was pioneered by Heinz Kohut, a psychoanalyst at the Chicago Institute of Psychoanalysis in the early 1960s. Kohut (1977), trained as a classical psychoanalyst became discouraged with the treatment outcome of traditional analysis with the narcissistically vulnerable patient. He became concerned with the artificial distance created by therapists who provided a blank screen for their patients' free associations. Kohut found this therapeutic approach to be less helpful in treating narcissistically vulnerable patients. He advocated a more empathic approach that he considered better suited to this group of individuals. Kohut's self-psychology offered a theory of personality and a different focus in psychoanalysis (Kohut, 1984).

Contemporary psychoanalysts have attempted to find common themes among the major schools while also highlighting their differences (Eagle, 1984; Pine, 1990; Bacal & Newman, 1990). Today it is common to find analysts and psychodynamic therapists who adhere to one model and others who integrate concepts from a variety of these models.

BASIC PRINCIPLES

Drive Conflict Theory

Freud was the first to develop a psychodynamic theory of personality. He described four models of the mind: topographical, structural, economic, and genetic. His early topographical model of the mind proposed three layers of experience—the conscious, preconscious, and unconscious. The conscious part of the mind is in the individual's awareness. The preconscious contains ordinary memories that although outside awareness, can be brought into conscious experience. The unconscious is hidden and not in the individual's awareness and can be accessed or inferred through psychoanalysis. The unconscious has a significant effect on everyday behavior. This topographical model Freud viewed as an iceberg, with the largest section, the unconscious, being hidden from view (Freud, 1915; Guntrip, 1961; Symington, 1986).

It was the unconscious that was given supreme status in Freud's early theory of personality, and it was one of his major contributions to psychology. The unconscious housed the sexual desires and instincts that were unacceptable to the conscious mind. Impulses and desires of a sexual or aggressive nature were repressed in the unconscious, and at times found their way forward toward active expression through dreams, slips, forgetting, and accidents. For Freud, understanding the unconscious was the key to understanding personality and psychopathology. However, Freud later de-emphasized the role of the unconscious, referring to it as an aspect of mental phenomena (Freud, 1915; Hall, 1954).

The structural model divides the personality into three parts: the id, the ego, and the superego. The id (Latin for "it") contains all the instinctual drives, primarily sex and aggression, and is the driving force that seeks expression and gratification of the basic needs. The id is present at birth, and contains all the inherited aspects of personality. The id is seen as operating primarily in the unconscious and is the source of all psychic energy. The sole pursuit of the id is to gratify all needs for sex, hunger, thirst, and other instinctual drives. Societal pressures do not permit the id to operate on this "pleasure principle" to gratify all needs; it therefore needs to be modified and brought under control. The inability to immediately gratify needs increases tension, and alternative ways to discharge this tension are pursued (Freud, 1915; 1923: Symington, 1986; Hall, 1954).

This task of pursuing other methods for discharging this tension is carried out by the ego. The ego operates under the reality principle and diverts id's energies to more appropriate places and delays gratification until it can be more appropriately discharged. The ego mediates between the "real" outside world and the internal instinctual world of the id. The ego (Latin for "I") having developed from the id, utilizes some of id's energy for its own use. The ego is the rational, logical mediator that finds more appropriate means for discharging id's energy. The ego is pragmatic but has no moral sense. Morality is provided by the superego (Freud, 1923; Symington, 1986).

The superego (over "I") is the moral overseer that carries the parental or societal rules for conduct. It strives for perfection and has clear rules for conduct. The superego gives the ego an "ideal" to strive for, providing it with goals for acceptable behavior. The prime task of the superego is to control id impulses, and provide the ego with a moral code that maintains "acceptable" behavior (Freud, 1923; Hall, 1954).

The id, ego, and superego are in constant interaction, dealing with conflicts created by id's desires and superego's morals. The ego is responsible for resolving these conflicts, and with increasing ego strength, there is greater ability to function independently despite the pulling forces from the id and the superego. The ego uses various mechanisms to deal with anxiety surrounding conflictual issues. These defense mechanisms were originally described by Freud and later elaborated by his daughter, Anna. These include repression, denial, projection, rationalization, intellectualization, reaction formation, regression, displacement, sublimation, and suppression (Freud, 1966). The use of defense mechanisms to transform psychic energy into a less threatening form is part of Freud's economic model of the mind. The focus of this model is on how psychic energy is discharged and distributed, and how this influences the expression of ideas and feelings.

Along with the topographical, structural, and economic models of the mind, Freud was the first to present a developmental or "genetic" theory of personality. He described five stages of development that reflected different parts of the body through which libido was discharged, referred to as the psychosexual stages. Each stage is associated with a specific conflict, and failure to resolve this conflict results in a fixation at that stage. Fixation at any stage could be due to overindulgence or to frustration of unmet needs, and is associated with certain personality characteristics.

The five psychosexual stages include the oral, anal, phallic, latent, and genital stage. The oral stage (0–18 months) is the first developmental stage where the mouth is the major focus, since it is the part of the body that most interacts with the environment, primarily through breast feeding. Conflict develops when weaning takes place and the infant has to let go of mother. Freud described two substages, the oral incorporative phase (0–6 months) and the oral sadistic phase (6–18 months). The former is associated with the development of trust, dependency and optimism. The second is involved with biting, chewing, and weaning from the breast. Fixation at this stage leads to a preoccupation with food and drink and to oral habits such as smoking and nail biting in times of stress (Freud, 1905; Hall, 1954; Carver & Scheier, 1992).

The next stage of development is the anal stage. Fixation at the anal stage (18 months–3 years) occurs if the infant is punished or shamed while being toilet trained, leading to the anal retentive, rigid, obsessional personality. Children with encopresis have been described as fixed at this stage. The anal triad of stinginess, obstinacy, and orderliness has also been described in compulsive personality disorders (Freud, 1905; 1915; Hall, 1954).

In the phallic stage (3–5 years) there is a shift to the genitals and masturbation begins. This initial autoerotic focus moves to the opposite sex parent and leads to the oedipal complex in boys and the electra complex in girls. In the oedipal complex the young boy becomes attracted to his mother and wishes to replace his father. However, castration fears inhibit this attraction to mother and leads to an identification with the father. The identification process precedes the development of the boy's superego, as he takes in or internalizes (introjects) his father's values. By becoming like father he can fantasize about being in his place (Freud, 1905; 1915; Hall, 1954).

A similar process occurs in the young girl, who as a result of blaming mother for castrating her penis, wishes to share father's penis—producing "penis envy." Resolution of the electra complex occurs when the young girl identifies with her mother, producing a more acceptable means by which she can increase her access to father (Freud, 1905; 1915; Hall, 1954).

Fixation at the oedipal stage results in either an excessive need for success, assertiveness, promiscuity, or intentional failure in sexual relationships and occupations secondary to guilt. In women, provocative, flirtatious behavior with excitement and then intentional withdrawal may predominate. The approach to resolution of this conflict affects subsequent sexual and interpersonal relationships (Freud, 1905; 1915; Hall, 1954).

In the following stage known as latency, there is a greater need to pursue social and intellectual needs, and teachers become important figures with whom to identify. Sexual and aggressive drives become less important in the early latency period (early teens) but become more active at the end of latency (Freud, 1905; 1915; Hall, 1954).

The genital stage begins in late adolescence and early adulthood. This stage marks the beginning of early relationships where mutual sexual gratification is sought. There is a shift from being more self-focused to being more socialized. If earlier stages are resolved, the young adult enters this phase with a focus on the genitals. However, even though the genital personality is pursued, it is never truly reached in its entirety (Freud, 1905; 1915).

In summary, Freud provides a view of personality that attends to developmental conflicts that center on the resolution of basic instinctual drives. Most of these conflicts and their resolution are experienced at an unconscious level. The main task for the individual is to develop sufficient ego strength so that the forces of id and superego can be reconciled, and genitally focused relationships can be pursued.

British Object-Relations Theory

Although Freud was the first to use the term "object," the object was viewed as an end point for the gratification of needs; any other gains were considered secondary to this primary function (Freud, 1905; Greenberg & Mitchell, 1983). According to Freud, the object was a person or anything that satisfied instinctual desires. Beyond this he did not give the object any special status. However, it is possible to view the superego as an internalized object that relates to parts of the ego.

It was Melanie Klein who pioneered the object-relations movement within psychoanalysis and wrote extensively on the importance of the object outside of meeting instinctual drives. Klein's contribution to psychoanalytic theory is considerable and many excellent sources are available for a full discussion of her work (Klein, 1946; 1959; Segal, 1964; Greenberg & Mitchell, 1983; Segal, 1992; Spillius, 1992). The purpose of this book is to present her key contributions that offer a unique understanding of personality and psychopathology. The four topics discussed here are "phantasy," the two developmental positions; the paranoid-schizoid and depressive positions; and the two major defenses of splitting and projective identification.

Although Melanie Klein adhered to Freud's formulation that sex and aggression were the driving forces of human nature, she became interested in how these instinctual drives were represented in the child's inner world. Her observations with children led her to develop an object-relations theory that attended to how the child perceived the object. Her focus, however, was on how the object was represented in the child's mind, rather than the actual quality of this relationship. Understanding the child's inner object world led her to develop a psychoanalytic theory that emphasized the child's "phantasy" of how these innate forces interacted. The major struggle for the child was to move from a position of feeling at oneness with the object, as an extension of itself, to later differentiating (or separating) from the object, viewing it as distinct from the self. Therefore, according to Klein the actual transactions between parent and child were not as significant (outside of exceptional circumstances), because the child's unconscious construction or phantasy of the world determined future development (Klein, 1946; Segal, 1964; Guntrip, 1961; Grotstein, 1991a).

Klein identified two positions in her developmental theory of personality that were universal to all individuals. Her preference for the term "position" instead of "stage," reflected her view that individuals oscillate from one position to the other, rather than succeeding sequentially through stages, as presented by Freud. These two positions were referred to as the paranoid-schizoid position and the depressive position. In the paranoid-schizoid position (0–6 months) the infant is consumed with its own aggression and overwhelmed with fears of annihilation. This aggression is "bad" in that it threatens the "good" (or nonaggressive part) inside the infant. In order to protect the "good" from annihilation, the infant separates these two parts. The process whereby good and bad are separated is known as splitting, a defense that is frequently used throughout adulthood, as is seen in the common experience of "falling in love," where the object is idealized and is not seen to possess any "bad" traits, until time provides a more realistic view.

In infancy, once splitting has occurred, the "bad" is projected out, thereby removing the annihilation anxieties from within. This leaves the infant with persecutory anxieties since the "bad" is now "out there," leading to the paranoid-schizoid position; paranoid as a result of projection and schizoid as a result of internal splitting. The most convenient object to receive this projection is the mother. The mother is expected to "contain" these projections, not to be destroyed by them, and to modify them so that they can be taken back in (reintrojected) and integrated within the individual, when it is ready to do so (Klein, 1946; Guntrip, 1961; Segal, 1992).

During the early phase of the paranoid-schizoid position the infant is seen as incapable of interacting with the whole object (mother) and is therefore seen as relating to fragments or parts of the object. In the case of the mother, the baby may sometimes see a good breast (that is forthcoming with milk) or a bad breast (that does not produce milk). Therefore, mother is also split into good and bad parts. It is this active splitting process applied to the baby's inner and outer experience that creates a "schizoid" world (Klein, 1946; Guntrip, 1961; Symington, 1986).

With increasing development the infant is able to perceive the mother as a whole object, and begins to see that she contains both good *and* bad parts. This perception of the simultaneous existence of both good and bad in mother leads to a major developmental change—the capacity to tolerate both good and bad experiences simultaneously, or more simply, to be able to tolerate ambivalence. If mother is capable of having both good and bad parts, then the infant must also contain both these parts. The realization that there is badness inside, leads to depressive anxiety—anxiety that centers around destroying mother. Discovering that one has sufficient aggression inside to destroy mother creates the anxiety of the depressive position (Segal, 1992; Greenberg & Mitchell, 1983; Symington, 1986).

In the depressive position (6 months to 2 years) the infant is more in touch with the newly acknowledged bad parts than the pre-existing good parts that were in awareness in the paranoid-schizoid position. If the mother has been able to contain or hold the infant's bad projections in the earlier stage, (without being destroyed by them), then the infant is able to, in the depressive position, re-accept some of this badness without fear of destruction. The mother's ability to "contain" these bad parts is crucial to the infant's later ability to internalize (or introject) them.

According to Melanie Klein it is the capacity to tolerate ambivalence in the self and others that promotes healthy personality development. This ability decreases the need for persistent splitting mechanisms that prevent an integrated experience of self and others. Although these developmental positions are experienced in the first two years of life, they remain significant throughout life. Individuals continue to struggle between these two positions, some remaining more in one position than the other (Segal, 1992; Guntrip, 1961). Psychopathology is determined by the extent to which splitting mechanisms are used by the individuals in their interactions with their inner and outer world. Individuals with schizoid, borderline, and paranoid disorders are more likely in the paranoid-schizoid position, given their regular use of this defense (Fairbairn, 1940; Kernberg, 1975).

Perhaps one of Klein's most significant contributions was her concept of projective identification. This concept has received widespread discussion with the definition of the term varying throughout history and with more interpersonal dimensions being added to the original definition. Klein's original definition stated that in projective identification, the parts that are projected onto the object are later identified with and reacted to by the sender (Klein, 1946). This is an intrapsychic definition that does not involve the object. The sender projects the material onto the object and then identifies with this part in order to control it, which is different from simple projection where an individual perceives an attribute in another that is really a self-attribute. This situation lacks the intense identification process that goes on with the attribute in an attempt to control it. In Klein's projective identification the projection and identification occur intrapsychically in the same individual. For example, the infant may project its bad parts to mother, identify with these parts and react violently to them in order to control them. Good parts can also be projected in order to preserve them and protect them from being destroyed by the infant's aggression. The good part is then identified with through a process of idealization. Projective identification permits the infant to "get rid of" whatever part is difficult for it to contain, be it good or bad (Guntrip, 1961; Segal, 1992; Gabbard, 1990).

Later definitions of projective identification changed from Klein's original definition to include a more interpersonal dimension. Ogden

(1979) described this additional dimension which created some controversy by those who viewed this process as strictly intrapsychic, and not interpersonal (Grotstein, 1991a; Sandler, 1987). The main difference between the two definitions is *where* the identification takes place. In the original definition identification takes place in the sender, in the latter it takes place in the object. In the new definition the object is perceived as accepting the projection and reacting to it (or identifying with it). In other words, the receiver is "provoked" into accepting the projection and acting it out, creating a powerful interpersonal dynamic that binds the sender and the receiver into a "projective identification interaction."

This definition, despite the modification, is intriguing, and is useful in understanding interpersonal relationships in individual and couple therapy. Individuals who project their disowned parts onto others may find themselves in intense situations if others accept their projections and react to them. These individuals may select relationships where significant others are receptive to accepting these projections, allowing them to continue to disown these parts. In individual therapy it is expected that the patient will develop a similar interaction with the therapist; however, in this case the therapist is trained to be a poor receptacle for these projections, forcing the patient to work through and reinternalize these disowned parts. In couples, it becomes a very useful and illuminating construct when attempting to understand complicated interpersonal dynamics. There is, however, little empirical support for this construct, and few attempts have been taken to measure it. The numerous articles devoted to this construct, including nonpsychoanalytic journals, may attest to its clinical usefulness when understanding complex interpersonal relationships.

Following Melanie Klein, others expanded object-relations theory (Symington, 1986; Guntrip, 1961; Grotstein, 1991b). However of all object-relations theorists, Ronald Fairbairn is credited with having described the first true object-relations theory of personality (Greenberg & Mitchell, 1983; Eagle, 1984). Fairbairn's psychoanalytic theory represented a radical departure from Freud's drive-conflict theory, and for this he received much criticism (Greenberg & Mitchell, 1983; Symington, 1986). Fairbairn took a step further than Klein, he completely disregarded instincts as the primary motivator of human experience, and stated that the organism is primarily "object seeking" not "pleasure seeking." By object seeking Fairbairn viewed the individual as *relationally focused* rather than pleasure focused, in that the motivational force driving human behavior was based on the need to relate with the object, a relationship considered essential for human survival (Fairbairn, 1944).

Based on this view Fairbairn offered a new theory of personality and psychopathology that he never wrote as a unifying theory but rather as a collection of ideas. Various writers have attempted to provide a coherent, cohesive object-relations theory of personality based on Fairbairn's writings (Guntrip, 1961; Greenberg & Mitchell, 1983). One criticism of Fairbairn is that he continued to use Freudian terminology, but redefined these terms, adding confusion to an area already fraught with varied jargon. Despite these criticisms, Fairbairn's contributions were original and unique with respect to a theory of personality and psychopathology. Fairbairn's theories of libido as object seeking versus pleasure seeking, the internal splitting of the ego and the object, attachment to bad objects, and mature dependence, provided a rich object-relations theory of personality. Fairbairn, like Klein, focused on the "inner object world," but was the first to describe the quality of the individual's relationship with the object. Fairbairn retained the concept of the ego and libido, but to him the ego was whole and intact from birth. He also did not distinguish drives (energy) from structure (ego), stating that this distinction was artificial. Energy and ego were one, the former representing the means toward the object (Fairbairn, 1940; 1944; 1949; 1951).

According to Fairbairn the primary task for the developing infant is to ultimately separate from the object and experience self and other as two distinct whole objects. This task is seldom if ever completed successfully, given our tie and attachment to the object; mainly to our "internal objects." This distinction is important, because through development, the attachment is really to an "internal representation" of the object, not to the *real* object. What is represented inside, however, is a fragmentary experience since the object is split into parts before it is internalized (introjected) in order to preserve the good, and control the bad, a process described earlier by Melanie Klein.

According to Fairbairn, the object is split into three parts that represent ideal, rejecting, and exciting aspects of the mother. The ideal part is the gratifying part of the mother that is nurturing and comforting to the infant. The rejecting part is the painful, depriving aspects of mother that are difficult to tolerate. The exciting part is the enticing, alluring aspects of mother that offers hope of a satisfying relationship. When these three parts are internalized, they then become attached to three corresponding parts of the ego: the central ego, antilibidinal ego, and libidinal ego (Fairbairn, 1944; 1949).

This splitting of the object and the ego into various parts creates a fragmentary internal experience. The good or ideal object that is attached to the central ego is the only part available to relate to the external world. The libidinal and antilibidinal egos and their corresponding object parts (exciting and rejecting), are unavailable for interaction with the external world as they are experienced as the "bad objects" and need to be controlled and repressed from consciousness. The bad object is bad because it is not gratifying. However, the child's need for the parent is so great that rejecting the bad object is intolerable, for without the object the child would be abandoned and objectless. Therefore, these parts are internalized, and this need remains attached to them. According to Fairbairn only the exciting and rejecting objects are internalized; he did not see the need to conceptualize an internal good object (Fairbairn, 1943).

This repression and attachment to bad objects is according to Fairbairn (1943) the core of psychopathology. The degree of psychopathology is determined by (1) the "badness" of the object, (2) the extent to which bad objects have been internalized into the unconscious, (3) the ego's identification with the internalized bad object, and (4) the defenses that are available to protect the ego from internal bad objects. These factors determine the degree to which one is available to have a "real relationship" with a real object. This tie to the internalized bad object is strong, and despite repeated suffering, the individual has difficulty giving it up, for loss of the bad object is intolerable. It is the exciting aspects, and hope for a truly satisfying relationship that maintain this attraction and attachment to bad objects (Fairbairn, 1943).

Fairbairn's discussion on the attachment to bad objects has been illuminating to many analysts and psychotherapists who see individuals who suffer in repeated destructive relationships. Fairbairn's theoretical contributions here are invaluable and unique in that his explanation of "repetition compulsion" explains why individuals are attracted to and unable to give up bad objects (Fairbairn, 1943; Greenberg & Mitchell, 1983).

Healthy functioning according to Fairbairn requires that one renunciate attachments to internal bad objects, which allows a less fragmented ego to relate with an object that can be perceived as separate, whole, and distinct from the self. This permits a mature relationship with the object, where giving and receiving are mutually experienced, and the capacity for true intimacy is possible. To Fairbairn the fundamental developmental task is to move from an infantile dependence to a mature dependence. In the former one is only able to take, and is in constant need to merge with the object. After a transitional phase of giving up the attachment to the internal bad object the individual is able to have a relationship where one is able to give and receive in an interdependent fashion (Fairbairn, 1949; 1951).

What is different about Fairbairn's model is its focus on environmental deficit rather than conflict. The prerequisite for attaining healthy object relationships is a relationship with mother where the child feels accepted in its own right and experiences mother as accepting his or her love. If this is experienced in childhood, it will permit the process of separation and differentiation from parents, as well as ease the renunciation or ties to internal bad objects that encourage infantile dependence. Fairbairn explains in more detail his "Endopsychic Structure" of Personality, but for the purposes of this book what has been presented is sufficient to be useful clinically in formulation and treatment (Fairbairn, 1943; 1944; Greenberg & Mitchell, 1983; Guntrip, 1961).

Others within the object-relations school are Michael Balint, Donald Winnicott, Margaret Mahler, and John Bowlby. Balint, Winnicott, and Mahler will be briefly discussed, Bowlby in more detail. Michael Balint, an analysand of Ferenzi, maintained loyalty to Freud's instinct theory and criticized Fairbairn for his total disregard of the importance of drives in understanding human behavior (Greenberg & Mitchell, 1983). For Balint libido was object seeking *and* pleasure seeking. He also coined the term the "basic fault," the unmet needs of childhood that influenced later personality development (Balint, 1968). Winnicott (1965), working with children, further expanded on the environmental conditions necessary in the mother-infant relationship in order for the child to develop independence, creativity, and a true self that was able to interact with others playfully. This decreased the necessity for the development of a false self, an armor that protects the true self from the harsh environment, while at the same time inhibiting creativity, play, and the capacity to engage in a true relationship. Winnicott described the importance of a "holding and containing environment" that allowed the infant to explore its true capacity without interruption or direction. During this period mother becomes slowly internalized and minor separations are possible. "Transitional objects" are used to replace mother during these periods of separation, and are frequently a toy, such as a teddy bear or a blanket. These articles act as substitutes during this internal attempt at separation from mother. Successful separation requires that the mother provide a "good-enough" experience (Winnicott, 1965).

The process of separating from the object was further elaborated by Mahler who originally described three phases of development: autistic (0–2 months), symbiotic (2–6 months) and separation-individuation (involved four subphases from 6 months to 3 years). In order to separate from mother and work through "separation anxiety" the child needs to internalize the soothing aspects of mother so that her inner presence can comfort the child in times of need. This emphasis on separation, individuation and differentiation has been the major focus of object-relations theory (Greenberg & Mitchell, 1983; Guntrip, 1961).

A more contemporary object-relations theorist is John Bowlby. Bowlby is perhaps the only one to have systematically researched his theory on infant development and the primary relationship. Through numerous studies grounded by theory, Bowlby showed that a secure attachment early in life influenced later development and later relationships (Bowlby, 1976; 1988). Ainsworth and associates (Ainsworth, Blehar, Waters, & Wall, 1978) went on to empirically investigate attachment and described three attachment patterns: secure, anxious, and avoidant, that described the infant's interaction with the mother after a brief period of separation. The secure infants were able to explore their environments in the presence of their mothers and when their mothers were no longer visible. After a brief period of distress at their mothers' departure they were eventually able to once again explore their environment. The mothers' return produced an immediate physical reconnection and later exploratory behavior in their mothers' presence. The anxious child experienced extreme distress in mother's absence and was unable to explore the environment in her absence. These infants became clingy and strongly attached to their mothers when they returned, and maintained proximity to them with little evidence of further exploratory behavior. The avoidant child showed some distress after mother's departure but ignored her and avoided contact with her upon her return (Ainsworth et al., 1978; Bowlby, 1976; 1988).

These three attachment patterns have been investigated by Ainsworth and her followers and have shown remarkable stability over time, and they are considered predictive of later relationships (Ainsworth et al., 1978; Bowlby, 1988). Ainsworth's research showed that a secure relationship with the mother gave the child an internal sense of security when mother was absent. One could say that this attachment experience is somehow internalized so it can continue to provide an internal sense of comfort and security when mother is no longer visible, hence the internalization of the good object. Those children who did not show a secure attachment to mother were unable to maintain any internal sense of security when mother was absent and displayed anxious or avoidant behaviors indicative of a poor internalization of a soothing mother.

Attachment theory can be applied to the understanding of separation problems in children and anxiety and agoraphobic conditions in adults (Free, Wingnet, & Whitman, 1993). Both conditions involve intense anxiety when one is alone, hence the lack of ability to self-soothe, indicating an insecure attachment history with the primary caretaker. Children that appeared detached also presented as "affectionless," and speculations were made regarding whether or not such a pattern preceded a tendency toward psychopathy. Attachment problems have also been described in depression (Pettem, West, Mahoney, & Kellar, 1993).

Attachment research will no doubt continue to illuminate us with the significance of the early relationship and its effects on later life. The object-relations theorists focus on this relationship and use it as a template for predicting future relationships, including the therapeutic relationship.

In summary, object-relations theory shifted the focus from drives and intrapsychic conflict to a deficit model where certain environmental antecedents predicted future personality development and psychopathology. The emphasis on the object and the object-relationship offered a "relational" and interpersonal dimension, illustrating our inherent human longing to connect and relate with another. The study of the object continued through self-psychology although the emphasis given to the object is viewed quite differently.

Self-Psychology

Whether self-psychology is part of object-relations theory or a separate movement within psychoanalytic theory has been heatedly debated (Greenberg & Mitchell, 1983; Bacal & Newman, 1990; Eagle, 1984; Ornstein, 1991). Historically it was not identified with the British-Object-Relations School and the thrust of the movement occurred in a country several thousands of miles away. Heinz Kohut, having been trained in classical drive-conflict theory and considered an ego psychologist, became dissatisfied with these two approaches in dealing with a particular group of patients—the narcissistically vulnerable. As a result, he developed a "Psychology of the Self" he considered more accurate, psychologically more meaningful, and clinically more useful. This led him to expand his theory and therapy (Kohut, 1971).

To understand self-psychology and its contributions to a theory of personality and psychotherapy, it is important to consider Kohut's (1) model of the self, (2) developmental antecedents necessary for healthy personality development, (3) theory of psychopathology, and (4) therapeutic focus. The last area will be elaborated in the treatment section and will be briefly mentioned here.

Having been influenced by ego-psychology Kohut maintained that the ego was active, and participated in the struggle of life experiences. His focus on the "self" was therefore a natural extension of his prior interests in ego-psychology. According to Kohut, the core of healthy human functioning originated from a "self" that was consolidated, cohesive, and able to creatively interact with the environment. This permitted the individual to explore life and relationships freely, with minimal anxieties, due to a strong inner experience of the self functioning in harmony. This fundamental tenet of healthy personality Kohut described after working with narcissistically damaged individuals. While working with these patients, he became acutely aware of the vulnerability of the self and evolved a developmental theory of personality that identified the prerequisites in the early environment that would produce a cohesive sense of self (Kohut, 1971; 1977; Wolfe, 1988; Greenberg & Mitchell, 1983).

Therefore, like object-relations theory, self-psychology is a deficit model; psychopathology is understood in terms of environmental deprivation. Also, like object-relations theory, Kohut views the object and the relationship with the object as crucial for development. The object's role in the creation of the personality and the quality of this relationship is perceived differently by self-psychology (Greenberg & Mitchell, 1983; Ornstein, 1991), although others see similarities (Bacal & Newman, 1990).

According to Kohut there is a "rudimentary self" that is present from birth. However, in order for the full development of an integrated self, a vital relationship with the object is necessary. This relationship provides the nutrients for growth and development through empathic responsiveness and careful attunement to phase appropriate developmental needs. Relatedness is essential for survival, and the object is needed to provide certain developmental functions that the child cannot carry out independently. In self-psychology the purpose of the object relationship is *to provide these functions,* not *for relating per se*; this is its key difference from object-relations theory. Kohut distinguishes between the object, which is the true independent individual separate from the self, from the self-object, which is experienced as part of the self (Kohut, 1977). The self-object refers to the *experience* provided by the relationship between the self and the object, rather than to the relationship itself (Wolfe, 1988). Therefore, the object is defined according to how it serves the self rather than by its own independent characteristics (Kohut, 1971; 1977).

As a developmental theory Kohut proposed two necessary functions that the self-object needs to provide to ensure the cohesive development of the self—mirroring and idealizing functions. Both these functions fulfil narcissistic needs essential for "healthy narcissism" to develop in the young child. In the first phase the child looks to the parent (primarily mother) like a mirror, in search of an admiring response. In many instances the child will look to the mother for validation after a task is completed seeking a confirming response such as "see—aren't I great?" This exhibitionistic, grandiose need is considered healthy and necessary if the child is to develop positive self-esteem. Therefore, it is normal and important at this stage for the child to feel omnipotent and grandiose so that this feeling may be internalized as positive aspects of the developing personality (Kohut, 1971).

The second developmental event involves idealization. In this phase the child needs to idealize the parent, to put him (usually father) on a pedestal and perceive him as possessing positive attributes the child longs to have. This idealization leads to a longing to merge with the parent and become "like him." The merger permits the child to become part of the parent and possess these attributes him- or herself which helps the child develop values and ideals that become part of the developing personality (Kohut, 1971).

Over time, with repeated mirroring and idealizing responses from parents, these functions become internalized through a process called "transmuting internalizations" (Kohut, 1977). Through this process the self-object functions provided by the parents are assimilated by the self, allowing the child to provide these functions for itself. However, the capacity to self-sustain self-object functions is rare, and there is a lifelong need for self-object relationships (Kohut, 1977).

If there is sufficient mirroring, idealizing, and emphathic responsiveness from parents, there is a greater chance that the child will develop a cohesive sense of self. Of course, the child does not need a "perfect environment" for the development of a healthy personality. On the contrary, Kohut also stated that optimal frustrations in attempting to meet mirroring and idealizing needs were essential for the child to achieve a more realistic view of the self and the object. However, *sufficient* empathic responsiveness has to be present in the child's earlier development to tolerate these optimal frustrations of sporadic parental empathic failures (Kohut, 1977; Bacal & Newman, 1990).

Psychopathology develops if there is chronic empathic failure in the child's early environment, leading to a fragmentary experience of the self. During stress this self is more vulnerable to disintegration, and needs constant self-object functions to maintain cohesiveness, because these functions were absent in early life and were therefore not internalized. This vulnerable self is more prone to anxiety, depression, psychosis, and other psychological difficulties (Kohut, 1971; 1977; Wolfe, 1988).

The disintegration of the self during distressing periods produces "disintegration products," the instinctual drives of sex and aggression. These instincts are activated when the child experiences frustration in obtaining self-object functions. Therefore, for Kohut, drives and instincts were not primary but secondary, a more regressive means of obtaining a satisfactory self-object experience (Kohut, 1977; Greenbergt & Mitchell, 1983). Like Fairbairn, Kohut viewed drives such as aggression as secondary to frustration with the environment. For Kohut, aggression is narcissistic rage following narcissistic injury, and is a result of the individual's frustration at the inability to experience the healthy, assertive self. Aggression then indicates fragmentation (Kohut, 1971; 1977; Greenberg & Mitchell, 1983).

Although Kohut discussed drives in this context, he also advocated that Freud's drive-conflict model and his self-psychological model could be viewed as complementing each other; the former being more appropriate for the neuroses and the latter being more appropriate for the narcissistic personality disorders. This mixing of models has been viewed critically by Greenberg and Mitchell (1983) who see a contradiction in Kohut's view that drives are both disintegration products and complementary with self-theory. In addition to these criticisms, Kohut has also been attacked for describing his theory as "unique," when it has obvious similarities to Sullivan, Fairbairn, and other object-relation theorists, many of whom are not mentioned in his writings. He is, however, credited with having placed more focus on the "self-experience" and advocating an empathic-introspective frame of reference in therapy that has been clinically useful and therapeutically valuable. His analytic approach will be discussed in more detail in the treatment section. Many followers of Kohut have continued to develop this area, leading to new developments in the field (Ornstein, 1991; Stolorow, Brandchaft, & Attwood, 1987; Wolfe, 1988; Bacal & Newman, 1990).

In summary, self-psychology advocates that reasonably successful early experiences promote the development of a self that is integrated and less vulnerable to fragmentation during times of stress. If these early functions are not provided, there will be a constant need to be in proximity to an object who can provide these functions. For example, an individual who constantly needs external approval may not have been successfully mirrored so that these functions could have been internalized and maintained by the self. Therefore there will be a constant need to have these functions provided. Certain difficulties in adult relationships may be associated with an arrest in development at a particular stage either in the mirroring or idealizing phase.

Contemporary Psychoanalysis

The discussion presented so far represents the work of the major psychoanalytic schools that have played an important role in current psychoanalytic thinking. Contemporary psychoanalytic thinkers have provided us with a critical synthesis of the original theories. It is not possible to provide a comprehensive review of contemporary psychoanalysis, but two sources are recommended. Fred Pine (1990) in *Drive, Ego, Object and Self* describes four psychologies as distinct intrapsychic organizations which are present in early life and evolve through specific developmental lines. They are also perceived as integrating through development and are therefore viewed as equal in their contributions to personality concepts in drive psychology, ego-psychology, object relations theory and self-psychology. Pine provides a unifying model which preserves the unique contributions of each school.

A thoughtful critique of the major psychoanalytic schools, and their ability to deal with various concepts such as needs, wishes, narcissism and other concepts has been provided by Morris Eagle (1984). Eagle dissects self-psychology, object-relations theory, and drive-conflict theory and identifies similarities, differences, and deficiencies in each theoretical model. Eagle (1984) disagrees with Greenberg and Mitchell's (1983) claim that drive-conflict theory and object relations theory are incompatible, advocating instead that both models can be integrated to provide a more comprehensive psychoanalytic theory.

The work of Pine and Eagle reveals the new move toward integrating schools which have maintained separateness, due to conceptual differences, such as "pleasure-seeking" versus "object-seeking," and object versus self-object. Contemporary psychoanalytic thinkers advocate that it is not one or the other, but both; that we are inherently object seeking and pleasure seeking and the experience of one does not negate the other.

Other developments in contemporary psychoanalytic theory include the incorporation of infant development research. Daniel Stern (1985) has challenged some of the concepts of object relations theory that perceive the child as much more primitive than has actually been discovered. Stern offers developmental research evidence to challenge some of the ideas that the child is cognitively unable to see the object as whole, and that it is consumed in fantasy. Stern argues that the preoedipal child is actually more in touch with reality, and that the capacity to emerge in fantasy develops much later. Stern and others have attempted to integrate these findings to develop a more contemporary psychoanalytic theory.

ASSESSMENT

The psychodynamic perspective as a result of its focus on subjective experience and unconscious mechanisms, places less emphasis on standardized methods of assessment. The initial sessions are viewed as assessment interviews to determine suitability for analysis or psychodynamic psychotherapy. Although not clearly articulated, certain variables such as age, verbal ability, introspectiveness, and ego strength are implicitly screened to select the most appropriate patient. There is no standard assessment interview or instruments used, because most of the relevant data are considered inaccessible to the individual and can only be inferred by the therapist. In addition, each patient is seen as an individual, having unique experiences that are difficult to tap with standardized instruments or assessment devices.

The interest in subjective experience and the inaccessibility of relevant data led to the development of instruments that attempt to tap the unconscious. These instruments are known as projective techniques, the name implying that unconscious material can be projected onto ambiguous stimuli and then interpreted. Two well-known techniques are the Rorschach Inkblot Test and the Thematic Apperception Test (Carver & Scheier, 1992). In the former test, 10 inkblots are presented to patients who are then asked to describe what they see. These inkblots are ambiguous in that they do not conform to any specific pattern and are therefore subject to individual interpretation. A complicated scoring method provides results consistent with certain unconscious themes. Although initial studies showed low internal consistency, low test-retest reliability, low inter-rater reliability, and low validity, investigators have continued to study this technique and have improved its psychometric properties (Carver & Scheier, 1992).

In the Thematic Apperception Test (TAT) the patient is presented a series of pictures representing ambiguous situations. On these cards various scenes are depicted (e.g., two people looking at each other with no specific expression) involving individuals interacting in a manner that is vague and open to interpretation. Attention is paid to the presence of specific themes in the content, and this information is viewed as representing unconscious material (Carver & Scheier, 1992).

Despite the difficulties inherent in assessing this area, investigators have continued to find more reliable and valid methods of assessing the significant relationship themes important for therapy. The Core Conflictual Relationship Theme (CCRT) describes the significant relationship themes that are the focus of therapy as well as the transference relationship (Luborsky & Crits-Christoph, 1990). Luborsky and Crits-

Christoph (1990) have been able to show good inter-rater reliability once a standardized method of measuring the CCRT was established.

Other investigators have continued to develop more reliable methods of measuring these psychodynamic constructs; attempting to operationally define these constructs has been difficult. Marziali and Olenuik (1990) have measured patients' object-relationships as represented in their inner world, and have devised a method of obtaining and coding this information. Despite the great difficulty associated with assessing this perspective, many enthusiastic therapists have gone on to explore and develop various methods of measuring the complex constructs in this area. Future research will help to define these constructs more clearly, making them more amenable to study. Given that this material is subject to divergent interpretations, therapists and researchers need to develop a common language.

Outside of these more specific assessment tools, there are key areas that need to be assessed before a psychodynamic formulation can be made. They include (1) historical developmental events, (2) relationship with primary caretakers, (3) perception of self and others, (4) relationship history, (5) use of defensive operations, and (6) the transference and countertransference in the clinical assessment interview.

First, the significant developmental history is obtained. This includes biographical information of the patient's parents, quality of their marital relationship prior to and after the birth of the patient, circumstances surrounding the patient's birth (wanted or unwanted child, birth order, post-partum complications), and the family environment in the early years. This includes a history of separations and loses through death or divorce, significant illnesses, presence of physical, sexual or emotional abuse, and other stressors or traumatic events in the patient's early life.

Second, and probably most important, is the relationship between the patient and his or her parents. How the patient describes the relationship with each parent is important to note. These primary relationships need to be assessed for their nurturing, comforting, and containing aspects through the difficult developmental processes the child encountered through maturation. How the patient viewed the parents, including their positive and negative qualities, is also important to assess. A father who was seen as hostile, critical and emotionally unavailable suggests a very different relationship from one who was viewed as warm, empathic and accepting.

Third, the parents' perception of the patient, described from the patient's point of view is also important to assess. This will provide information about whether the patient felt valued and accepted as a child. The degree to which the patient can tolerate both positive and negative qualities in him- or herself is also important to assess as an indication of the capacity to tolerate ambivalent experiences. Similar information regarding the perceptions of others will help in developing an initial hypothesis of the patient's experience of the self, the object, and the object-relationship.

Fourth, more detailed information on the patient's relationship history is essential in identifying repetitive themes with respect to selection of partners, and specific relationship dynamics that tend to recur in relationships. The patient's awareness of these repetitive themes will provide information regarding their availability for psychodynamic psychotherapy.

Fifth, the ego and its use of defensive operations needs to be explored. Specifically, ego strength and resilience can be assessed by examining how the individual has coped in the past when confronted with difficult situations. The specific defenses utilized whether they are primitive, mature, or immature, will also indicate the level of ego development, and further alert the interviewer to the availability for psychodynamic psychotherapy.

Sixth, and finally, and probably unique to the psychodynamic perspective is the assessment of transference and countertransference in the initial interview. The psychodynamically oriented interviewer will note how the patient is reacting to the interviewer and will be aware of his or her own feelings toward the patient.

All this information will provide additional data about the "intrapsychic" world of the patient, since this is the major focus of the initial assessment along with the individual's experience of self, other and significant object-relationships. The psychodynamic assessor is also attuned to the fact that unconscious material unfolds during therapy, and that a complete assessment of this area is not possible in the initial interview. However, a good initial assessment can aid in the development of a psychodynamic hypothesis that will be modified as therapy evolves.

THE FOUR PS

In completing the psychodynamic column one can use general psychodynamic themes as outlined by Cleghorn and associates (Cleghorn, Bellissimo, & Will, 1983) or focus on a particular theory that may be the most applicable and helpful for treatment (see Table 8.1). If using Cleghorn's "central enduring themes" **predisposing** dynamic factors could be significant past key relationships, past conflicts, and past experi-

Table 8.1
Psychodynamic Perspective

Predisposing	* fixation or arrest in a specific psychosexual stage * inadequate holding/containing environment * arrest in the paranoid-schizoid position * insecure attachment to primary caretaker * attachment to bad objects * lack of good object experiences * infantile dependence with primary object * inadequate mirroring/idealizing functions * extensive use of splitting; other defenses * traumatic/abusive early environment
Precipitating	* loss of a relationship * death of a significant other * failures in social, occupational, interpersonal situations * traumas * new relationship * change events—births, occupations, friends, etc.
Perpetuating	* compulsive attachments to bad objects/destructive relationships * chronic use of maladaptive defenses * chronic involvement in destructive projective identification interactions * chronic dependence on self-objects for sustaining functions * lack of insight * chronic use of splitting
Protective	* secure attachment with primary caretaker * "good enough" mothering received as a child * holding/containing environment in early years * internalization of good object * good mirroring/idealizing experiences * capacity to engage in mature relationships * minimal use of splitting mechanisms

ence of the self that predispose an individual toward a particular condition. If selecting a particular theoretical framework, it is important to choose the theory that best describes the individual and outlines a treatment plan. If considering a major psychiatric disorder, an excellent resource is available that examines the psychodynamic perspective in clinical psychiatric disorders (Gabbard, 1990). ***Predisposing*** psychodynamic factors, regardless of the particular psychodynamic theory, almost always center on the early primary relationships. As described in the basic principles section, predisposing factors include fixation at a particular psychosexual stage, defensive styles, inadequate holding or containing environments, arrest in the paranoid-schizoid position, extensive past use of splitting mechanisms, infantile dependence, attachment to bad objects, destructive projective identification interactive styles, insecure attachment, and inadequate mirroring and/or idealizing self-object experiences. All these predisposing conditions can lead to the development of emotional and interpersonal problems, major psychiatric disorders or personality disorders. For example, insecure anxious attachment to mother may increase vulnerability to anxiety disorders. Also, an individual whose experience of self is contingent on being in a relationship may be more vulnerable toward anxiety when this relationship is threatened.

Individuals with a strong attachment to bad objects are prone to repeat similar unsuccessful relationships throughout adulthood. Other psychodynamic mechanisms may make an individual vulnerable to depression. These include a history of difficulty dealing with anger ("anger turned inward"), fixation at the depressive position with guilt about destroying the good internal object, and lack of a self-soothing capacity secondary to inadequate early self-object experiences. Each theory offers an explanation for a specific vulnerability. For example, self-psychology may be more useful in describing the narcissistically vulnerable patient while object-relations theory may be more applicable to borderline and schizoid-personality disorders. These theories were originally applied to these populations, respectively.

Precipitating psychodynamic factors activate or trigger dynamic issues. Most commonly, these are losses of relationships, but can include other events such as initiating a relationship, a change in life that leads to reexamination of intrapsychic issues such as trauma, illness, separation, divorce, death and others. A loss of a relationship may precipitate depression in a sensitized individual. Failure in social, occupational or interpersonal relationships may also activate repressed negative experiences of the self.

These precipitants can go on to become ***perpetuating*** factors, as is evident in individuals experiencing chronic interpersonal difficulties with a significant other. Ongoing intrapsychic conditions which may perpetuate a condition or disorder are compulsive attachments to bad objects, frequent use of splitting, chronic involvement in destructive projective-identification interactions, complete dependence on self-objects for sustenance, and poor insight.

Protective psychodynamic factors provide a shield against stressful events and prevent the development of major psychological disorders. These include good psychological insight, capacity to engage in mature relationships, minimal use of primitive defense mechanisms, and any corrective experience that may have compensated for early negative experiences. An example of the latter is the presence of at least one nurturing figure in the earlier years juxtaposed with trauma. The availability of good objects which can be internalized or can provide good self-object experiences can offset the impact of psychological trauma. The ability to engage in healthy relationships throughout development is especially protective. These individuals are better able to engage in a therapeutic relationship.

COPING-RESPONSE STYLE

Introspection and self-analysis during stressful times are considered a psychodynamic coping-response style. Individuals with this coping style may reflect and focus inward to develop an understanding of "why" they are experiencing their current difficulties. This motivation towards self-understanding may have developed as a result of previous successful outcomes utilizing this coping style. Understanding is often relieving and enables better self-management.

Individuals with this coping-response style are more likely to benefit from psychodynamic psychotherapy. Although these individuals are not the only ones who will benefit from this form of therapy, they may be a good match for this particular approach because it is consistent with their existing coping-response style. Individuals with limited introspective capabilities may move toward this style as a result of insight gained from other forms of therapy.

Individuals who seek out others to "talk" about their feelings and experiences may also be good candidates for psychodynamic psychotherapy, being accustomed to using relationships to explore inner experiences. Of course, this also illustrates a capacity to engage in a relationship, to receive support as well as enhance self-understanding. These individuals will do well in any form of therapy which involves a supportive therapeutic relationship. Whether or not psychodynamic therapy is chosen as the treatment of choice will depend on the patient's coping-response style and motivation to explore intrapsychic issues. Other therapies (e.g., behavioral) can be integrated as therapy progresses (Wachtel, 1977).

TREATMENT

Classical Psychoanalysis

Treatment according to this perspective includes psychoanalysis and psychodynamic psychotherapy. Psychoanalysis as described by Freud was carried out four or five times a week with the patient lying on the couch and the analyst sitting behind the patient, out of the patient's view. This arrangement was designed to permit the patient to freely associate without being influenced by any verbal or nonverbal behaviors of the analyst. The analysand was instructed to say whatever came to mind, without censoring any material. The analyst was to remain a blank screen in order to promote "free" associations from the patient. The analyst could clarify and offer interpretations of the material presented, but remained at a distance from the patient. Unfortunately this "blank screen" recommendation was carried to such a degree that the analyst became a distant, detached, unempathic, ingenuine therapist (Carver & Scheier, 1992). Freud himself was described as being very empathic, genuine and human with his patients, and this distant stance was somehow incorrectly perpetuated by his followers. Fortunately, this approach to analysis has been challenged, and more contemporary psychoanalysts have been dispelling the blank screen, and replacing it with a more human, genuine therapist (Greenberg & Mitchell, 1983; Kohut, 1971).

Classical psychoanalysis is an open-ended therapy that is carried out for several years. The sessions are confidential and an agreement is made for at least four 50-minute sessions a week. The nondirective, unguided therapy begins by analyst and analysand establishing a working relationship and agreeing together on the details of the number of sessions, length of treatment, fees, and general rules of the therapeutic contract as it pertains to missed sessions and other issues. During the early phases of treatment the analyst pays close attention to numerous details, such as the patient's dress, mannerisms, what is said, what is not said, interactions with the analyst, and other nonverbal behaviors. The analyst looks for themes in the analysand's content and pays attention to how the patient's difficulties and everyday experiences reflect unconscious repressed fantasies or conflicts from childhood. Responses in the form of interpretations are made initially at a superficial level and are consistent with the patient's conscious experience. Interpretations regarding deeply repressed material are not usually made early in treatment (Symington, 1986; Freud, 1910; Brenner, 1955).

As therapy evolves a relationship develops between analysand and analyst. This relationship, known as "transference," is the major vehicle through which therapeutic change occurs. In the transference the patient develops feelings toward the analyst and an interpersonal relationship develops. According to psychoanalytic theory this relationship is a repetition of an earlier relationship with mother or father, which becomes reignited with the analyst in therapy. Intense feelings develop toward the analyst, creating a more conflictual relationship. Working through the transference relationship is considered the active ingredient of change in psychoanalysis. The analyst becomes increasingly more important to the patient which leads to an increase in the patient's demands upon the analyst (Brenner, 1955; Hollender & Ford, 1990; Greenberg and Mitchell, 1983).

The "working through" process is a rather long, affectively charged, complicated journey that is sometimes the most difficult time in therapy. The analyst also explores other unconscious themes in the analysand's free associations, and together they come to appreciate how traumatic childhood experiences with the primary objects contribute to present day difficulties. As insight into these early experiences increases, the analysand gains deeper understanding of significant past events and is able to see how these events have influenced his or her life and have contributed to present day difficulties (Freud, 1910; Brenner, 1955).

The working through process also involves the analysis and resolution of the transference. The patient's understanding of the transference deepens through therapy and by itself promotes an even deeper understanding of past and present conflictual issues. The working through is considered to have three stages: repetition, elaboration, and amplification. The analysis of the transference facilitates recall of significant memories from the past. The transference is a repetition of significant past relationships and as it unfolds and becomes more elaborate; it heightens the patient's experience by amplifying core dynamic issues that had prior to this point, been unavailable for conscious experience (Freud, 1910; Carver & Scheier, 1992).

As the analysis of the transference nears completion the termination phase begins. During this phase the patient's attachment to the analyst is reexamined. The patient usually experiences anxiety over this impending termination, and often there is a relapse of the symptoms that were present at the beginning of treatment. As this stage is worked through, the patient offers additional memories or insights that confirm the interpretations offered earlier. This response is often interpreted as the patient wanting to present a gift to the therapist, a way of saying thank you for the positive effect therapy has had on the analysand's life. In addition, the final phases of therapy involves the patient revealing wishes that have been kept secret from the analyst, wishes that portray the analyst as an omnipotent character. These fantasies are analyzed along with the patient's fantasies of what might happen after termination (Freud, 1912).

The key ingredients of psychoanalysis according to Freud is the development of a certain atmosphere that permits the analysand to freely explore whatever comes to mind in the therapeutic situation. The focus is on making the unconscious fantasies and conflicts from childhood conscious. The relationship with the therapist reenacts these early relationships and the conflicts of childhood are worked through in the transference. The basic premise here is that it is the repressed, ungratified sexual fantasies of childhood that lead to difficulties in later life. Unconscious wishes are made conscious through free association, interpretation, and analysis and resolution of the transference. The primary intervention practiced is interpretation. Interpretations facilitate insight, and insight alone is curative. The therapist always remains neutral, so as not to interfere with the analysand's unconscious. Any countertransferential feelings are considered to represent the analyst's own unresolved conflicts, and an interference to the analysis. This therapeutic process is described as a journey that takes place without any specified rules or format, and is unique to each individual (Freud, 1912; Brenner, 1955; Symington, 1986; Greenberg & Mitchell, 1983).

Object-Relations Psychotherapy/Analysis

The above description illustrates psychoanalysis carried out according to Freud. Current psychoanalysis may be carried out as described above or it may vary with respect to the number of visits, the use of a chair instead of a couch, and the particular theoretical model. Psychodynamic psychotherapy is conducted once or twice a week, and does not conform to all the strict rules of analysis. In many cases the therapist is not a trained analyst, but similar theoretical and clinical principles may be followed by an analyst and a psychodynamic therapist practicing from the same theoretical framework. Since Freud, there have been numerous changes, with today's analysts and psychodynamic therapists focusing on different issues in therapy. For example, object-relations therapists will concentrate on different developmental processes, depending on the specific model within object-relations theory that is adhered to. A Kleinian analyst may pay more attention to themes consistent with the paranoid-schizoid or depressive position and deal with the internal and external splitting mechanisms that the patient uses, while providing a containing environment for the patient's projections (Guntrip, 1961; Greenberg & Mitchell, 1983; Segal, 1992).

The major goal of therapy if one is following Fairbairn, is to help the individual give up his or her attachments to internal bad objects. To do this the analyst needs to become a sufficient good object so that these bad objects can be released in the context of a safe therapeutic environment (Fairbairn, 1943). How this is to be done, Fairbairn does not fully explain (Greenberg & Mitchell, 1983). By helping the patient give up these ties to internalized bad objects, he or she is moved from an infantile method of relating to a more mature form, permitting the individual to participate in a "real relationship," the ultimate goal of therapy.

Object-relations therapies vary depending on the specific model being followed; however, there are common themes that can be identified across all these models that are the focus of therapy. Generally, object-relations therapists and classical analysts are similar in the value they give to the unconscious and to the analysis and resolution of the transference; they differ in what they emphasize. The object-relations therapist attends to primitive splitting, internal and external good and bad objects, projective identification, attachment to internalized bad objects, differentiation, symbiosis, and other unconscious mechanisms that have developed as a result of the individual's frustration in relating with the primary object. Except for the Kleinian analyst, attention is on relational rather than psychosexual issues (Cashdan, 1988; Greenberg & Mitchell, 1983). The analysis of transference in object-relations therapy involves the interpretation of this relationship as symbolic of the early primary relationship. Focus is not limited to sexual fantasies but involves the exploration, interpretation, and working through of projective identification issues with the therapist. The therapist must be available to accept and contain the patient's projected good and bad parts. With the resolution of the transference the patient is able to tolerate both good and bad parts in the therapist and within him- or herself, enabling him- or herself to perceive the therapist as a whole object, capable of containing both these parts simultaneously. Toleration of ambivalence and resolution of primitive splitting makes the patient available for more mature relationships that allow giving and receiving to be experienced simultaneously. The ultimate goal of object-relations therapy is the diminution of splitting of inner and outer world experiences so that individuals can engage in relationships as a integrated whole objects (Greenberg & Mitchell, 1983; Guntrip, 1961).

There are, however, some key differences between classical psychoanalysis and object-relations therapy that are important to mention. First, classical therapy's emphasis is on attending to and interpreting intrapsychic conflict in order to provide information to the patient about unconscious motivators of behavior. In object-relations therapy the focus is on *the relationship* with the patient, and it is this relationship that provides the active ingredient of change. In object-relations therapy the therapist engages in a relationship with the patient, and it is the management of this relationship over time that leads to change. Therefore, in object-relations therapy the analyst is a participant, not a neutral bystander; the analyst is equally responsible for the creation of the transference (Greenberg & Mitchell, 1983).

Countertransference is also viewed differently, it is seen as essential to the analytic process as it provides useful information about the patient's relationship dynamics; it is not an interference, it is inevitable. Interpretations are utilized to work through transference not just to provide information (Greenberg & Mitchell, 1983). These differences are significant, and have shifted the attention of psychoanalysis from an insight-focused, to a relationally focused therapy. This shift has been positively viewed for it has created a "real" more genuing therapeutic relationship between the therapist and the patient. This attention given to the quality of the therapeutic relationship has also been emphasized in self-psychological psychotherapy.

Self Psychological Psychotherapy/Psychoanalysis

An analyst or therapist who is working from a self-psychological model will attend to developmental issues that reveal arrests in the mirroring or idealizing phase. The therapist is actively empathic and genuine and considers this attitude an essential ingredient that promotes change. The therapist's subjective introspectiveness allows a deeper understanding of the patient that is not possible if the therapist remains a distant observer or object for containing projections. The analyst's empathic attunement not only creates a safe, trusting, therapeutic relationship but also allows the patient to be more attuned with the vulnerable, frightened self that is terrified of disintegration. The therapist, according to this model, permits the patient to use him or her as a self-object who will provide the mirroring and idealizing experiences that were absent in childhood. With the therapist providing these "functions" the patient is able to internalize them, and develop cohesive sense of self (Basch, 1988; Wolfe, 1988; Kohut, 1971; 1977; 1979; 1984; Rowe & MacIsaac, 1991).

Once again, this process is regarded as a journey undertaken by the therapist and the patient. The difference in self-psychologically oriented therapy is that defense mechanisms are viewed as protecting the self from disintegration. Therefore, interpreting these defenses in the absence of a trusting, empathic, self-object relationship only serves to strengthen these defenses. The analyst's empathic attunement decreases the patient's defenses, which facilitates the exploration of unconscious material. This different stance developed as a result of Kohut's disillusionment with the traditional psychoanalytic school. Therapy, however, progressed in the same fashion, from the early phase to the analysis of the transference, to transference resolution.

The goal (of self-psychological therapy, like object-relations therapy) is to develop more differentiated relationships with significant others. However the focus is on the development of a cohesive sense of self that is not vulnerable to fragmentation and has developed internal self-soothing capacities. The ability to have good self-object experiences is considered a good outcome in therapy but the ability to sustain these functions individually is considered the ultimate goal of therapy.

Like object-relations therapy, self-psychology stresses the interpersonal dimension in the therapeutic relationship, and it is through this relationship that change occurs. The difference is in the focus of therapy. Object-relations therapists concentrate on bad objects and projective identification, and the therapist permits him- or herself to be used as a container for projections, without identifying with them, the goal being to permit the patient at a later point to achieve integration. The self-psychological therapist provides functions that were missing in childhood so that they can be internalized and contribute to a more cohesive sense of self. Both approaches are considered relational in their therapeutic focus (Greenberg & Mitchell, 1983).

It is difficult to clearly describe the step-by-step process that occurs and needs to occur in psychoanalysis and psychodynamic psychotherapy. For the most part this has been considered a unique, subjective experience not amenable to research. However, an increasing body of research has attempted to study the conceptual and therapeutic issues in psychodynamic psychotherapy. Various terms are being operationally defined and research is showing good outcome with transference interpretation interventions (Luborsky & Crits-Christoph, 1990; Marziali & Olenuik, 1990). As process research in psychodynamic psychotherapy continues, the active ingredients of a good therapeutic outcome will be identified.

Brief Psychodynamic Psychotherapy

Perhaps more researched and gaining significant popularity is short-term psychodynamic psychotherapy. This abbreviated form of long-term therapy has been showing promising results (Crits-Christoph, 1992). A variety of brief dynamic therapies have been described by Davanloo (1980), Luborsky (1984), Sifneos (1972), Strupp and Binder (1984), and Mann (1973). Future research should aid in identifying specific populations for these therapies.

Humanistic Therapies

Other therapies can be considered under this column. Some of these include the humanistic therapies and interpersonal therapy. Humanistic therapies include client centered, gestalt, and existential (Corsini & Wedding, 1989). The humanistic view, however, does not pay attention to assessment and formulation prior to therapy, and for this reason it is not discussed in a separate chapter. Nevertheless, an ongoing formulation of the therapy process is attended to, and it is therefore discussed in the treatment section. Although differences exist across the humanistic therapies with respect to how therapy is conducted, they all share certain fundamental principles considered unique to the humanistic perspective. First, clients are viewed as experts of their own experience and a certain therapeutic environment involving a genuine, empathic therapist is considered essential to promote inner exploration (Rogers, 1965). This environment is more important than providing interpretations to facilitate the experience of insight. In some cases, as in gestalt therapy, specific interventions (e.g., empty chair dialogue) are used to enhance the clients' awareness of their own experience. This view of therapy is known as the phenomenological approach (Rice & Greenberg, 1992).

Second, the humanistic perspective does not believe "pathology" explains psychological disturbances, but rather views all individuals as possessing the capacity for growth and development, referred to as the individual's "actualizing tendency." Blocks to self-growth occur as a result of certain learned self-concepts that operate under "shoulds," rather than needs and wants. The goal of therapy is to free the individual from these shoulds, and promote healthy functioning, growth, and development (Rice & Greenberg, 1992).

Third, the humanistic therapies focus on constructing new meaning, and clients are encouraged by the therapist to engage in an experiential search in order to arrive at a heightened perceptual awareness of themselves and their inner experiences. This realization is accomplished by the therapist carefully attending, empathically responding, differentiating and integrating a specific client experience. Interpretive interventions are not utilized (except in some of the existential therapies) given the fundamental belief that the client, and not the therapist, is the expert on his or her own experience (Rice & Greenberg, 1993).

Finally, all humanistic therapies are person centered in that a real relationship develops between the client and the therapist, rather than a transferential one based on past relationships with primary caretakers. More attention is paid to the present and the future, and the prime purpose of the relationship is to allow the client to pursue more deep self-exploration. Greater attention is also given to affect to facilitate this process. More recently process-experiential therapy (Greenberg, 1993) has integrated client-centered, gestalt, and existential approaches in a marker-guided therapy that is currently being investigated in the treatment of depression. Preliminary results indicate a positive outcome with this approach.

Given the basic therapeutic principles discussed above, some may question the inclusion of this form of therapy under the "psychodynamic" perspective. The historical development of the humanistic perspective with its negative reaction to psychoanalysis, its negative view of interpretive interventions, its deemphasis of past experiences as a focus in therapy, and its disregard for any "transferential" aspects to the therapeutic relationship all suggest a different perspective. Despite the differences the fundamental approach in these therapies is to promote "self-exploration of inner experiences." Regardless of what is considered the active therapeutic ingredients necessary to promote change, the search for meaning is the primary goal of therapy. Therefore, the humanistic approach is dynamic, in that the ultimate goal of therapy is to promote greater self-understanding and freedom to experience life more fully. Unlike the cognitive perspective that considers thoughts as distortions, the psychodynamic and humanistic approaches both view thoughts as important in the individual's attempt to construct meaning, and are considered valid and not "distortions" of reality. Therefore, both approaches share similar views of what is considered the ultimate goal of therapy.

Interpersonal Therapy

The second form of therapy to be addressed under the psychodynamic perspective is interpersonal therapy. This therapy has been recently investigated and found effective in the treatment of depression. The approach as it applies to depression was originally developed by Klerman, Weissman and Rounsavalle (1984). The theoretical basis of this form of therapy is based on Sullivan's Interpersonal theory (1953), Meyer's (1957) psychobiological approach, and Bowlby's (1976) attachment theory. Although early developmental issues are important, attention is directed toward present interpersonal difficulties accompanying depressive symptoms. Symptom reduction through education and medication precedes interpersonally focused interventions. Working through unresolved grief, interpersonal role disputes, role transitions, and interpersonal deficits, are the primary problems identified in depressed individuals and one or two of these issues become the focus of treatment. Specific strategies that involve exploration, clarification, facilitation of affective expression, and examination of communication styles, are used to resolve some of these issues. The therapeutic relationship is also used to deal with interpersonal interactions that lead to difficulties. However, defensive styles and internal conflicts are not the focus of therapy.

Given the deemphasis on self-exploration, defenses, internal conflicts, and the focus on present relationships make interpersonal therapy appear somewhat divergent from the psychodynamic perspective. Given its historical roots in interpersonal theory (a branch of object-relations theory) and attachment theory, and its concentration on the individual's struggle in relationships, it is considered under the psychodynamic perspective.

SUMMARY

Psychodynamic theory and therapy have provided us with a rich understanding of personality and psychopathology. The last few decades have stimulated many to apply empirical methods to studying this intriguing form of therapy, leading to refinements in definitions and measurements of various constructs such as transference (Luborsky & Crits-Christoph, 1990) and object representations (Marziali & Oleniuk, 1990). Although some criticize this search for operational definitions, arguing that it distorts the original meaning, it is important that if we are to develop further understanding and refinement in psychodynamic theory and therapy, we need to develop a common language, so that communication within fields can improve and move the entire field forward. If psychodynamic theory and therapy are to advance, there will be continuing pressure for the field to demonstrate reasonable psychometric properties for the constructs described and for their role in therapy. There is evidence that this process is already happening, and producing promising results (Strupp, 1992).

REFERENCES

Ainsworth, M. D., Blehar, M. C., Waters, E., & Wall, S. (1978). *Patterns of Attachment Assessed in the Strange Situation and at Home.* Hillsdale, NJ: Lawrence Erlbaum.

Bacal, H. A., & Newman, A. M. (1990). *Theories of Object Relations: Bridges to Self-Psychology.* New York: Columbia University Press.

Balint, M. (1968). *The Basic Fault.* London: Tavistock.

Basch, M. F. (1988). *Understanding Psychotherapy: The Science Behind the Art.* New York: Basic Books.

Bowlby, J. (1976). *Attachment and Loss: Volume I. Attachment.* New York: Penguin Books.

Bowlby, J. (1988). *A Secure Base.* New York: Basic Books.

Brenner, C. (1955). *An Elementary Textbook of Psychoanalysis.* Garden City, NY: Doubleday Anchor Books.

Carver, C. S., & Scheier, M. F. (1992). *Perspectives on Personality* (2nd ed.). Needham Heights, MA: Allyn and Bacon.

Cashdan, S. (1988). *Object Relations Therapy: Using the Relationship.* New York: W. W. Norton.

Cleghorn, J. M., Bellissimo, A., & Will, D. (1983). Teaching Some Principles of Individual Psychodynamics through an Introductory Guide to Formulations. *Canadian Journal of Psychiatry, 28,* 162–172.

Corsini, R. J., & Wedding, D. (1989). *Current Psychotherapies* (4th ed.). Itasca, IL: F.E. Peacock.

Crits-Christoph, P. (1992). The Efficacy of Brief Dynamic Psychotherapy: A Meta-Analysis. *American Journal of Psychiatry, 149,* 151–158.

Davanloo, H. (1980). *Short Term Psychotherapy.* New York: Aronson Press.

Eagle, M. N. (1984). *Recent Developments in Psychoanalysis: A Critical Evaluation.* Cambridge, MA: Harvard University Press.

Fairbairn, W. R. D. (1943) 1952. Repression and the Return of Bad Objects. In *An Object Relations Theory of the Personality.* New York: Basic Books.

Fairbairn, W. R. D. (1940) 1952. Schizoid Factors in the Personality. In *An Object Relations Theory of the Personality.* New York: Basic Books.

Fairbairn, W. R. D. (1944) 1952. Endopsychic Structure Considered in Terms of Object Relationships. In *An Object Relations Theory of the Personality.* New York: Basic Books.

Fairbairn, W. R. D. (1949) 1952. Steps in the Development of An Object Relations Theory of the Personality. In *An Object Relations Theory of the Personality.* New York: Basic Books.

Fairbairn, W. R. D. (1951) 1952. Addendum to Endopsychic Structure Considered in Terms of Object Relationships. In *An Object Relations Theory of the Personality.* New York: Basic Books.

Free, N. K., Wingnet, C. N., & Whitman, R. M. (1993). Separation Anxiety and Panic Disorder. *American Journal of Psychiatry, 150,* 595–599.

Freud, S., & Breuer, J. (1974). *Studies on Hysteria.* Harmondsworth, Middlesex, England: Penguin Books.

Freud, A. (1966). *The Ego and the Mechanisms of Defense.* New York: International Universities Press.

Freud, S. (1905) 1977. On Sexuality: Three Essays on the Theory of Sexuality. Harmondsworth, Middlesex, England: Penguin Books.

Freud, S. (1910) 1957. The Future Prospects of Psychoanalytic Therapy. In J. Sutherland, (Ed.), *Collected Papers 2.* London, England: Hogarth Press.

Freud, S. (1923) 1984. The Ego and the Id. In *On Meta-Psychology: The Theory of Psychoanalysis.* Harmondsworth, Middlesex, England: Penguin Books.

Freud, S. (1915) 1985. The Unconscious. In *On Meta-Psychology: The Theory of Psychoanalysis.* Harmondsworth, Middlesex, England: Penguin Books.

Freud, S. (1912) 1990. The Dynamics of Transference. In A. H. Esman, (Ed.), *Essential Papers on Transference.* New York: New York University Press.

Gabbard, G. O. (1990). *Psychodynamic Psychiatry in Clinical Practice.* Washington, DC: American Psychiatric Press.

Greenberg, J. R., & Mitchell, S. A. (1983). *Object Relations in Psychoanalytic Theory.* Cambridge, MA: Harvard University Press.

Greenberg, L. S. (1993). *Change Processes in the Experiential Therapy of Depression.* (NIMH Depression Study in progress). Toronto, Ontario: York University.

Grotstein, J.S. (1991a). The Kleinian School. In O. Weininger, J. Cutcher, & J. Townsend, (Eds.), *Melanie Klein and Object Relations, 9*(2), 16–33.

Grotstein, J. S. (1991b). The Contributions of the British Object Relations Schools. In O. Weininger, J. Cutcher, & J. Townsend, (Eds.), *Melanie Klein and Object Relations, 9*(2), 34–62.

Grotstein, J. S. (1991c). An American View of the British Psychoanalytic Experience: Psychoanalysis in Counterpoint. The Americanization of Psychoanalysis. In O. Weininger, J. Cutcher, & J. Townsend, (Eds.), *Melanie Klein and Object Relations, 9*(2), 1–15.

Guntrip, H. (1961). *Personality Structure and Human Interaction: The Developing Synthesis of Psychodynamic Theory.* New York: International Universities Press.

Hall, C. S. (1954). *A Primer of Freudian Psychology.* San Francisco: New American Press.

Hall, C. S., & Lindzey, G. (1985). *Theories of Personality* (3rd ed.). New York: John Wiley and Sons.

Hollender, M. H., & Ford, C. V. (1990). *Dynamic Psychotherapy: An Introductory Approach.* Washington, DC: American Psychiatric Press.

Jones, E. (1953). *The Life and Work of Sigmund Freud. Vol I.* New York: Basic Books.

Kernberg, O. (1975). *Borderline Conditions and Pathological Narcissism.* New York: Aronson Press.

Klein, M. (1946) 1975. Notes on Some Schizoid Mechanisms. In *Envy and Gratitude.* New York: Delacorte Press.

Klein, M. (1959) 1975. Our Adult World and Its Roots in Infancy. In *Envy and Gratitude.* New York: Delacorte Press.

Klerman, G. F., Weissman, M. M., & Rounsavalle, B. J. (1984). *Interpersonal Psychotherapy of Depression.* New York: Basic Books.

Kohut, H. (1979). *How Does Analysis Cure?* In A. Goldberg, & P. Stepansky, (Eds.). Chicago: Chicago University Press.

Kohut, H. (1984). Introspection, Empathy, and the Semi-Circle of Mental Health. *International Journal of Psychoanalysis, 63,* 395–407.

Kohut, H. (1971). *The Analysis of the Self: A Systematic Approach to the Psychoanalytic Treatment of Narcissistic Personality Disorder.* Maddison, CT: International Universities Press.

Kohut, H. (1977). *The Restoration of the Self.* Maddison, CT: International Universities Press.

Luborksy, L. (1984). *Principles of Psychoanalytic Psychotherapy: A Manual for Supportive Expressive Treatment.* New York: Basic Books.

Luborsky, L., & Crits-Christoph, P. (1990). *Understanding Transference: The CCRT Method.* New York: Basic Books.

Mann, J. (1973). *Time limited psychotherapy.* Cambridge, MA: Harvard University Press.

Marziali, E., & Olenuik, J. (1990). Object Representations in Descriptions of Significant Others: A Methodological Study. *Journal of Personality Assessment, 54,* 105–115.

Meyer, A. (1957). Psychobiology: A Science of Man. In E. Winters & E. M. Bowers, (Eds) *Psychobiology: A Science of Man.* Springfield, IL: Thomas.

Ogden, T. H. (1979). On Projective Identification. *International Journal of Psychoanalysis, 60,* 357–373.

Ogden, T. H. (1983). The Concept of Internal Object Relations. *International Journal of Psychoanalysis, 64,* 227–241.

Ornstein, P. (1991). Why Self-Psychology is not an Object-Relations Theory: Clinical and Theoretical Considerations. In A. Goldberg, (Ed.), *The Evolution of Self-Psychology: Progress in Self-Psychology.* Hillsdale, NJ: Analytic Press.

Pettem, O., West, M., Mahoney, A., & Kellar, A. (1993). Depression and Attachment Problems. *Journal of Psychiatry and Neuroscience, 18*(2), 78–81.

Pine, F. (1990). *Drive, Ego, Object and Self: A Synthesis of Clinical Work.* New York: Basic Books.

Rice, L. N., & Greenberg, L. S. (1992). Humanistic Approaches to Psychother-

apy. In D. K. Freedheim, (Ed.), *History of Psychotherapy: A Century of Change.* Washington, DC: American Psychological Association.
Rowe, C. E., & MacIsaac D. S. (1991). *Empathic Attunement: The Technique of Psychoanalytic Self-Psychology.* Northvale, NJ: Aronson Press.
Rogers, C. R. (1965). *Client-Centered Therapy: It's Current Practice, Implications and Theory.* Boston: Houghton Mifflin.
Sandler, J. (1987). *Projection, Identification, and Projective Identification.* Maddison, CT: International Universities Press.
Segal, H. (1964). *Introduction to the Work of Melanie Klein.* New York: Basic Books.
Segal, J. (1992). *Key Figures in Counselling and Psychotherapy.* London: Sage Publications.
Sifneos, P. (1972). *Short Term Psychotherapy and Emotional Crisis.* Cambridge, MA: Harvard University Press.
Spillius, E. B. (1992). *Clinical Lectures on Klein and Bion.* Tavistock, London: New Library of Psychoanalysis.
Stern, D. N. (1985). *The Interpersonal World of the Infant.* New York: Basic Books.
Stolorow, R., Brandchaft, E., & Attwood, G. (1987). *Psychoanalytic Treatment: An Intersubjective Approach.* Hillsdale, NJ: Analytic Press.
Strupp, H. H., & Binder, J. (1984). *Psychotherapy in a New Key.* New York: Basic Books.
Strupp, H. H. (1992). Future of Psychodynamic Psychotherapy. *Psychotherapy, 29,* 21–27.
Sullivan, H. S. (1953). *The Interpersonal Theory of Psychiatry.* New York: Norton.
Sutherland, J. D. (1980). The British Object Relations Theorists: Balint, Winnicott, Fairbairn, and Guntrip. *Journal of the American Psychoanalytic Association, 28,* 829–860.
Symington, N. (1986). *The Analytic Experience.* New York: St. Martin's Press.
Wachtel, P. L. (1977). *Psychoanalysis and Behavioral Therapy: Towards an Integration.* New York: Basic Books.
Winnicott, D. W. (1965). *The Maturational Process and the Facilitating Environment: Studies in the Theory of Emotional Development.* Madison, CT: International Universities Press.
Wolfe, E. (1988). *Treating the Self: The Science Behind the Art.* New York: Guilford Press.

SYSTEMIC FACTORS

CHAPTER 9

THE COUPLE/MARITAL SYSTEM

THE PERSPECTIVES

A variety of perspectives represent the couple system; many of these were discussed in the individual section. In this chapter the "couple perspective" refers to a frame of reference that examines dyadic relationships. Emphasis is placed on the individual's most important relationship, as this relationship is considered to have a significant impact on psychological functioning. Attention is on relationship variables and how they contribute to psychological problems and disorders. Adopting a couple perspective in addressing an individual problem can provide important information that may be unobtainable if taken only from an individual frame of reference. In some cases relationship distress may be the presenting problem, necessitating a couple formulation and treatment plan. In other cases an individual problem may be precipitated, exacerbated, or maintained by relationship factors. The major perspective taken in this chapter is that one's significant relationship has an important effect on psychological well being, making it an important area to attend to in the assessment, formulation, and treatment of mental health problems.

Several couple perspectives are discussed in the literature that offer conceptual frameworks to understand relationship difficulties. The same theories that have been applied to individuals, such as the psychodynamic, behavioral, and cognitive perspectives, have been applied to couples. Alternate schools of thought not previously discussed under the individual heading are Emotionally focused or Experiential theories (Greenberg & Johnson, 1988) Structural-Strategic theory, and Bowen Family Systems theory (Jacobson & Gurman, 1986). The models differ in how they conceptualize couple distress and by the techniques that are used in therapy.

In addition to providing an alternate perspective, there are other reasons for developing an approach to understanding significant dyadic relationships. Difficulty in relationships is cited as the most common reason individuals give for seeking psychotherapy (O'Leary, 1987). Marital and couple problems account for 40% of mental health clinic intakes in the United States. Others have found (Chamberlaines, Barnes, Waring, Wood, & Fry, 1989) that those who seek psychiatric help in outpatient clinics perceive less intimacy in their marriage than those who do not seek help, matched for the same presenting problem. In this study, women were more likely to seek psychiatric help than their male counterparts for relationship difficulties. Other researchers have examined marital relationships and their influence on the outcome of certain psychiatric disorders. A number of researchers have found a relationship between marital intimacy and depression in women (Chamberlaines et al., 1989; Beach, Sandeen & O'Leary, 1990). A recent study (Goering, Lance, & Freeman, 1992) found that the depressed woman's perception of marital support at time of admission was a strong predictor of post-hospital recovery. Marital adjustment has also been considered in the etiology or at least in the course and treatment of anxiety disorders such as phobias, panic disorder, and obsessive compulsive disorders (Barlow, 1981), and in childhood emotional and behavioral disorders (Reid & Crisafulli, 1990).

In addition to the influence of marital discord on individual disorders, marital distress by itself is a major concern given the high rate of divorce, domestic violence, and crime associated with domestic disputes (Babcock, Waltz, Jacobson, & Gottman, 1993). The prevalence of marital distress is unknown given the lack of epidemiological research in this area; however, given the common presentation of marital and relationship distress in mental health clinic referrals, it is a growing concern among many mental health professionals.

This perspective is probably the most familiar to the social work student who is exposed to the systemic perspective early in training. Psychology graduate students may receive some training in this area depending on the available supervision. Therefore, the majority of marital or couple therapists are social workers or psychologists. Psychiatrists are underrepresented in the field, likely due to a lack of emphasis on this subject in training, and limited supervision experiences available in residency. However, because of recent interest in marital and family issues in the outcome of psychiatric disorders, psychiatry residents are beginning to be exposed to the systemic areas.

BRIEF HISTORY

The history of this perspective began with the marital therapy movement. This movement is a relatively recent one, developing 60 years ago when marital therapy was carried out by the clergy, social workers, physicians, and lawyers. At that time there was no formal training in this area, since marital therapy was not an identified discipline. In the 1920s the first institute to offer marital counseling was a New York City community church. Shortly after this Paul Popenoe developed the American Institute of Family Relations in California. Emily Mudd is credited with having developed the Marriage Council of Philadelphia, and soon after this, in the 1930s the Groves Conference on the Family and the National Council on Family Relations were held. In 1942 these two groups formed the American Association of Marriage Counselors making this a distinct professional field. Since the marital relationship was viewed as an integral part of the family, the name was changed to the American Association of Marriage and Family Counselors (AAMC). In 1963 California law required marital and family therapists to be licensed, leading to the AAMC changing its name to AAMFT—the American Association of Marital and Family Therapy. In 1978 the U.S. commissioner of education designated the AAMFT as the official body to accredit training programs (Prochaska & Prochaska, 1978).

Marital therapy also developed in other countries including Italy (Selvini-Palazzoli, Boscolo, Cecchin & Prata, 1978) and England (Dicks, 1967). Palazzoli developed a family therapy which was later applied to couples. Dicks was one of the first to describe a psychodynamic theory of marital relations emphasizing an object-relations perspective. Although marital therapy continued to develop its own theories, it was considered a form of family therapy that did not have the status of a separate, distinct field of study. For many years marital therapy was discussed under family therapy, and many felt that the marriage somehow became lost in the family. However, this situation changed over the next 30 years, and marital therapy obtained separate status as a distinct form of therapy that was no longer viewed as a subheading of family therapy. Textbooks and journal articles became available that were devoted solely to the study of the marriage and marital therapy. Today marital therapy is a separate therapy that is practiced primarily by social workers and psychologists, and a few psychiatrists. Extensive research has accumulated over the last two decades to lend support to this form of therapy. There are many forms of marital therapy that have been discussed in the literature, some have been empirically investigated. For those unfamiliar with this area a general approach that can be used with all couples will be presented first. Following this will be a discussion of the different theoretical models that have been applied to understanding and treating marital distress.

BASIC PRINCIPLES

A General Approach

Marriage and marital distress can be understood from a variety of theoretical models including psychodynamic, cognitive-behavioral, systemic, and others. Even though each theory offers a rich framework for understanding marital and couple distress, it is usually difficult for the trainee to grasp and utilize these concepts when first exposed to them. A simple framework or approach that is atheoretical and that can be applied to virtually all couples is needed. A variety of relational constructs discussed in the literature can provide useful frameworks for understanding relationships, the most popular, however, is intimacy.

In marriage there is an emotional bond that is shared by husband and wife; this bond has been described as intimacy. This relational construct of intimacy has been of great interest to therapists and researchers who wish to study close relationships. An intimate relationship is one in which there is sharing of personal information at many levels, which includes sharing of activities, common goals, and interests. However, it is the sharing of feelings that is considered the most important variable in the experience of intimacy in a relationship. In addition to the experience of mutual sharing, *each* partner needs to feel heard and validated by the other. In order to experience a truly intimate relationship both partners need to be able to maintain a balance between closeness and separateness. Both individuals in the relationship must be able to feel separate from their partner, as well as close to them. In other words intimacy implies an interdependence between two people who can also function separately. Most couple therapists agree that the struggle to maintain intimacy without sacrificing autonomy is the major theme that characterizes most relationships, distressed and nondistressed (Scharff & Scharff, 1991; Greenberg & Johnson, 1988; Jacobson, 1989; Waring & Chelune, 1983).

Schaefer and Olson (1981) suggest five different areas in which couples can share an intimate relationship: (1) intellectual, (2) emotional, (3) physical/sexual, (4) recreational, and (5) social.

To share intimacy in these areas requires not only the ability to communicate but the feeling that it is safe to do so. Intellectual intimacy refers to sharing thoughts and ideas and conversing on the same intellectual level. Emotional intimacy, considered the most important area, involves sharing feelings, from the superficial to the most vulnerable deeply felt affective experiences. Physical and sexual intimacy involves the capacity to be physically intimate as well as sexually intimate. Recreational intimacy refers to sharing activies, such as sports, hobbies, vacations, and other planned activities, while social intimacy involves sharing common friends with whom to enjoy joint activities. Different patterns of intimacy are likely experienced across all relationships, and the degree of agreement between partners with respect to the type of intimacy they consider most important, likely determines relationship satisfaction. If both partners agree that the expression of emotional intimacy is the most important factor in the relationship, then they may be more likely to work together to achieve this. Problems arise when there are differences between partners with respect to the type of intimacy that is most valued. Differences in the need for various intimate experiences will determine the types of difficulties a couple will experience.

These five areas of intimacy can also be evaluated by using the PAIR, an assessment instrument devised by Schaefer and Olson (1981) that will be discussed in the Assessment section. This is a simple yet comprehensive approach to understanding a couple and identifying their specific area of difficulty. Therapies can then be selected to deal with the particular problem area identified. For example, sex therapy is indicated for couples with difficulties with sexual intimacy, increasing social and recreational activities to foster social and recreational intimacy, and couple communication skills to improve communciation on an affective and intellectual level. Several models of therapy offer assistance in enhancing intimacy in relationships (Greenberg & Johnson, 1988; Guerney, 1988; Jacobson, 1989). The McMaster model also offers the beginner a helpful general approach to conceptualizing couple relationships (Epstein, Baldwin, & Bishop, 1983).

The general approach described above is a good place to start. For those who wish a more thorough understanding of the variety of theories and corresponding therapies in this area, a discussion is presented below. A general introduction to some of these models may provide the reader with an appreciation of the marital therapy literature. It may also help the reader to apply the basic principles learned in the individual section to the couple section. The three major models of marital therapy that will be described are psychodynamic theory, cognitive-behavioral theory, and systems theory.

Psychodynamic Theories

The psychodynamic theory of marriage and marital therapy is based on the application of individual psychodynamic principles to the couple relationship. The major focus of this theory as it applies to marriage is on mate selection, individual intrapsychic issues, and marital conflict (Paolino & McCrady, 1978). Within psychodynamic theory are three schools of thought that have been selectively applied to the understanding of marriage and marital conflict. These include drive conflict theory, object-relations theory, and self-psychology. Only the important concepts of each theme as it applies to marriage will be discussed, since these concepts have been described at length in the psychodynamic chapter. The reader is referred to this chapter if a quick review is needed.

A popular psychodynamic view of marriage is that "marriage is not made in heaven, but in the unconscious," implying that the process of mate selection is determined by significant unconscious mechanisms. According to drive-conflict theory (Ackerman, 1958) this choice is analytically or narcissistically based. In the first case the object is chosen for its ability to gratify dependency needs and to protect and nurture. The narcissistically chosen object represents the individual's "ideal-self," so that the relationship allows the individual to recapture or maintain the ego-ideal. What is unconscious is the recognition of certain traits in the partner that are reminiscent of unresolved conflicts. This unconscious recognition creates an attraction toward the spouse who is viewed as a potential object with whom to resolve infantile conflicts. Marriage also allows the individual to identify with the loving aspects of the parents through the spouse, and to express repressed sexual desires. Thus according to Freud the marriage provides an opportunity to work through unresolved conflicts from childhood.

Object-relations theory, because of its focus on the relationship, has also contributed to the understanding of marriage and marital conflict (Scharff & Scharff, 1991). The main developmental task according to this theory is to individuate and differentiate from the early primary object and to be able to integrate both good and bad parts within the self and in the other. The difficulty in marriage is for the partners to accept their significant others as an individual in his or her own right, as a person with both good and bad parts. Ideally each partner should tolerate the other's dependency needs and be able to return to some regressive states without feeling threatened. This creates an atmostphere of trust, and promotes an affectionate bond between partners. The ability to express early repressed infantile needs without denigration decreases the need for defensive operations that deny these dependency needs. The goal then for the couple is to develop a mature relationship that allows both to give and to receive, creating an interdependent truly intimate relationship (Fairbairn, 1952).

The main operating unconscious mechanism in marriage according to object-relations theory is projective identification. In the marital relationship each partner projects either good or bad parts on to his or her spouse, who then accepts these parts and in turn acts them out. This creates an interactional cycle that allows each spouse to keep conflictual disowned parts out of consciousness by placing them on to the spouse. A clinical example illustrates this point. A wife complains that the husband has difficulties with emotional intimacy and blames him for not being more affectively available. The husband accepts this as a result of his own feelings of inadequacy regarding his capacity to be emotionally intimate, and therefore acts in a manner to confirm his wife's accusation. However, the wife although unaware, has her own difficulties with emotional intimacy, and by projecting this on to her husband she is free from dealing with it herself.

In a healthy relationship individuals are able to grow and differentiate, even if they entered the marriage in a less differentiated state. In an unhealthy or highly conflictual relationship individual growth is inhibited, dependency needs are unmet, and defenses continue to operate to repress these needs. Conflict or symptoms of underlying conflict present when one spouse becomes more aware of his or her own neediness which cannot be tolerated by the other. This new awareness and acknowledgment of previously repressed infantile wishes changes the relationship because the spouse who was originally chosen to help in this repressive process (by not meeting these needs) is now asked to meet them; a shift from the original collusive projective identification process. It is the working through of this process that constitutes the bulk of the work in object-relations couple therapy.

Another psychodynamic model that has been applied to couples is self-psychology. As discussed in chapter 8, mirroring and idealizing functions need to be internalized in the early years so that these functions may be maintained as an adult. In addition, individuals select others to provide these functions, and it is considered adaptive to be able to find self-objects who can continue to maintain those earlier internalized functions (Feldman, 1982). Both individuals enter marriage with their own unique self-object experiences. If both have internalized these functions to a sufficient degree, there will be less reliance on the partner to provide these functions.

Some dependence on the partner to maintain these functions is acceptable and considered healthy. However, if one needs the other to be a constant self-object, then difficulties will arise when the partner is unable to provide these functions on a constant basis, an inevitable outcome. Partners may select each other to provide these functions, and the degree to which the partners need each other to provide them will determine the level of marital conflict. Conflict will occur if each spouse operates on a different self-object need. That is, conflict is inevitable if one spouse relates with mirroring expectations and the other spouse relates with idealizing expectations and neither is able to provide these for the other. These expectations make it difficult for each spouse to see the other as an independent, separate person who has his or her own needs and wants. This perspective sounds similar to the object-relations theory of couples described above, and in reality there is great overlap among all the psychodynamic models. Feldman (1982) has developed an integrated model that takes into account all the perspectives described above as well as some that will be discussed below.

Social Learning-Cognitive Theory (Cognitive-Behavioral)

The cognitive-behavioral model of marriage and marital distress was originally described by Stuart (1969) who was the first to apply behavioral principles to understanding distressed relationships. The original focus was strictly behavioral, but later principles derived from social psychology, cognitive theory, and systems theory were integrated to produce a Social Learning-Cognitive theory of marriage and marital distress (Jacobson & Margolin, 1979).

According to this model the marital relationship can be understood by examining (1) the development of behavioral response chains, (2) the rate of positive reinforcement, (3) reciprocity and behavioral exchange, (4) cognitive appraisal of spouse's behaviors, and (5) competency in communication and problem solving skills (Jacobson & Margolin, 1979; Jacobson & Gurman, 1986). Each of these will be discussed separately.

Explaining the development of couple behavior is much more complicated than that of individuals. Interactions between two individuals involve many stimuli that have been classically conditioned and predict a particular behavioral response from each spouse. Over time completed sequences of behaviors known as behavioral response chains develop between spouses. For example, when a wife comes home from work, quiet and withdrawn, this behavior serves as a discriminative stimulus (SD) for the husband to approach his wife and offer support. The husband's response serves as a discriminative stimulus for his wife to explain the reasons for her present behavior. Her explanation may elicit supportive behaviors from her husband which will in turn increase the frequency of further self-disclosing behaviors from his wife. Therefore, each partner's behavior serves as a stimulus for the spouse's subsequent behavior, leading to the development of a behavioral response chain between husband and wife (Jacobson & Gurman, 1986).

The second significant behavioral factor that affects couple behavior is the rate of positive reinforcement in the relationship. Social reinforcement which includes acceptance, praise, attention, and sufficient demonstrations of physical affection is an important reinforcer in a relationship. The level of satisfaction in the relationship is determined by the reward/punishment ratio; that is, there should be a consistent, predictable high rate of reinforcement in order for spouses to feel satisfied with their partner and the relationship. Research has shown (Stuart, 1969; Jacobson & Gurman, 1986) that nondistressed couples have a high rate of reinforcement in their relationship that is consistent and predictable. Nondistressed couples are also able to tolerate a delay in receiving reinforcement since they have learned that there is a high probability of receiving it at some time. Distressed couples on the other hand reward each other in a sparse, unpredictable manner, thereby necessitating the need for reinforcement, since uncertainty exists as to when reinforcement will occur. Therefore, distressed couples have a reduced reward/punishment ratio.

The second issue involves the natural process of reinforcement erosion that occurs in any relationship. Over time as a result of habituation, there is a decrease in a spouse's ability to reinforce his or her partner. In habituation repeated presentations of the same reinforcer lead to a decrease in response as a result of the reinforcer eventually losing its novelty and potency. Therefore, it is necessary for couples to develop a variety of long-term reinforcers in order to prevent reinforcement erosion, which leaves each partner feeling bored with the relationship.

The third important variable in understanding distressed relationships is behavioral exchange or reciprocity. This concept is based on social exchange theory and systems theory. The exchange model is a model of behavioral economics that stipulates that each individual in a relationship will work toward maximizing benefits and minimizing costs (Thibaut & Kelly, 1959). This theory advocates that spouses exchange behavior, so that if one spouse rewards his or her partner, he or she will in turn be rewarded. Punishment is also exchanged, leading to an interdependency and reciprocity created between spouses for receiving reward and punishment. Research indicates that all couples reciprocate positive exchanges whether they are distressed or nondistressed. Consequently, one can say that there is a law of reciprocity that states that couples tend to reward each other at the same rate, whether they are distressed or not. Interestingly however, punishment is reciprocated more in distressed than nondistressed relationships, a finding that has significant implications for therapy (Jacobson & Gurman, 1986).

It is not the behavior itself that predicts a specific spousal response, but the interpretation or appraisal given to the spouse's behavior that determines whether the behavior is perceived as rewarding or punishing (Baucom & Epstein, 1990). That is, spouses make attributions of their partners' behavior, which are not always shared with each other. This cognitive variable has been added to the behavioral theory of marriage in order to create a cognitive-behavioral model of marriage and marital therapy. How the relationship is appraised in comparison to outside influences will determine if an individual will continue in the relationship. An unsatisfied spouse may remain in a distressed marriage if he or she does not see positive outcomes outside of the relationship. A spouse who perceives more positive outcomes outside the relationship, may be more likely to leave the relationship unless this condition changes. A spouse's evaluation of the relationship is constantly being modified as information about the relationship and partner is processed and appraised.

The final factor that determines a couple's ability to maintain a satisfactory relationship is their level of skills in communication and problem solving. These skills are essential for couples to help them deal with all the demands placed on them in an ongoing relationship.

In summary, couple distress presents as a result of reinforcement erosion, increase in displeasing behaviors, negative attributions of spouse's behaviors, and poor communication and problem-solving skills. In the early phase of a relationship there is a high exchange of reward, more pleasing behaviors, and more potential reinforcers leading to a positive evaluation of the relationship. As time goes on more displeasing behaviors occur in conjunction with reinforcement erosion, leading to the inevitable disappointment in the relationship. Also more demands are placed on the relationship due to finances, household issues, and children, which change the relationship. During these periods those couples who have good communication and problem-solving skills will be in a better position to cope with these new demands, and eventually their relationship will deepen. Those who cannot, will accumulate resentment and a list of unresolved conflicts that eventually lead to marital distress. The cognitive-behavioral model of marriage is then able to predict the marital conditions necessary for a successful marriage and those that lead to marital distress.

Systems Theory

Systems theory has been described as a certain "style of thinking" (Steinglass, 1978). This style of thinking has been extensively applied to the understanding and treatment of dysfunctional families. Some systemic family therapists do not consider a couple a system, because they are a dyad, and are therefore an unbalanced system. To balance the dyad a third person is needed, usually a child, parent, friend, or therapist. Even though some systemic thinkers do not describe a couple as a system, others view the couple as a subsystem of the large family system. Therefore, the fundamentals of systems theory as it applies to couples will be presented in this section. Systemic couple therapy will not be discussed in this chapter, since a more elaborate discussion of this approach and its therapeutic application will be discussed in the family chapter.

Systems theory, as it has been applied to the study of families and other systems, is based on General Systems Theory developed by Bertalanaffy (1968), who challenged the linear reductionistic thinking of natural science and offered an alternate "style of thinking" that took into account the complex interactions between elements that belong to an organization or group. A simple analysis of each element is insufficient if one is trying to understand how the group or organization functions, since the whole is greater than the sum of its parts. Most of early systems theory was applied to living organisms, and four key concepts were described that can be applied to couples and families. They are the concepts of organization, control, energy, and the dimension of time and space (Steinglass, 1978). Elements are organized in a system, and this organization implies that the elements are interacting in some consistent manner. This organization infers a property of wholeness that cannot be understood by analyzing each part. Also implied in this concept of organization is the idea of boundaries and hierarchies. Boundaries exist between elements or between a group of elements (subsystem) within a system. Hierarchies create order and maintain levels within the organization. Control in the system is achieved by homeostasis, promoting growth and differentiation. Homeostasis is regulated through a variety of mechanisms, called feedback loops. Feedback loops maintain a circular relationship between two events. A positive feedback loop is self-destructive in that an increase in one part of the system leads to an increase in another part of the system, sending the system out of control. A negative feedback loop balances the system, for an increase in one part of the system, creates a decrease in another part of the system, thereby creating homeostasis. In couples and families a symptom or problem is considered to maintain the system. In these systems communication patterns represent the feedback loops. The third concept of energy refers to the tendency of living systems to increase their energy and level of organization. The final concept refers to how the system organizes itself in time and space, which leads to the development of certain processes and structures.

These are the basic concepts of systems theory that have been extensively applied to couples and family systems. However, different therapists have focused on different aspects of systems theory, leading to the development of a variety of systemic models of couple and family therapy. There are, nevertheless, couple and family therapists who do not consider systems theory a true theory of causality because attention is not given to the historical root of the problem, but rather to the here and now. The dysfunctional symptoms or behaviors are understood with respect to how they maintain the system. Individual behavioral, cognitive or intrapsychic issues are not attended to.

According to systems theory, in a healthy marriage, partners should be able to communicate clearly, develop clear boundaries between each other and between themselves and the children, occupy a higher level in the family system from the children, and be able to work within the larger family system to achieve homeostasis and adapt to change. Marital interactions between husband and wife are understood in terms of circular causality. For example, if the husband behaves in a manner x, then his wife reacts with response y, which in turn increases husband's behavior x, which in turn increases his wife's response y, and so on. Some of these interactive cycles have been called pursue-withdraw, and withdraw-withdraw. In the first case one spouse pursues and the other withdraws. The more the second spouse withdraws the more the first spouse pursues, hence repeating the cycle. In the second instance both partners withdraw sometimes creating a much more difficult situation. Dysfunctional marriages occur when there is (1) pathological communication between partners, (2) poor boundaries and lack of hierarchy between the marital and child subsystem, (3) poor adaption to internal and external stressor as a result of a closed marital system, and (4) dysfunctional interactive cycles.

The greatest attention has been given to communication, and many systemic models have been applied to help couples learn to communicate on many different levels (Nichols, 1988).

In summary the marriage is seen as an important subsystem of the larger family system. The role of marital partners is expected to change throughout the life cycle and new demands will pressure this subsystem to adapt, change, and grow, in order to maintain satisfactory marital and family functioning. Many consider the marriage as the central subsystem within the family that determines family life. It is therefore the most important subsystem in the family that needs to be understood and maintained in order to increase the probability of optimal family functioning.

ASSESSMENT

Couple and marital assessments are more complicated than individual assessments because assessing a marriage or relationship requires three separate assessments—the couple, the husband, and the wife. In some cases a brief family assessment may be needed in order to obtain additional information from children, especially if marital discord has contributed to family dysfunction.

How the assessment is conducted and what is emphasized usually depend on the therapist's style and orientation. A general approach that can be used with all couples can be isolated by examining the literature. First, a couple assessment requires at least four sessions. In the first interview the couple are seen together and the therapist obtains the necessary information from each spouse and the couple and observes how the couple interacts. Two separate sessions are held with each spouse in order to gather further information and to provide a safe, private, confidential environment for the disclosure of any sensitive material concerning violence, extra-marital relations, and commitment to the relationship. In the final session the therapist clarifies and collects additional information and gives the couple feedback regarding the identified relationship difficulties and whether marital/couple therapy is indicated.

This format is common in clinical practice but is certainly not universal, although it does provide a comprehensive assessment. Some therapists do not conduct individual sessions with each spouse claiming that this places the therapist in a difficult position if "secrets" are disclosed that the other spouse is unaware of. Nevertheless, many couple therapists accept this position and see it as essential in carrying out a comprehensive, accurate assessment, and respect each individual in the couple and their right to privacy. This continues to be a controversial topic.

The first couple session provides the therapist with an opportunity to form a first impression. In this session the therapist initially inquires if both parties agreed to attending the assessment. The response to this question provides information regarding motivation for therapy and identifies which spouse is more distressed in the relationship. Both spouses are then asked to describe how they view their relationship, what difficulties they have experienced and for how long, and if either is currently considering separation or divorce. After the presenting problem is identified, further information regarding past relationship difficulties, the history of the relationship including how they met, and what attracted them to each other, the courtship period, decision to marry, and other historical information concerning the relationship is obtained. Each spouse is asked for his or her own view of the relationship and the degree of agreement between the spouses is noted.

Once the relationship history is assembled, attention shifts to each spouse's individual developmental history, which involves gathering information about each spouse's childhood experience, relationship with parents, family life, their parents' marriage, previous relationships, and sexual history prior to meeting their spouse. Attention is paid to traumatic developmental events involving any form of abuse, and to dysfunctional family of origin experiences.

Having presented a general format and approach, we now turn to some additional methods that can enrich the assessment process. As mentioned earlier, the therapist needs a framework to guide the assessment process and to gather data. In addition to what has been discussed, the following may help provide a conceptual schema to the couple assessment. Following the general approach to couples that was discussed earlier, one can assess the relationship by examining the couple's experience of emotional, intellectual, social, recreational, and sexual intimacy in their relationship. Other important relationship dimensions to assess are power and commitment. Power is determined by asking who makes the decisions in the relationship or family. In some cases one spouse may hold the power and in other cases it may be divided between the two. Past and present motivation to remain and work in the relationship provides an indication of each spouse's commitment to the relationship.

The relationship can also be assessed according to the theoretical constructs discussed earlier. A psychodynamically oriented therapist will attend to each individual's developmental histories, degree of differentiation from the primary object, past object choices, attachments to bad objects, need for self-object functions, vulnerability to certain projective identification interactions, and capacity to be involved in a mature relationship. Attention will also be focused on the couple's projective-identification patterns and their mutual ability to be self-objects for each other.

A cognitive-behavioral couple therapist will assess the frequency of displeasing and pleasing behaviors, spousal negative attributions, communication and problem-solving skills, and reinforcement erosion. A systemic therapist will be less likely to get involved in any lengthy assessment process and will determine the problem at the first session by observing the couple system. The historical roots or development of the problem are ignored and the initial assessment consists of observing the couple's communication style, their maintenance of boundaries and hierarchies within their subsystem and the larger family system, and their contributions to achieving homeostasis.

It is not essential that one assess a couple through every perspective. All these approaches provide rich models to conceptualize relationship difficulties and one or two models may be sufficient for a given case. In addition to the clinical interview, several objective assessment instruments that assess various dimensions of the relationship can also be utilized. Instruments are available that measure intimacy, such as the PAIR, (Schaefer & Olson, 1981) or the Waring Intimacy Questionnaire (Waring & Reddon, 1983). General marital instruments that measure overall distress include the Dyadic Adjustment Scale (Spanier, 1976), the Locke-Wallace Scale (Locke & Wallace, 1959) and others (see Fredman & Sherman, 1987). Numerous other instruments have been devised for assessing the couple/marital relationship and many of these can be found in the cognitive-behavioral marital therapy texts (Jacobson & Margolin, 1979; Baucom & Epstein, 1990) and in other sources (Fredman & Sherman, 1987). A good clinical assessment and well-chosen assessment instruments can provide the therapist with a comprehensive assessment that will be helpful in planning treatment.

THE FOUR PS

In order to consider the important predisposing, precipitating, perpetuating and protective couple factors, a frame of reference is needed before this column can be completed. Couple factors may be identified according to how they impact on an individual problem, or the relationship itself may be the presenting problem. When formulating an individual the important couple factors are considered with respect to how they affect the individual's presenting problem. If the presenting problem is a couple problem, then the relationship is the frame of reference. Couple factors include individual factors that contribute to relationship distress or success. Important couple factors can originate from within the relationship (e.g., difficulties with intimacy) or from outside the relationship (e.g., extrarelationship factors such as difficulties with in-laws).

Predisposing couple factors that increase the chance of relationship difficulties are destructive projective identification patterns, dysfunctional interactional styles, poor communication and problem-solving skills, and a history of ambivalent feelings regarding commitment to the relationship (see Table 9.1). Any significant individual pathology in either spouse that limits their capacity to engage in a mature relationship will predispose the couple toward a dysfunctional relationship. Extrarelationship factors that can predispose a couple toward relationship problems include difficulties with in-laws, financial problems, poor living conditions, and a history of limited social relationships with other couples with whom they can exchange confidences and share recreational activities.

Throughout a relationship couples experience many life events that can act as important ***precipitants*** in triggering relationship difficulties. Within the relationship these include a significant change in one of the spouses, such as illness, career, or individual growth that imposes certain demands on the other spouse to accommodate to these changes. Conflict may develop if the spouse who is asked to accommodate is resistant. A good example here is when a wife goes from housewife to working mother and requests that her husband share in the household duties that she has up to now carried out on her own. The new situation requires that a couple renegotiate their roles and duties in the home. Other significant precipitants that impact on the relationship include pregnancy, arrival of the first child, decrease in shared activities, and decreased interest in sex. These are a few examples of changes within the relationship that can precipitate relationship problems.

External precipitants that impact on the relationship can originate from extended families (e.g., sickness or death of a parent), other systems (work, friends), and from society (poor housing, unemployment). All these extrarelationship factors potentially can upset the couple especially if the relationship is distressed. Therefore, any event or change that disrupts either partner or the relationship and leads to couple difficulties can be viewed as a precipitating negative couple factor.

Perpetuating factors are those that become chronic and continue to impact on the relationship. Once again these chronic factors may affect only one spouse, thereby affecting the relationship, or they may affect the couple directly. Within the relationship this can be any difficulty in a spouse such as a chronic physical or mental illness that stresses the couple on an ongoing basis. Chronic difficulties with emotional, sexual, or any other form of intimacy can stress the relationship until these problems are resolved. Ongoing physical or emotional abuse can also perpetuate significant couple distress. Persistent child behavior problems and inconsistent parenting can also perpetuate marital problems.

Protective couple factors enable spouses to form a secure intimate bond with each other that promotes individual growth as well as relationship satisfaction. In addition to the affective bond, couples need to be

Table 9.1
Couple/Marital System

Predisposing	* dysfunctional interactional styles * destructive projective identification patterns * poor self-other differentiation * poor communication/problem-solving skills * pathology in either spouse * family of origin problems * financial problems * poor living conditions
Precipitating	* change in either spouse –illness –occupation –growth –roles * pregnancy * children * financial problems * child behavioral problems * in-law problems * extra-marital affairs
Perpetuating	* chronic spousal difficulties (e.g., chronic illness, etc.) * chronic difficulties with intimacy: emotional, intellectual, sexual, recreational, social * chronic parent-child problems * chronic physical/emotional/verbal abuse * chronic lack of support * ongoing extramarital affair * chronic communication problems
Protective	* spousal capacity for mature, differentiated relationship * secure intimate bond * good communication/good conflict resolution * strong commitment to relationship * supportive spouse

able to communicate, negotiate, and problem solve in order to decrease conflict and tension in the relationship. Individuals who are committed to the relationship and are willing to expend the energy required to maintain it, are more likely to protect the relationship from deterioration. In addition, each spouse's prior experience in their family of origin may offer some protection for their own relationship. Individuals who have witnessed a secure, parental marital relationship may have had some of the necessary relationship skills modeled for them, that can be protective in their own marriage. A couple's capacity to identify difficulities and work through them, will not only protect the relationship, but will provide a buffer for each spouse from the daily stresses they experience outside the relationship. Having a supportive spouse in whom one can confide has been identified as a major factor in the course of psychiatric disorders (Brown & Harris, 1978; Keitner & Miller, 1990; Goering, Lance & Freeman, 1992).

COPING-RESPONSE STYLE

Although not discussed as a specific coping-response style, the availability of at least one intimate relationship or confidant has been considered a protective factor against depression and other psychological difficulties. There is accumulating evidence that the marital relationship may be an important source of support, and the presence of marital conflict or poor spousal support may have an impact on psychological well being.

Therefore, what is important to note in this column is the degree to which the dyadic relationship is used as a support or coping system. The capacity to have an intimate supportive relationship is likely confounded with individual factors, in that a certain amount of individuation and differentiation is neccessary before one can engage in a relationship. However, being in a relationship is not synonymous with having an intimate supportive relationship. The latter requires a feeling of safety and security in the relationship so that vulnerable feelings can be expressed without fear of criticism and retaliation. The ability to trust another with our most vulnerable feelings is a difficult task, and may be more likely to occur if prior relationships including the primary relationship with parents were comforting and secure. Individuals who use their intimate relationship to cope may be more vulnerable when this relationship is stressed or is unable to provide support. Therefore, this "turning to an intimate other" can be seen as a coping-response style, in that self-disclosing, ventilating, being listened to, comforted, and validated by a significant other, may increase the chance of an adaptive response in times of stress. This could be called a confiding-coping-response style in that the act of confiding attenuates the experienced distress. An individual who has used a significant relationship to cope previously may be more receptive to a dyadic intervention that focuses on strengthening this relationship if this relationship is currently dysfunctional. An individual approach although helpful may not access the dyadic relationship thus indicating couple therapy.

TREATMENT

Over the last three decades several forms of marital therapy have been described and researched. They include psychodynamic, cognitive-behavioral, systemic, marital enrichment, communication workshops, emotionally focused, and many other forms of therapy. However, before discussing some of these therapies in more detail a somewhat simpler approach that follows the general approach covered in the basic principles section will be described.

Before beginning any treatment, it is imperative that the therapist develop a good therapeutic alliance with each spouse and with the couple. Such an alliance permits both spouses to express those feelings and thoughts that they have been unable to express prior to therapy. A positive alliance creates a safe environment that facilitates self-disclosure. The safety experienced in the therapeutic environment will eventually generalize to their own relationship outside the therapist's office. The alliance is built by empathically validating each spouse's position in the relationship so that they perceive the therapist as truly understanding their point of view. When working with couples, it is important to validate each partner so that the therapist is not seen as taking sides. Once there is a reasonable alliance between the therapist and the couple, specific interventions can be implemented.

General Approach to Treatment

As mentioned above the construct of intimacy has been used to assess relationship satisfaction, and five areas of intimacy were described. If the assessment identifies specific deficits in one or several areas of intimacy, then treatment is directed toward improving these areas. For example, if there are difficulties in emotional intimacy improvement can be facilitated by helping the spouses to communicate their feelings to each other. It is important that spouses learn to communicate positive and negative feelings to one another, something that requires good communication skills and a feeling of safety in the relationship. Facilitating emotional disclosure in the session helps spouses reveal their feelings to each other in a safe environment, and moves the couple toward a more emotionally intimate relationship.

Sexual intimacy, an area identified as problematic in at least 80% of distressed couples, can be treated by sensate focus and other exercises that promote physical intimacy and enhance sexual enjoyment (O'Leary, 1987). Specific interventions are needed to deal with sexual problems, because relationship therapy alone does not improve the sexual relationship (Jacobson & Gurman, 1986). Sex therapy, however, should be integrated with relationship therapy and tailored according to the couple's needs.

Distressed couples spend very little time together in recreational activities, partly due to the mutual avoidance that develops over time in a distressed relationship. Having couples plan weekly positive activities together helps reverse this trend, which not only increases the time couples spend together, but also increases the probability of more positive experiences in the relationship necessary to correct negative spousal attributions. Obtaining a list from each spouse regarding his or her preferred couple recreational activities is a good starting point.

A similar strategy can be used to facilitate intellectual intimacy. In this case couples can be asked to spend 10 minutes a day sharing their thoughts regarding nonrelationship issues. Discussions about careers, friends, and current events can help couples express their ideas to each other, enhancing intellectual intimacy in the relationship.

Social intimacy can be encouraged by helping couples plan activities with friends and other couples. In some cases specific skills (e.g., social skills) may need to be taught to ensure a good outcome.

These five areas of intimacy can be the focus of treatment, and interventions can be aimed at facilitating the couple's experience of intimacy in each area. A variety of techniques such as communication skills training can be borrowed from specific approaches to carry this out. The goal is not to enhance intimacy in all five areas but to focus on those areas that have been identified by the couple as needing attention. This approach although simplistic can be very useful in helping couples and therapists identify the areas that need attention so that specific techniques can be used in a focused, goal-directed manner. Most couple therapists agree that the ultimate goal of couple or marital therapy is to restore the intimate bond between partners. However, important issues may need to be considered during therapy that might impede progress. Understanding the meaning of some of these blocks in therapy and utilizing interventions to overcome them requires some knowledge of the more specific therapeutic approaches. Only two approaches will be presented here: psychodynamic and cognitive-behavioral couple therapy. Systemic marital therapy will not be discussed as this form of therapy is covered in detail in the family chapter.

Psychodynamic Couple Therapy

Psychodynamic couple therapy, like individual therapy, is usually an open-ended, nondirective, unstructured, long-term therapy. Sessions are held weekly and homework assignments are rarely given unless other approaches are integrated. The primary interventions used are exploration, clarification, and interpretation. As discussed above the psychodynamic approach to marital/couple therapy focuses on mate selection, individual intrapsychic issues, and the dynamics of the marital conflict. The main therapeutic intervention in the psychodynamic couples approach is to explore the individual intrapsychic issues of each spouse with respect to how they impact on the relationship. Interpretation of early developmental issues encourages each spouse to take ownership for their own contributions to the relationship. Understanding their early developmental history may also help in working through destructive projective identification processes. Interpreting and working through projective identification is the main task of the psychodynamic couple therapist who adheres to an object-relations model (Scharff & Scharff, 1991).

Common to all psychodynamically oriented couples therapy is the attention given to the interpretations of transference. Unlike individual therapy, however, there are several transference relationships in couple therapy. They include the therapist-husband, therapist-wife, husband-wife, and therapist-couple transference. Attention is paid to all four transference relationships and interpretations of these various relationships are made later in therapy, after a therapeutic alliance has been developed and both spouses have been allowed to express and explore their identified relationship difficulties.

In addition to the interpretation of projective identification and transference, the therapist also interprets the various pathological defenses used by both spouses that contribute to their difficulties. Identifying and modifying certain defensive styles may help both spouses be more available for an intimate relationship (Nadelson, 1978). A self-psychological approach to the treatment of couples attends to each spouse's ability to provide certain self-object functions for each other. Both spouses will be encouraged to provide a certain amount of mirroring and idealizing functions, as these are considered essential throughout life. Initially the therapist will provide these functions for each spouse, especially in those cases where one spouse is narcissitically vulnerable. By providing these functions the therapist aims to promote a cohesive sense of self in both spouses, and increases each spouse's capacity to provide mirroring and idealizing functions for his or her partner. The therapist also encourages each spouse to seek additional sources to provide these functions so that they do not rely completely on each other.

These are some of the main psychodynamic principles that have been applied to the treatment of couples. These therapies have not always been described in a manner that allows one to easily carry them out. Training in individual psychodynamic therapy is probably necessary before one can apply it to couples. More research using this form of couple therapy is needed in order to clearly describe the therapeutic process and the active ingredients of change. Therapy progresses until the underlying conflicts are worked through and the presenting symptoms are resolved. Once this is accomplished termination is addressed. Since psychodynamic couple therapy can go on for one to three years, an intense attachment will develop to the therapist that will make termination difficult. These feelings are worked through as in individual therapy and the couple's fears of leaving therapy are openly discussed. Although research in psychodynamic couple therapy is limited, there is some evidence to suggest that it has a better long term outcome than the brief nondynamic therapies (Jacobson & Addis, 1993). There is a great need for more research using this model of therapy with couples. Future research should identify those couples best suited for this approach.

Cognitive-Behavioral Marital Therapy

The integration of cognitive and behavioral marital therapy is a recent development. Prior to this integration behavioral marital therapy offered couples a brief, highly structured, well researched therapy that was found to be very effective in reducing marital distress. Behavioral marital therapy involves at least 12-20 sessions that are preceded by a lengthy assessment phase. After the assessment process, the therapist gives the couple feedback on the identified areas of difficulty and a therapeutic contract is offered that specifies the number of sessions, length of sessions, compliance on homework assignments, and agenda for each session. The issue of completing homework assignments is overemphasized in this therapy and couples are made aware of the importance of unlearning old behavioral patterns, learning new behavioral interactions, and most important, learning new skills relevant to maintaining a long-term relationship. This process has been extensively described by Jacobson and Margolin (1979), and will be briefly reviewed here.

After the first few assessment sessions the idea of a "collaborative set" is put forward by the therapist to encourage each spouse to take equal responsibility for relationship difficulties. Following this, the therapy is individualized for each couple taking into account their unique differences. Since few positive behaviors are exchanged between distressed couples this is one of the first areas attended to. After completing the Behavior Exchange checklist (Jacobson & Margolin, 1979), specific desired behaviors are identified and both spouses are asked to predict how modifying their own behavior will alter their spouse's behavior. This exercise increases the occurrence of positive behaviors which are considered necessary for each spouse to develop a more positive attitude toward their partner.

With each session, an agenda is set, homework assignments are reviewed, and any obstacles to completing homework assignments are analyzed. Emphasis is always on the positive, in that the therapist reinforces the couple for their progress, positive changes, and effort. The therapist also models positive behaviors to each spouse before prescribing any exercises to the couple in various skills training programs.

In cognitive-behavioral therapy communication training receives the most attention, because poor communication is identified as the number one couple problem. Initially the therapist models the two skills of communcation—reception and expression. Under the receptive area couples are taught how to (1) listen and attend to each other, (2) validate their partners' experience, (3) empathize, (4) para-phrase, and (5) check out their interpretation of what has just been said. Expressive skills taught include (1) being specific about what the issues are, (2) stating feelings directly, and (3) using "I" statements such as "when you do this I feel like . . ." (Jacobson & Margolin, 1979).

After these basic communication skills are learned attention shifts to problem solving and conflict resolution. Specific communication skills are modeled that help couples define conflicts, specify problems, and state the emotional impact of the problem. Various problem-solving skills such as troubleshooting and brainstorming are also taught. Once again these exercises are first modeled by the therapist using an identified couple problem. Following this, each spouse is asked to practice these skills in the session and at home. These skills help couples discuss their conflicts clearly and ensure that both partners are able to express their difficulties and work together toward a common solution. Once the couple has learned problem-solving and conflict resolutions skills, attention shifts to areas of intimacy, affection, and sexuality. Specific therapies are prescribed for sexual difficulties such as sensate focus exercises. Affectional expression is encouraged once again through modeling and practicing. Intimacy is facilitated by increasing communication skills in the emotional area.

The final phases of therapy deal with issues of termination, but in behavioral marital therapy this focuses on reviewing the original presenting problem, evaluating progress, increasing the probability of generalization to the relationship on a daily basis, anticipating future difficulties, and considering possible solutions. Booster sessions may be prescribed if needed to ensure that gains made in therapy are maintained.

The cognitive component of cognitive-behavioral marital therapy was integrated as a result of research findings that spousal positive behavioral exchange did not necessarily change each spouse's perception of the other in a positive direction. It became apparent that the interpretation each spouse gave to the behavior determined whether or not there was an attitudinal shift (Baucom & Epstein, 1990). In other words, if a wife's recent increase in positive behavior toward her husband is interpreted by him as manipulative, it is unlikely that he will view her behavior in a positive manner. This finding emphasized the importance of cognitive factors in the marital relationship and has been extensively described by Baucom and Epstein (1990), Jacobson and Holtzworth-Munroe (1986) and Waring (1989), and will be briefly described here.

The cognitive component of this therapy involves the following: (1) first teaching the couple the cognitive model of marital distress; (2) helping spouses to identify those cognitions that affect how they perceive their spouse and the relationship in a dysfunctional fashion; and (3) modifying cognitive distortions once they are identified through cognitive restructuring (described in the individual session).

One of the difficulties with the cognitive component in this form of marital therapy is that spouses tend to attribute relationship difficulties to deficiencies in their partner, and are therefore more resistant to modifying their own beliefs in contrast to depressed individuals who are able to see the relationship between their negative automatic thoughts and their mood. The therapist must supportively explore each spouse's perceptions and interpretations and identify cognitive distortions in a nonblaming, nonpathologizing manner. Homework exercises are prescribed to enhance each spouse's ability to be self-aware of affective experiences that impact on the relationship, reflect on thought processes associated with these affective states, and identify subsequent behavioral responses that follow from these "cognitive-affective processes."

Cognitive-behavioral marital therapy has provided an integrated approach that takes advantage of principles and techniques from cognitive and behavior therapy. This approach has been extensively investigated with favorable results (Jacobson, 1993).

SUMMARY

Adopting a couple perspective can provide a unique view of individual problems and also lead to the identification of relationship difficulties. An individual's significant relationship has an important influence on psychological well being, and this relationship needs to be considered when individual psychological distress is being assessed. Individually focused therapies may be ineffective in the presence of severe relationship distress. In those cases where the relationship is the identified problem, dyadic interventions are preferred as the first line of treatment (Garfield & Bergin, 1986). Since couple therapy has been found to be effective in alleviating relationship distress, this form of therapy needs to be considered as a viable option (Gurman & Kniskern, 1992). Recent interest in the relationship between marital distress and psychiatric disorders, such as depression, will continue to emphasize this perspective as an important one in the mental health profession (O'Leary & Beach, 1990).

REFERENCES

Ackerman, N. W. (1958). *The Psychodynamics of Family Life*. New York: Basic Books.

Babcock, J. C., Waltz, J., Jacobson, N. S., & Gottman, J. M. (1993). Power and Violence: The Relationship Between Communication Patterns, Power Discrepancy and Domestic Violence. *Journal of Consulting and Clinical Psychology, 61,* 40–50.

Barlow, D. H. (Ed.). (1981). *Behavioral Assessment of Adult Disorders*. New York: Guilford Press.

Baucom, D. H., & Epstein, N. (1990). *Cognitive-Behavioral Marital Therapy*. New York: Brunner/Mazel.

Beach, S. R. H., Sandeen, E. E., & O'Leary, K. D. (1990). *Depression in Marriage: A Model for Etiology and Treatment*. New York: Guilford Press.

Bertalanaffy, L. V. (1968). *General Systems Theory: Foundation, Development, Applications*. New York: New Brazillier.

Brown, G. N., & Harris, T. (1978). *Social Origins of Depression*. London: Tavistock.

Chamberlaines, S., Barnes, S., Waring, E. M., Wood, G., & Fry, R. (1989). The

Role of Marital Intimacy in Psychiatric Help Seeking. *Canadian Journal of Psychiatry, 34,* 3–7.

Dicks, H. V. (1967). *Marital Tensions.* New York: Basic Books.

Epstein, N., Baldwin, L., & Bishop, S. (1983). The McMaster Family Assessment Device. *Journal of Marital and Family Therapy, 9,* 171–180.

Fairbairn, W. R. D. (1952). *Psychoanalytic Studies of Personality.* Tavistock, England: Routledge Press.

Feldman, L. B. (1982). Dysfunctional Marital Conflict: An Integrative and Interpersonal-Intrapsychic Model. *Journal of Marital and Family Therapy, 8,* 417–428.

Fredman, N., & Sherman, R. (1987). *Handbook of Measurements for Marriage and Family Therapy.* New York: Brunner/Mazel.

Garfield, S. L., & Bergin, A. E. (1986). *Handbook of Psychotherapy and Behavior Change* (3rd ed.). New York: John Wiley and Sons.

Goering, P. N., Lance, W. J., & Freeman, S. J. J. (1992). Marital Support and Recovery in Depression. *British Journal of Psychiatry, 160,* 76–82.

Greenberg, L. S., & Johnson, S. M. (1988). *Emotionally Focused Therapy for Couples.* New York: Guilford Press.

Guerney, B. G. (1988). *Relationship Enhancement.* San Francisco: Josey-Bass Publishers.

Gurman, A. S., & Kniskern, D. P. (1992). The Future of Marital and Family Therapy. *Psychotherapy, 29,* 65–71.

Jacobson, N. S., & Holtzworth-Munroe, A. (1986). Marital Therapy: A Social Learning-Cognitive Perspective. In N. S. Jacobson & A. S. Gurman, (Eds.), *Clinical Handbook of Marital Therapy.* New York: Guilford Press.

Jacobson, N. S. (1989). The Politics of Intimacy. *The Behavior Therapist, 12*(2), 29–32.

Jacobson, N. S., & Gurman, A. S. (1986). *Clinical Handbook of Marital Therapy.* New York: Guilford Press.

Jacobson, N. S., & Addis, M. E. (1993). Research on couples and couple therapy: What do we know? Where are we going? *Journal of Consulting and Clinical Psychology, 61*(1), 85–93.

Jacobson, N. S., & Margolin, G. (1979). *Marital Therapy.* New York: Brunner/Mazel.

Keitner, G. I., & Miller, I. W. (1990). Family Functioning and Major Depression: An Overview. *American Journal of Psychiatry, 147*(9), 1128–1137.

Locke, H., & Wallace, K. (1959). Short Marital Adjustment and Prediction Tests: The Reliability and Validity. *Marriage and Family Living, 2,* 251–255.

Nadelson, C. (1978). Marital Therapy from a Psychoanalytic Perspective. In T. J. Paolino Jr., & B. S. McCrady, (Eds.), *Marriage and Marital Therapy: Psychoanalytic, Behavioral and Systems Theory Perspectives.* New York: Brunner/Mazel.

Nichols, W. C. (1988). *Marital Therapy: An Integrative Approach.* New York: Guilford Press.

O'Leary, D. K. (1987). *Assessment of Marital Discord: Integration for Research and Clinical Practice.* Hillsdale, NJ: Lawrence Earlbaum.

O'Leary, D. K., & Beach, S. J. H. (1990). Marital Therapy: A Viable Treatment for Depression and Marital Discord. *American Journal of Psychiatry, 147,* 183–186.

Paolino, T. J., & McCrady, B. S. (Eds.). (1978). *Marriage and Marital Therapy: Psychoanalytic, Behavioral and Systems Theory Perspectives.* New York: Brunner/Mazel.

Prochaska, J., & Prochaska, J. (1978). Twentieth Century Trends in Marriage and Marital Therapy. In T. J. Paolino, & B. S. McCrady, (Eds.), *Marriage and Marital Therapy: Psychoanalytic, Behavioral and Systems Theory Perspectives.* New York: Brunner/Mazel.

Reid, W. J., & Crisafulli, A. (1990). Marital Discord and Child Behavior Problems: A Meta-Analysis. *Journal of Abnormal Child Psychology, 18,* 105–117.

Schaefer, M. T., & Olson, D. H. (1981). Assessing Intimacy: The PAIR Inventory. *The Journal of Marital and Family Therapy, 1,* 47–60.

Scharff, D. E., & Scharff, J. S. (1991). *Object Relations Couple Therapy.* New York: Aronson Press.

Selvini-Palazzoli, M., Boscolo L., Cecchin, C. F., & Prata, G. (1978). Paradox and Counter-Paradox. New York: Aronson Press.

Spanier, G. B. (1976). Measuring Dyadic Adjustment: New Scales for assessing the quality of marriage and similar dyads. *Journal of Marrige and the Family, 38,* 15–28.

Steinglass, P. (1978). The Conceptualization of Marriage from a Systems Theory Perspective. In T. J. Paolino, Jr., & B. S. McCrady, (Eds.), *Marriage and Marital Therapy: Psychoanalytic, Behavioral and Systems Theory Perspectives.* New York: Brunner/Mazel.

Stuart, R. B. (1969). Operant Interpersonal Treatment for Marital Discord. *Journal of Consulting and Clinical Psychology, 33,* 675–682.

Thibaut, J. W., & Kelly, H. H. (1959). *The Social Psychology of Groups.* New York: Wiley.

Waring, E. M. (1988). *Enhancing Marital Intimacy through Facilitating Cognitive Self-Disclosure.* New York: Brunner/Mazel.

Waring, E. M., & Chelune, G. J. (1983). Marital Intimacy and Self-Disclosure. *Journal of Clinical Psychology, 39*(2), 183–190.

Waring, E. M., & Reddon, J. R. (1983). Measurement of Intimacy and Marriage: The Waring Intimacy Questionnaire. *Journal of Clinical Psychology, 33,* 53–57.

CHAPTER 10

THE FAMILY SYSTEM

THE PERSPECTIVE

This chapter focuses on the family system. Many theoretical models offer a perspective on family functioning and family pathology. Common to all these models is the emphasis on the relationship between family functioning and psychological well-being. There are two approaches that can be adopted when considering this perspective. First, an individual problem can be viewed primarily from an individual perspective, with family factors having varying degrees of influence on the course of the disorder or condition. In some cases family factors play a major role in the onset, maintenance, and course of a particular psychological disturbance. In such cases the family may be seen as part of a comprehensive assessment, with the major focus of treatment being tailored to the "individual." Alternatively, any problem experienced by an individual living in a family system is considered symptomatic of a wider systemic problem, necessitating a systemic intervention. In this case, the system is the "identified patient," not the individual. This systemic perspective is strongly represented in the family studies area and is unique in its approach to psychological problems.

The family perspective offers a different view of what causes and maintains symptomatic behavior in individuals and dysfunctional families. Individual and family psychological health is determined by family functioning. Dysfunctional families produce dysfunctional individuals, and family interventions are required to change the family system and the symptomatic individual. This family perspective then offers a broader view of individual problems, and provides a framework for understanding family pathology.

The family perspective is represented by the family therapy field, a discipline very familiar to social workers who receive significant exposure to theories of family functioning. Psychologists vary with respect to the training they receive in this area. Child and educational psychologists are more likely to see families than psychologists practicing in other areas. Psychiatrists receive some training in this perspective through their mandatory exposure to child psychiatry and may receive additional exposure working with adult psychiatric patients. All professionals may at some point see families as part of a child or adult assessment or for family therapy. Understanding the family context in which individuals experience their difficulties is the major focus of this chapter.

A family is usually defined as consisting of two parents and at least one child. However, this traditional definition does not hold today, given the many single parent and reconstituted families, adopted families, foster homes, and other systemic groupings. Therefore, a family is defined as a group of individuals who live and interact together in a manner to form a system. Over time individuals may leave the system but they will always be members of the family.

BRIEF HISTORY

Although Freud placed heavy emphasis on family influences in psychopathology he did not see families in his practice. Since the origins of psychopathology were traced back to the family, Freud's focus was on freeing individuals from their family of origin's influence. Any contact with a family member during therapy was viewed as "contaminating" the therapy. Psychoanalysis was for the individual, not the family. Nevertheless, family therapy has its roots in psychoanalysis, because most practitioners in psychotherapy received training in this area.

Nathan Ackerman (1958), credited by many as the grandfather of the family therapy movement, was the first to apply psychoanalysis to the understanding of families. Ackerman pioneered the psychodynamic family therapy movement that focused on intrapsychic developmental issue in the family. Other well-known family therapists to follow this tradition include James Framo, Boszomenyi-Nagy, Henry Dicks, Lyman Wynne, and others (Goldenberg & Goldenberg, 1991; Nichols, 1988). This movement began after the Second World War when families were reunited and faced new problems of reorganization. Two other movements also established the family as a legitimate area of study: the child guidance movement in the 1950s, and the marital therapy movement in the early 1940s (Nicols, 1988).

As the family therapy movement advanced additional models were explored and applied to the study of the family. The concept of the "system" was borrowed from Bertalanaffy's (1968) general systems theory and provided a new perspective on the family. Murray Bowen (1960; 1966), originally trained as a psychoanalyst, was the first to apply systems theory to the understanding of families, and spent considerable time developing this theory while working with families with a schizophrenic member. This work was furthered by a well-known group in Palo Alto, California, who integrated systems theory, communication theory, and cybernetics to develop strategic family therapy. Being students of Gregory Bateson, a well known anthropologist who applied communication theory to understanding families with a schizophrenic member, Jackson and Haley integrated these three disciplines and developed a coherent model of family functioning (Bateson, Jackson, Haley, & Weakland, 1956; Bateson, 1972). Jackson was influenced by both Freud and Sullivan, and is credited with establishing the Mental Research Institute (MRI). In addition to Bateson, Haley was also influenced by Milton Erickson and Salvador Minuchin, both known for their charismatic and unique styles in therapy. Others involved in the original staff who are well-known today include Virginia Satir, Donald Weakland, and Paul Watzlawick (Nichols, 1988; Goldenberg & Goldenberg, 1991).

Satir pioneered the Humanistic-Experiential Family therapy movement that was later developed by Carl Whitaker (Whitaker & Keith, 1981) and Walter Kempler (1981). Satir preceded her male colleagues in seeing families by developing the first family therapy training program in 1955 at the Illinois State Psychiatric Institute. This program predated the development of the MRI in Palo Alto and was instrumental in Jackson inviting Satir to help him develop the institute. This Humanistic/Experiential therapy was based on an integrated client-centered/gestalt approach, originally developed by Carl Rogers and Fritz Perls (Nichols, 1988).

The MRI group, led by Don Jackson, had a significant influence on the family therapy movement in its first decade by developing the first formal family training program funded by the National Institute of Mental Health. Similar strategic schools influenced by the MRI group developed in Milan, Italy, under the direction of Selvini-Palazzoli and Boscolo (Selvini-Palazzoli, Boscolo, Cecchin & Prata, 1978). In the late sixties with a shift in focus, the institute was renamed the Brief Therapy Center of the MRI. The center continued, however, to be influenced by Watzlawick, Weakland, Figg and Fisch (Watzlawick, Deavin, & Jackson, 1967).

Another significant figure in the family therapy movement is Salvador Minuchin, a psychoanalytically trained child psychiatrist who spent a great deal of time treating poor families in New York's inner city. Minuchin's interest in families developed after reading an article by Don Jackson in the late 1950s. Minuchin found his psychoanalytic training to be ineffective when treating difficult families; he therefore developed a briefer, more practical approach that he called Structural Family Therapy (Minuchin, 1974). His original approach had a significant impact on many students of family therapy. He is also credited with developing the Philadelphia Child Guidance Clinic that has continued to serve ghetto families.

Other developments in family therapy over the past 20 years include the Behavioral Family therapy movement, which involves the application of behavior therapy principles developed from individual therapy, to the family. One of the leaders in this area is the Oregon Social Learning Center headed by Gerald Patterson and John Reid who have focused on parent-child conflicts, and teaching parents parenting skills (Patterson, 1971). An integrated cognitive-behavioral-systemic approach known as Functional Family Therapy also developed in the early eighties by Alexander and Parsons and focused on the interpersonal significance of family behavior (Alexander & Parsons, 1982). The Behavioral Family therapy movement has, as in the individual area, contributed an empirical approach to family therapy, and is probably the only model to have been extensively investigated.

According to Goldenberg and Goldenberg (1991) family therapy has moved from a technique orientation to an increased emphasis on theory and professionalization. The challenge for the field in the future will be to integrate and consolidate the existing theoretical schools, and to develop better research tools that can measure core family constructs, process change events in therapy, and treatment outcome. Family therapy research needs to catch-up with individual psychotherapy research. It is possible that as our technology advances in individual psychotherapy research, some of these advances will transfer to the family therapy field, an area that deals with much more complicated data.

BASIC PRINCIPLES

Psychodynamic Theories of the Family

The psychodynamic approach to family therapy as discussed above was pioneered by Nathan Ackerman (1958) who developed a systemic psychoanalytic model for understanding families. The psychoanalytic model places emphasis on each member's own intrapsychic issues, while the systemic component focuses on the interaction of these personalities in the family. The marital system is viewed as the core of the family unit where unresolved intrapsychic issues are played out. The parents' unresolved conflicts, if not worked through, become displaced onto the children who are convenient receptacles for parental psychopathology. Therefore, the marital problem determines the parent-child problem, and the children's involvement in colluding with or accepting displaced projections will determine the family's overall psychological functioning. The family is considered to share unconscious processes that contribute to certain interactive styles. Conflicts arise as the family moves through developmental transitions and new demands are placed on the old system. Examples of developmental transitions include the birth of a child, children's increasing needs for autonomy, parental separation or divorce, and death of a family member. Conflict can arise from one member or several members, in either case affecting the whole system. Conflict can also develop between nuclear and extended family members across generations.

Specific developments within the psychodynamic school have influenced theories of family functioning. Object-relations theory, given its focus on "relating," can be conveniently applied to the study of the family. Dicks (1967) was the first to apply Fairbairn's object relations to the marital relationship, and James Framo (1982) focused on how parental object relations influenced the children. Since parents project their disowned parts onto their children, and children have little choice but to accept these projections, this projective identification interaction (see Individual-Dynamic chapter) is the basis of family functioning and conflict according to an object-relations model of family pathology. Other family therapists affiliated with the object-relations approach to understanding families include Skynner (1976) and Scharff and Scharff (1987).

The study of family relationships has been expanded to include the extended family and previous generations. According to Boszormenyi-Nagy and Spark (1973) present family functioning can only be understood in the context of previous generations. They described "invisible loyalties" that have originated from past generations and are transmitted from one generation to the next. These intergenerational issues are important to examine when attempting to understand present family difficulties. Family genograms or family maps are outlined to look for these transmissions across generations, so that the family can obtain a longitudinal perspective of the issues as well as become aware of the implicit rules and loyalties that have never been spoken of or acknowledged. Bowen (1978) instructs families to draw their family genogram on a blackboard in order to give the family a visual representation of their family tree.

The self-psychological approach, although applied to couples, has yet to be applied to families. A dynamically oriented group therapy has also been carried out by Bell, Wynne, and Beels (Nichols, 1988). Bell has developed a truly integrated approach that has incorporated psychodynamic, existential/humanistic, Bowenian, systemic and behavioral approaches (Bell, 1975).

Family Systems Theory

The original systems theory as described above was developed by Bertalanaffy (1968) to describe biological organisms. This theory challenged the reductionistic cause and effect model of Newtonian physics. It offered an interactional model to explain phenomena that focused on circular causality, a whole that was greater than the sum of its parts, and the interactive nature of elements within an organization. Systems theory attended to how elements within an organized complex interact and achieve homeostasis. The idea of elements interacting to form a complex organization could be easily applied to families. Systems theory focuses on the family as a homeostatic system with negative feedback loops that resist change (Nichols, 1984; Skynner, 1976). Therefore when there is an increase in one part of the system, a feedback loop is activated that causes a decrease in another part of the system in order to achieve homeostasis.

As mentioned above it was Bowen who was credited with applying general systems theory to understanding families, but other family therapists also developed and advanced the application of this theory to studying families. The three schools that adopted this new systemic approach focused on different aspects of the system. The three systemic schools of family therapy are known as the strategic/communications school, the structural school, and the Bowenian Systems school.

Strategic/communications theory

Strategic family therapy was based on communications theory, cybernetics and systems theory. It was Gregory Bateson who first applied general systems theory, cybernetics and information theory to understanding the communication patterns of families with a schizophrenic member (Bateson et al., 1956). The MRI group led by Jackson and Haley was responsible for developing a family therapy based on the integration of these theories.

The major focus of the strategic school is on communication. By understanding the patterns of communication in a family one is able to see the feedback loops that operate to maintain homeostasis. Therefore, understanding and analyzing the communication patterns leads to an understanding of the system and how it functions. Communication is what drives the system. Pathological forms of communication are identified that are associated with certain dysfunctional family systems. The double bind message is described as one of the pathological communication styles seen in families with a schizophrenic member. In this form of communication the ill member is given two opposing messages simultaneously such as "don't leave the house" and "get out of the house." This form of communication is considered to eventually contribute to psychosis. This theory, however, has since been refuted with pathological communication styles being seen as secondary to the disorder rather than primary with etiological implications (Bateson et al., 1956).

The communication/strategic approach ignores human motivation and inner experiences, viewing them as existing inside a black box that cannot be studied and is therefore irrelevant to understanding a system. Complete attention is given to communication input and output. Any interaction is said to be communicative, whether or not verbal language is used. Nonverbal messages and all behavior in any interaction are viewed as having communication value. Consequently, communication can be studied because it follows certain rules and has a command or report aspect that is significant in any interaction, especially in a family system where rules about what to communicate, how to communicate, and who to communicate with are established very early in the system (Jackson, 1959; Haley, 1971).

The systems perspective views all family behavior as achieving homeostasis. Attaining healthy family functioning requires that the system remain open so that it may respond and change as it meets the demands of the outside world. A family system that is closed and rigid cannot respond adaptively to any changes that come from within or outside the system, and will strive for homeostasis at any cost, even if the end result is a dysfunctional system.

In order for families to grow and develop, it is necessary that they experience some temporary disorganization while new more adaptive behaviors are being learned and integrated into the system. Successful families possess good problem-solving skills and accommodate to changing circumstances. Rigid families possess a narrow range of behaviors that are inflexible to change (Nichols, 1984).

Structural theory

Structural family systems theory as mentioned earlier was developed by Salvador Minuchin (1974). The focus of this systemic approach is on the organization of the family. Family members occupy particular positions, and these positions determine their roles and the rules they must follow in the family. The family rules are implicit and dictate which behaviors are and are not acceptable within the system. Family structure is maintained by hierarchical organization and boundaries. Parents assume a higher position in the hierarchy while children occupy a lower position. The family is divided into two subsystems: the parental subsystem and the sibling subsystem. Specific rules exist for members within a system. Subsystems can be organized according to gender, generation, and common interests. Clear boundaries between individuals and between subsystems are necessary in order for members to function independently and autonomously. Boundaries between members maintain a sense of separateness, whereas boundaries from the outside world emphasize a sense of belonging. Clear boundaries between the parental and the sibling subsystems provide privacy to the parental or marital system, necessary for the spouses to maintain a marital relationship. Healthy family functioning promotes individual well being as well as family cohesiveness.

According to this model, family dysfunction occurs when developmental changes or crises stress the family, and the old rules no longer maintain organization in the family. At this point rules need to be renegotiated, and the families' current structure is the focus of therapy. According to Minuchin, a family that is unable to cope and adapt to the stresses it encounters is considered to have a dysfunctional family structure. Minuchin (1974) describes two components of healthy family functioning: the maintenance of clear yet flexible boundaries between family members, and the maintenance of generational hierarchies between members with the parental subsystem at the highest level. Families with too rigid boundaries ("disengaged") sacrifice intimacy for individual autonomy. "Enmeshed" families with diffuse boundaries create difficulties for separation and individuation. If boundaries are too diffuse, individual privacy is sacrificed and members are experienced as being too intrusive and enmeshed with each other. "Alignments" and "coalitions" between members also affect family functioning. Coalitions sometimes develop when two family members align against a third member (e.g., mother and daughter may "gang up" against the father). "Triangulations" occur when parents demand that a child align with one of them, a strategy that usually prevents parents from dealing with their own marital issues.

One of Minuchin's greatest contributions was his development of the family map, a diagram of the family structure. His diagrams also illustrate boundaries, subsystems, family organization, coalitions, alignments, and triangulations within the family. This family schema is invaluable in that it can provide a very informative diagram of a family and how it is presently functioning. Minuchin's model is probably one of the easiest to understand, yet quite complete in its ability to take into account the complex interactions of family members.

Bowen's systems theory

As mentioned above Murray Bowen is credited with having been the first to apply systems theory to the study of the family. Bowen's theory (1966) is an integrated model that includes principles from both psychodynamic and systems theory. His systemic theory of family functioning clearly articulates the essential elements necessary for a family to promote individual growth and maintain family cohesiveness. Healthy family functioning allows individual members to differentiate and individuate from their family of origin. Because the family is seen as an "emotional unit," strong emotional ties bind individual members to each other, even after they have physically departed from the family. For Bowen it is the family emotional system that is the unit of study. He compared the family system to other living systems and preferred to view the family as a natural system rather than a mechanistic system with feedback loops. Bowen described eight interlocking concepts that influence family functioning. Some of the more familiar ones are differentiation of the self, triangles, family projection process, emotional cutoff, and intergenerational transmission process. The ability to differentiate one's self from one's family is the major task that allows members to free themselves from emotional family ties. Differentiation can be understood as existing on a continuum from fusion to complete differentiation of the self. The concept of triangles was discussed earlier, and once again according to Bowen, triangulation occurs when a twosome involves a third person in order to deal with dyadic instability. The family-projection process involves the triangular relationship between mother, father and child. The more undifferentiated the parents the greater the chance that they will rely on the child as an object of their projections in order to stabilize the system. In an attempt to disentangle from this family projection process, children as young adults may try to separate from their family of origin by imposing a large physical and emotional distance from their family. According to Bowen this is not true separation because the emotional issues remain unresolved and are avoided by the distance that is created. This false sense of freedom Bowen has called "emotional cutoff" and is most likely to occur in families where the child experiences excessive anxiety as well as intense emotional dependence, two experiences that push the child to artificially separate from the parents.

One of Bowen's unique contributions was his emphasis on the intergenerational transmission of dysfunctional family processes. Problems in differentiation, individuation, triangulations and other processes can be passed on from one generation to the other, repeating the cycle across generations. According to Bowen it may take as many as 8 or 10 generations in order to stabilize a dysfunctional family process. Bowen's Systems theory is a very rich theory of family functioning in which psychodynamic and systems theory principles have been integrated to produce one coherent theory of family functioning and family pathology.

Behavioral Family Theory

The application of behavioral principles to understanding the family is a relatively new development. According to the behavioral model, family members are involved in long sequences of behaviors that have developed as a result of learning. Behaviors that have been reinforced tend to remain in the family, while those that are not reinforced or punished tend to become extinguished, and eventually disappear. Despite the complexities encountered in family behavior, learning principles have been applied to the study of the family and have been found to be effective in changing dysfunctional family behavior.

There are two major schools within Behavioral Family theory: the Social Learning school developed by the Oregon Institute (Patterson, Reid, Jones & Conger, 1975), and a more integrated model known as Functional Family Analysis (Alexander & Parsons, 1982). The focus of the Oregon Group pioneered by Gerald Patterson and colleagues is on parent-child problems. Dysfunctional family behavior is considered to occur as a result of poor parenting skills. Because parents inadvertently reinforce negative behavior, these behaviors increase in frequency, creating behavioral problems in the family. The therapy, as will be discussed in the therapy section, teaches parents to reinforce positive behaviors and to ignore negative behaviors.

The Functional Analysis group integrates cognitive, behavioral and systems theory (Alexander & Parsons, 1982). Instead of placing a value on observable behavior, this approach views all behavior as adaptive in that the ultimate goal of behavior is to achieve a specific interpersonal outcome. The purpose of interpersonal behavior is to create closeness, distance, or some combination of the two. This approach examines "why" a particular behavior is occurring, and what is maintaining it.

Even though a behavior may have a negative outcome, it may also have a desired positive interpersonal effect. A common example of this is seen in families when parents only attend to a child when he or she is disruptive, thereby reinforcing the very behavior they are trying to decrease. Although the consequences of this behavior are negative, in that the child is reprimanded for it, he or she also receives attention from the parents, a very powerful reinforcer for a child. Over time parents only interact with children when they misbehave and do not interact with them at other times when they are not misbehaving. Therefore, from the child's perspective a more positive interpersonal outcome is associated with negative behavior than with positive behavior, leading to an increase in the negative behavior. The functional analysis approach to families places a greater emphasis on the interpersonal aspects of family behavior and once this is understood behaviors can be modified through behavior therapy.

Other Models of Family Functioning

Many other models of family functioning are present in the literature. These include the Experiential model (Nichols, 1988), the McMaster Model (Epstein, Bishop, & Baldwin, 1982), and the Circumplex model (Olson, Sprenkle, & Russell, 1979). Experiential family therapy grew out of the Humanistic movement in the 1960s and is an atheoretical model that attends to the present, here and now experience, and gives emphasis to individual awareness, expression, and self-fulfilment (Nichols, 1988). According to this school, denial of impulses and the suppression of feelings are seen as the root of many family problems. The McMaster model and the Circumplex model are excellent assessment models and will therefore be discussed in the assessment section.

ASSESSMENT

A family assessment can be conducted in two ways: by following a particular theoretical model, or by using specific assessment devices that attempt to assess some dimension of family functioning. If one is following the former approach, the assessment will be directed towards gathering data that confirm or disconfirm the underlying hypothesis. If following any one of the models that were discussed earlier, several areas of family functioning can be assessed. Some of these are (1) whether or not the family is an open or closed system, (2) how symptoms are achieving homeostasis in the family, (3) dysfunctional communication patterns, (4) family boundaries and hierarchies, (5) family reinforcement patterns, (6) family projection processes, (7) triangulation, and (8) integenerational transmissions of family rules and behaviors. The degree to which any one of these areas will be assessed depends on the theoretical orientation of the therapist. The latter approach delineates specific constructs that represent family functioning across all families and attempts to measure these using various instruments.

Several instruments have been devised to measure family functioning such as observational measures, structured interviews, self-report inventories, and analyses of family tasks (Fredman & Sherman, 1987). Perhaps the most well known models of family assessment are the Family Environment Scale (Moos, 1974), Olson's Circumplex model (Olson et al., 1979), and the Family Assessment Device of the McMaster Model (Epstein, Baldwin, & Bishop, 1983). The Family Environment Scale (FES) is a self-report inventory that assesses family "climate" or family functioning. It consists of 90 true/false items that measure three broad areas of family functioning: a relationship dimension, personal development and growth, and family maintenance. Ten subscales are also generated and include cohesion, expressiveness, and conflict (relationship dimension); independence, achievement, intellectual-cultural, active recreational, and moral religious (personal growth dimension); and organization and control (maintenance dimension). A score is derived from each subscale and an average score produces a family profile. The FES is probably the most extensively studied family assessment device that has been used in a wide variety of clinical situations including parent-child problems, families with medically ill members, alcoholic families, and abusive families. It has also been used with a variety of cultural groups. The scale has good psychometric properties and continues to be used as a research and clinic tool in many settings (Moos, 1974).

Olson's Circumplex model (Olson et al., 1979) measures family adaptability and cohesion. By studying over 100 families Olson described 16 types of families. The first dimension, adaptability, measures the family's ability to accommodate to changes and reorganize family structure with respect to family rules, power, and relationship roles. The cohesion scale measures the degree of emotional attachment in the family, and the degree to which the family is enmeshed or disengaged.

The Family Assessment Device (Epstein, et al., 1983) assesses the family system, the structure, and the family's coping skills. This is a 60 item self-report inventory that assesses six aspects of family functioning: problem solving, communication, roles, affective responsiveness, affective involvement, and behavior control. A family score is achieved through compiling the scores of individual members to arrive at an overall rating of general functioning. This scale continues to be investigated and has been found to be an effective assessment tool.

Basic assessment principles have also been discussed by Heller (1987) and Liddle (1983) and are excellent sources for the beginner. An alternate starting point is to draw the family genogram and then to redraw the family structure according to Minuchin's family map. Instructions on how to draw family genograms can be found in McGoldrick and Gerson's (1985) *Genograms and Family Assessment.* This gives a visual representation of the family dynamics that is descriptive and informative. Other assessment models focus on the key areas of family relating that need to be addressed. These are expressed clearly in the McMaster model.

Outside of the specific assessment models, when seeing a family, it is important to determine the degree to which the family is cohesive, able to provide a secure and nurturant base for its members, and able to provide intimacy without sacrificing autonomy. The families' capacity to express emotions to each other such as sadness, anger, joy, and others is also an important area to assess. The capacity of the parental subsystem to carry out the necessary marital as well as family functions within the system is important for healthy family functioning. All these areas need to be assessed either informally or formally using some of the assessment devices suggested above. For further family assessment devices see Fredman and Sherman (1987). For the beginner, Minuchin's structural family map in conjunction with some of the other assessment devices such as the Family Assessment Device or those discussed by Heller (1987) and Liddle (1983) are good places to begin.

THE FOUR PS

After becoming familiar with the different theoretical models of family functioning it becomes easier to identify the relevant predisposing, precipitating, perpetuating and protective family factors (see Table 10.1). ***Predisposing*** family factors are those factors that increase the likelihood of either healthy or dysfunctional family functioning. Such factors include significant parental psychopathology that leads to destructive family projection processes, transmission of strict family rules or family loyalties from past generations that constrict the family in some manner, and any chronic physical or mental illness in an individual or several family members. Poor instrumental or affective communi-

Table 10.1
Family System

Predisposing	* significant parental psychopathology * poor instrumental/affective communication * chaotic, disorganized family environment * lack of family structure * poor boundaries, lack of hierarchies * lack of family intimacy * closed family system
Precipitating	* separation, divorce, death of family member * illness in family member * change in individual in the family * financial problems * school problems * neighborhood problems * joining of new family member via birth, adoption, etc.
Perpetuating	chronic: * marital discord * psychiatric or physical illness in a member * child behavioral problems * financial, neighborhood problems * school problems * extended family problems
Protective	* minimal parental psychopathology * intergenerational transmission of strong commitment to the family * good communication—instrumental/affective * provides intimacy/permits autonomy * clear boundaries and hierarchies * open system * financial security * extended family support.

cation may predispose a family to certain difficulties such as a chaotic, disorganized life style or a vulnerability to somatization, depression, or anxiety disorders, especially in family members who are unable to safely express their feelings in the family. Families that are able to (1) deal with instrumental and affective issues, (2) allow individuation and yet provide intimacy, (3) keep boundaries clear yet not too rigid or loose, (4) remain an open system that is able to be flexible and adapt according to changing individual and family needs, are all important predisposing factors that increase the chance of healthy family functioning. Families with a predisposition towards individual or family pathology have been described as having poor boundaries, lack of a hierarchy or generational boundaries, poor communication, and poor self-other differentiation.

Precipitating family factors are usually acute events that occur either inside (intrafamilial) or outside the family (extrafamilial), that have a significant impact on the family system necessitating that the family respond in some manner to preserve homeostasis. Intrafamilial problems may be separation, divorce, death of a family member, and a psychological or physical problem in an individual member. Common extrafamilial crises include financial problems, moves, school problems, neighborhood problems, death of a relative, and others. All these events can be viewed as precipitating family factors in that they stress the family system to respond in some manner to restore equilibrium. How the family deals with these stressful events will depend on their prior functioning and potential to adapt and respond to change.

Perpetuating family factors maintain a dysfunctional family system. Sometimes a precipitating event can go on to become a perpetuating factor if it becomes chronic. Perpetuating factors can also be seen as occurring inside or outside the family. Perpetuating factors within the family include chronic marital discord, chronic psychiatric or physical illness in an individual member, chronic child behavioral problems, and any other problems that stress the family on an ongoing basis. Examples of outside-of-the-family perpetuating factors are chronic financial stressors, chronic extended family problems, poor housing, occupational stressors that impact on a particular member and school problems. It is the chronicity of the problem that determines whether or not it becomes a perpetuating factor.

Protective family factors are ones that promote optimal family functioning and individual growth, such as minimal parental psychopathology, intergenerational transmission of strong commitment to the family, good parental marital relationship, clear boundaries between members, an open family system with good communication, and good family organizational and problem solving skills. Other protective family factors are family emphasis on autonomy without sacrificing intimacy, good family psychological and physical health, family financial security, and good accessibility to family resources. A common protective factor described by many family therapists is a cohesive emotional bond that provides family members with a feeling of safety and security and encouragement to individuate and function independently outside of the family.

COPING-RESPONSE STYLE

An individual who uses his or her family as a secure base or major support is seen as having a familial coping-response style. If there is a change in the availability of this buffering system, the individual is more vulnerable to stress. These individuals may be more likely to benefit from family therapy if the presenting problem has important systemic issues relevant to the onset or maintenance of the disorder. Although not a specific response style, one could say that this systemic coping strategy is likely a common support for many individuals. Those who have a supportive family that they can rely on in times of stress may be protected during these difficult times. Alternate supports would need to be accessed if for some reason this system is no longer available. Dysfunctional families that are themselves the source of stress can be helped to become more functional and supportive to each other through family therapy. If severe family pathology is present that is resistant to therapy, then individual members must be discouraged from developing a familial coping-response style with their own family, and an alternate coping style should be accessed or developed.

TREATMENT

Psychodynamic Family Therapy

The focus of psychodynamic family therapy is to uncover each family member's individual contribution to the overall family dynamics. The therapy is usually long term and unstructured, with more attention being given to uncovering unconscious intrapsychic processes that become apparent as therapy unfolds. Various interventions such as exploration, clarification, confrontation, support, and interpretation are utilized in this form of family therapy. Family members are made aware of how their own individual psychodynamic issues get acted out in the family. Family projections are interpreted, and children are freed from parental projective identification processes. Once these conflictual issues are worked through, alternative ways of interacting with each other are explored. Individual and family defenses are identified and interpreted, and any suppressed or repressed affect is supportively encouraged expression in the family session. Psychodynamic family therapy was originally discussed by Nathan Ackerman (1958), who has been described as a very charismatic, warm, honest, yet provocative therapist who self-disclosed his own feelings in family sessions as a way of cutting through the family denial process.

Others have also been associated with this area. More recently object-relations family therapy has been described (Scharff & Scharff, 1987) that attends to working through family projective identification interactions, especially in the parental relationship. Attention is also given to each parent's own internalized good and bad objects, and how these play out in dysfunctional family transactions are interpreted and worked through in a family context.

Variability likely exists across psychodynamic family therapists with some adhering strictly to one particular model and others integrating techniques from a variety of forms of family therapy. There has been some concern regarding the suitability of most families for this form of therapy, especially in single-parent, low income, dysfunctional families that struggle with a variety of child, family, and economic problems. These families need a more structured, practical, skills-oriented approach to help them create some order in the family. Although evidence is limited, a psychodynamically informed family therapy may be very helpful in providing a richer conceptualization of the family, and dynamic interventions can be used when it is deemed appropriate. Those able to use these interventions will more than likely benefit, especially if parents are able to work through some of their own issues and minimize using their children as objects for their own projections. Helping children explore and express their feelings with their parents can encourage more affective exploration in the family and promote family intimacy. Therefore, a psychodynamically informed therapist can help the family work through some difficult issues that may be necessary before other interventions are considered.

Systemic Family Therapy

Strategic/communications family therapy

Although the three systemic areas are discussed separately above (in order to facilitate understanding of the subtle theoretical differences between them) in clinical practice there is a blending of interventions described by the major systemic schools. Strategic family therapy developed from the Communications Schools. Some texts discuss the strategic and communications schools as two separate therapies, while others integrate the two. Given their consecutive development and common theoretical base, they will be discussed together.

The application of Communication theory to family therapy led to the intense focus of family communication styles. Interventions were then developed to change dysfunctional communication patterns within families. As mentioned above, the focus was not so much on the content of the message but on the process of communication. In order to carry out communications family therapy the therapist first observes the family and identifies dysfunctional communication patterns (Jackson, 1959; Haley, 1971). Attention is focused on nonverbal and verbal communication. Once dysfunctional communication styles are identified, various techniques and strategies are used to change the communication patterns. While the family discusses the identified problem the therapist notices and points out problematic communications that may be leading to dysfunctional behaviors. Specific rules are clearly articulated to the family. For instance, members must speak for themselves and not for others, communication should be clear, not vague and diffuse, and individuals should speak directly to each other and not "about" each other. These are some of the communication rules discussed by Haley (1971), who argues that the goal of therapy is to improve family communication so that they may deal with the day to day problems in an efficient problem-solving manner.

As the name suggests family therapy involves designing various strategies to bring about change in the family. Attention is paid to the sequences of behaviors that precede the identified problem behavior. Interventions are directed at solving the presenting problem not on changing all aspects of family functioning. Focus is on changing the behavioral sequence and interrupting the vicious cycle that maintain the problem behavior.

Families are usually seen as a group but this approach does not insist that all members attend the session. Whoever chooses to come is encouraged to discuss how they see the problem. The lack of insistence on all family members attending is based on the theory that changing one member's actions will lead to a change in the family system. Once the problem behavior is identified, information is gathered with respect to how the family has been attempting to solve the problem. The strategic therapists know that ineffective solutions maintain the problem, and getting the family to understand this or gaining insight into the problem does not change the situation. Alternate strategies are suggested to create change. These include paradoxical interventions that instruct the family to do the reverse of what makes sense. For example, a mother who complains that her son's behavior is disruptive and yet allows him to misbehave is instructed to be lenient, tolerant, and even help her son misbehave. At the same time, the therapist instructs the child to misbehave even more. This paradoxical strategy leads to a change in the mother's behavior, who then ultimately takes control of the situation. The change is attributed to the mother's rebelling against the therapist's "ridiculous" prescription, leading her to alter her behavior (Nichols, 1988).

The reasons for this change are attributed to the tendency of individuals and families to adopt a defeatist attitude to common sense suggestions. Because these solutions have, according to the family, already been tried, they are unlikely to accept these suggestions from the therapist. As a result the strategic therapist suggests alternative interventions that paradoxically lead the family to change. Paradoxical interventions work by motivating the family to prove that the therapist is wrong, or by making obvious the "ridiculousness" of the prescription. These interventions are considered to produce more rapid change as a result of inducing significant behavioral change in the family (Haley, 1971).

"Reframing" is another technique used by strategic therapists that offers an alternate meaning to a problematic behavior. For example, if a husband complains of his wife as constantly "nagging" him, this behavior is reframed as his wife wanting to get "close" to him. A reframe offers an alternate, positive interpretation that is identified as problematic. Several other techniques are used by these therapists to bring about family change. These techniques have also been used by other schools and are useful in very dysfunctional families that are highly resistant to change (Haley, 1971).

Strategic therapy, practiced by the Mental Research Institute group, is considered brief, concrete and goal directed. Families are asked to operationalize their goals in therapy and to be specific regarding what they would like to see change in their family. The MRI brief approach uses a maximum of ten sessions. This therapy usually involves a treatment team that sits behind a two-way mirror, with the family's knowledge that they are observing and will be offering comments and suggestions. This procedure permits additional strategic interventions to be carried out that take into account that the therapist is also part of the system. For example, a family that is highly resistant to change, may be given feedback that the team behind the mirror is unsatisfied with the therapist's interventions. This intervention engages the family to defend the therapist's competence by bringing about the very behavioral change that up to now has been resisted. The family unites to show the team that it is wrong, and that the therapist has in fact helped the family.

These are some of the interventions used by strategic family therapists. Different strategic therapists pay attention to different interventions. Haley (1971), having been influenced by Minuchin, focuses on structural and strategic interventions. Selvini-Palazzoli (1980) and her colleagues in Italy developed a once-a-month session therapy, initially constructed to accommodate families who came from long distances. It was later discovered that this time lag between sessions was actually beneficial in that it gave the family members sufficient time to change their interactional sequences. Numerous variations to the original strategic therapy are practiced today with many eclectic family therapists using these interventions during difficult therapeutic situations. Although intriguing, their has been limited research conducted to evaluate the effectiveness of these interventions. Nevertheless, many clinicians have found these interventions to be useful, especially in very difficult resistant cases.

Structural family therapy

In structural family therapy the prime focus is structural reorganization. Minuchin (1974; Minuchin & Fishman, 1981) describes three phases of therapy; joining, mapping, and intervening. The first task of the therapist is to join the family, which according to Minuchin is essential if one is to obtain any leverage to implement change. The attempt to join the family is usually initiated in the first session by asking all members how they see the problem. All members are given ample time to articulate their view of the problem, and the therapist takes time to listen to each member making sure all have been heard. Joining the family is facilitated by engaging each member, a process that permits the therapist "into" the family as a visiting member. The therapist gains a firsthand view of what it is like to be in the family and experience its organization.

Once the therapist has joined the family, he or she is in a position to observe the interactional dynamics. These behavior patterns are recreated by getting the family members to interact through an enactment rather than asking them to describe how they usually interact. In an enactment the therapist instructs the family to discuss an issue that comes up in the session. By observing their discussion the therapist is able to delineate boundaries between members and to ascertain who is in power and who makes decisions. Parents are observed to see if they maintain a higher position in the hierarchy and if clear boundaries exist between them and the children.

After observing these transactions, the structural therapist arrives at a diagnosis that describes how the family structure, the subsystems, and the boundaries between these subsystems interact to produce a dysfunctional family system. A tentative formulation is made based on the presenting problem and the structural dynamics that are displayed. This initial formulation is revised as therapy progresses and further information is acquired.

Interventions are used thoughtfully, sometimes shaking up the existing structure so that a more functional system is created. Minuchin has been described as an intense therapist who sometimes shocks the family into making a shift that is necessary for producing structural change. Structural change also requires paying attention to interactive cycles so that the circularity of various behavioral sequences are identified. Sometimes parents are instructed not to give in to a child's tantrum behavior so that they can resume their rightful authority and hierarchy in the family. The structural therapist also refrains from blaming the parents, and whenever possible, encourages a feeling of competence and confidence that is needed for parents to function in their role. Interventions in the session focus on empowering the parents to carry out the necessary actions themselves without the help of the therapist. At times the therapist will intervene to strengthen diffuse boundaries between enmeshed subsystems or individuals, or conversely to loosen boundaries between disengaged, detached members and subsystems. The overall goal of the therapy is to create a family structure that provides clear boundaries between its members and between the important subsystems, and to resolve family conflicts that contribute to a dysfunctional family system.

Bowen's systems therapy

According to Bowen (1978) resolving family attachments is the key to developing a mature differentiated self. In the first session, a clear definition of the problem is obtained. All members are asked how they see the problem, what maintains it, and why they are seeking help at this particular time. Through these assessment questions the therapist obtains information about the family's emotional system, the differentiation of its members, how the family handles anxiety, and the functioning of each individual member. Stressors are identified and each member's reaction to these stressors is assessed.

The goal of therapy is to reduce anxiety and tension, and to increase differentiation among family members. For Bowen family therapy begins with the two most important members of the family, the parents, even if the child is the identified patient. Since family dysfunction occurs as a result of poor differentiation of the parents from their family of origin, Bowen helps the parents through this process. Therefore, family therapy according to Bowen is carried out with the parents or with individuals within the family. If both parents are able to differentiate from their own family of origin, they will be able to create change in their own families. In order to promote tension reduction the therapist encourages each spouse to speak to the therapist and not to each other in an attempt to get each to listen to the other and think about what is being said, rather than reacting to it.

Very early in the sessions Bowen instructs each spouse to draw their family genogram so that intergenerational transmission of family patterns are identified. The couple is encouraged to take a wider systemic look at their extended families, identify emotional cutoffs that create distances in families, and recognize family conflicts that are passed on from generation to generation. Both spouses acquire a picture of their family of origin's emotional system.

The therapist must also be careful not to become triangulated with the couple, which will prevent each member from achieving further differentiation. For Bowen, the therapist must remain outside the system in order to effectively work with the couple. This approach is more likely if the therapist has also achieved a significant level of differentiation from his or her own family of origin. Bowen has also discussed the importance of trainees dealing with their own family of origin in order to help others with this same task.

In therapy, Bowen acts as a coach and encourages individuals to "go home" and interact with their family of origin to increase their understanding, de-triangulate from old relationships, and to ultimately differentiate as an individual. Contact with the family of origin is not encouraged if one is interested in blaming parents or resolving long-standing issues. The main purpose is to separate from the family of origin without an emotional cut off. If separation is achieved, significant changes can be made in the individual's immediate nuclear family. According to Bowen this produces long-term changes unattainable through other therapies.

Behavioral Family Therapy

Behavioral family therapy like other forms of behavior therapy is a highly structured, goal oriented, brief, directive therapy. Patterson

(1971) and colleagues at Oregon have developed a variety of techniques for dysfunctional families with child behavioral problems. After a family assessment has been completed, the specific ways in which parents reinforce their children's behavior are recorded. These reinforcement patterns are pointed out to the parents and alternative strategies are suggested. Parents are taught how to ignore disruptive "bad" behaviors and to reinforce nondisruptive, "good" behaviors. Parental attention is viewed as a powerful reinforcer with children, and this information is conveyed to the parents.

Patterson and colleagues spend a great deal of time teaching parents various parenting skills so that they may consider alternatives to punishment. Some of these include using time out and negative reinforcement (removal of a reinforcer) instead of punishment. As part of a skills-orientated approach, parents are taught how to communicate with their children, negotiate family rules, maintain an organized household, and most of all be consistent and together in their parenting. Different techniques are suggested for dealing with young children and adolescents, the former requiring much more structure and very clear rules. Adolescents on the other hand need to be part of the negotiation process in the development of family rules.

This therapy has been found to be very effective in cases of highly dysfunctional families where there are significant parent-child problems (Patterson et al., 1975). Unique to this approach is the home visit, where objective data is gathered before, during, and after treatment, providing an accurate picture of the day to day family life and allowing the therapist to monitor progress in treatment. This approach has also been used with couples who engage in coercive interactive cycles that effect overall family functioning.

The functional behavioral group (Alexander & Parsons, 1982) as discussed above takes into account the interpersonal outcome of all behavior and does not place a value on behavior as being either good or bad, but rather interpersonally significant for the family. Because it is an integrated approach it examines the systemic effect of behavior and the cognitive factors associated with that particular behavior. Behavioral approaches as described above are used to deal with dysfunctional behavior, but how each member perceives the behavior and how it is interpreted, are explored in therapy.

SUMMARY

The family perspective adds a unique dimension to understanding individual problems. Family factors can play an important role in the onset, course, and outcome of individual psychological disorders. In some cases the family system is the problem, and the symptomatic individual is identified as the patient. Having an understanding of the family system will help differentiate what is primary—the individual or the family. Families can be involved in some part of individual therapy or the family can be *the focus* of therapy; the decision is based on how the presenting problem is formulated.

Although selecting a particular approach is difficult, the presenting problem, the family's characteristics and the available research should guide the clinician in selecting the most suitable form of therapy. Behavioral approaches have been studied extensively by Patterson (et al., 1975) and have been found to be useful in families with child behavior problems. Little evidence is currently available to support the other therapies, however one might assume that the family needs to be able to use the therapy that is offered to them. Psychodynamic family therapy may be more appropriate for the more "psychologically minded" family. Experiential therapy may be more helpful for families that have a great deal of difficulty expressing affect. Strategic, structural, and systemic therapies may be more helpful for families that need to change dysfunctional interactional patterns and communication problems. As family researchers continue to develop more sophisticated instruments, family therapy research will flourish and provide clinicians with more specific guidelines regarding which type of therapy is best for certain family problems (Gurman & Kniskern, 1992).

REFERENCES

Ackerman, N. W. (1958). *The Psychodynamics of Family Life*. New York: Basic Books.

Alexander, J., & Parsons, B. V. (1982). *Functional Family Therapy*. Pacific Grove, CA: Brooks/Cole.

Bateson, G., Jackson, D. D., Haley, J., & Weakland, J. (1956). Towards a Theory of Schizophrenia. *Behavioral Science, 1,* 251–264.

Bateson, G. (1972). *Steps to an Ecology of Mind*. New York: Dutton.

Bell, J. E. (1975). *Family Therapy*. New York: Aronson Press.

Bertalanaffy, L. V. (1968). *General Systems Theory: Foundation, Development, Applications*. New York: Braziller Press.

Boszormenyi-Nagy, I., & Spark, G. M. (1973). *Invisible Loyalties: Reciprocity in Inter-Generational Family Therapy*. New York: Harper and Row.

Bowen, M. (1966). The Use of Family Theory in Clinical Practice. *Comprehensive Psychiatry, 7,* 345–374.

Bowen, M. (1960). A Family Concept of Schizophrenia. In D. D. Jackson (Ed.), *The Etiology of Schizophrenia.* New York: Basic Books.

Bowen, M. (1978). *Family Therapy in Clinical Practice.* New York: Aronson Press.

Dicks, H. V. (1967). *Marital tensions.* New York: Basic Books.

Epstein, N., Bishop, D. S., & Baldwin, L. M. (1982). The McMaster Model of Family Functioning: A View of the Normal Family. In F. Walsh, (Ed.), *Normal Family Processes.* New York: Guilford Press.

Epstein, N., Baldwin, L. M., & Bishop, D. S. (1983). The McMaster Family Assessment Device. *Journal of Marital and Family Therapy, 9,* 171–180.

Framo, J. L. (1982). *Explorations in Marital and Family Therapy: Selected Papers of James L. Framo.* New York: Springer Publishing.

Fredman, N., & Sherman, R. (1987). *Handbook of Measurements for Marriage and Family Therapy.* New York: Brunner/Mazel.

Goldenberg, I., & Goldenberg, H. (1991). *Family Therapy: An Overview* (3rd ed.). Pacific Grove, CA: Brooks/Cole.

Gurman, A. S., & Kniskern, D. P. (1992). The Future of Marital and Family Therapy. *Psychotherapy, 29,* 65–71.

Haley, J. (1971). Approaches to Family Therapy. In J. Haley (Ed.), *Changing Families: A Family Therapy Reader.* New York: Grune and Stratton.

Heller, J. H. (1987). The Beginner's Guide to the First Family Interview. *The American Journal of Family Therapy, 15,* 291–303.

Jackson, D. D. (1959). Family Interaction, Family Homeostasis, and Some Implications for Conjoint Family Therapy. In J. Masserman, (Ed.), *Individual and Family Dynamics.* New York: Grune and Stratton.

Kempler, W. (1981). *Experiential Psychotherapy with Families.* New York: Brunner/Mazel.

Liddle, H. W. (1983). Diagnosis and Assessment in Family Therapy. A Comparative Analysis of Six Schools of Thought. In J. D. H. Hansen, (Ed.), *The Family Therapy Collections.* Rockville, MD: Aspen Publishers.

McGoldrick, M., & Gerson, R. (1985). *Genograms and Family Assessment.* New York: W. W. Norton.

Minuchin, S. (1974). *Families and Family Therapy.* Cambridge, MA: Harvard University Press.

Minuchin, S., & Fishman, H. S. (1981). *Family Therapy Techniques.* Cambridge, MA: Harvard University Press.

Moos, R. H. (1974). *Combined Preliminary Manual: Family, Work, and Group Environment Scales.* Palo Alto, CA: Consulting Psychological Press.

Nichols, M. (1984). *Family Therapy: Concepts and Methods.* New York: Gardner Press.

Nichols, W. C. (1988). *Marital Therapy: An Integrative Approach.* New York: Guilford Press.

Olson, D. H., Sprenkle, D. H., & Russell, C. S. (1979). Circumplex Model of Marital and Family Systems: Cohesion and Adaptability Dimensions, Family Types and Clinical Applications. *Family Process, 18,* 3–28.

Patterson, G. R. (1971). *Families: Application of Social-Learning to Family Life.* Champaign, IL: Research Press.

Patterson, G. R., Reid, R. B., Jones, R. R., & Conger, R. E. (1975). *A Social-Learning Approach to Family Intervention. Vol 1: Families with Aggressive Children.* Eugene, OR: Castalia Publishers.

Scharff, D. E., & Scharff, J. S. (1987). *Object Relations Family Therapy.* New York: Aronson Press.

Selvini-Palazzoli, M., Boscolo, L., Cecchin, G. F., & Prata, G. (1978). Paradox and Counter-Paradox. New York: Aronson Press.

Selvini-Palazzoli, M. (1980). Why a Long Term Interval Between Sessions? The Therapeutic Control of the Family Therapist's Supra-System. In M. Andolfi, & I. Zwerling, (Eds.), *Dimensions of Family Therapy.* New York: Guilford Press.

Skynner, A. R. C. (1976). *Systems of Family and Marital Psychotherapy.* New York: Brunner/Mazel.

Watzlawick, P., Deavin, J. H., & Jackson, D. D. (1967). *Pragmatics of Human Communication.* New York: W. W. Norton.

Whitaker, C. A., & Keith, D. V. (1981). Symbolic Experiential Family Therapy. In A. S. Gurman, & D. P. Kniskern (Eds.), *Family Therapy.* New York: Brunner/Mazel.

CHAPTER 11

THE OCCUPATIONAL/SCHOOL SYSTEM

THE PERSPECTIVE

Most individuals spend their waking hours involved in some form of activity. Preschool children involve themselves in play, older children and adolescents attend school, young adults attend college, university, or are employed, and adults of all ages until retirement, engage in some form of occupation either outside or within the home. Since the greatest proportion of an individual's time is spent in these activities, they will no doubt have an impact on an individual's psychological well-being. The relationship between occupational factors and psychological health is the focus of this chapter.

How occupational factors influence mental health has been studied by several disciplines. These include occupational therapy, industrial psychology, occupational psychiatry and organizational psychology. Although they are distinct professsions, their perspective is similar; occupation is considered to be a central aspect of human experience and the propensity toward activity is viewed as a basic human need (Creek, 1990). Several definitions of occupation have been offered in the literature, the most comprehensive by Kielhofner (1980a). According to Kielhofner, "occupation is the purposeful use of time by humans to fulfil their own internal urges toward exploring and mastering their environment that at the same time fulfils the requirement of the social group to which they belong and personal needs for self-maintenance" (Kielhofner, 1980a, p. 659). This definition emphasizes both the individual and social benefits that are received through an individual's occupation.

Positive occupational functioning is considered to psychologically benefit the individual. Dysfunction occurs when occupational roles cannot be maintained effectively. Occupational factors (such as occupational stress) can contribute to psychological distress on their own, or they can exacerbate or retard the recovery from psychological and psychiatric disorders. It is important to note that the term "occupation" does not simply refer to employment. It can include unpaid employment, play, leisure, and any variety of activity that occupies an individual's time. The importance of these activities and how they effect psychological functioning will be discussed in this chapter.

BRIEF HISTORY

The historical roots of this perspective can be traced by exploring the development of three major fields: occupational therapy, industrial and organizational psychology, and occupational psychiatry. Prior to any formal professional movement, engagement in activity as a therapeutic maneuver can be traced to 2600 B.C., China. Hippocrates also advocated the use of activity and strenuous exercise in treating the mind and the body. A more formalized exploration of the use of occupational exercises developed in 1100 A.D. in university medical schools. As the disciplines of psychology, anatomy, and physiology rapidly developed in the eighteenth and nineteenth centuries, the physiotherapy and occupational therapy movement began. Important figures during this period include C. J. Tissot and Philipe Pinel; the former advocated the use of occupational exercises as therapy and the latter introduced work therapy and physical exercises for the "insane" (Morrison, 1990).

The Occupational Therapy movement developed in Britian and the United States in the 1850s and 1750s respectively. In 1882, Adolf Meyer, a psychiatrist, emphasized the importance of activities in mental institutions. In the early 1900s occupational therapy developed in Boston, Chicago, and Baltimore. The man identified as the father of the occupational therapy movement was William Rush Dunton, a psychiatrist whose seminal paper "Occupational Therapy: A Manual for Nurses" earned him this title (Wilson, 1987).

The term "occupational therapy" (OT) was coined by George Edward in the early 1900s. Throughout this period the occupational therapy movement progressed, and in 1923 Dunton established the American Occupational Therapists' Association. Occupational therapy schools developed throughout the United States, Britain, and Scotland, and in 1986, 28 countries were represented in the World Federation of Occupational Therapy. In less than a century the OT field grew to include general hospital and psychiatric populations. More recently, there has been a movement away from the hospitals into the community (Wilson, 1987; Morrison, 1990).

The occupational psychiatry movement began during World War I. In 1917 a Boston psychiatrist, Herman Adler, published an article that identified psychiatric symptoms in unemployed individuals. In 1927 a review of Industrial Psychology was published in the *American Journal of Psychiatry* that emphasized the importance of vocational counseling during early developmental years, to prevent later occupational problems. In the 1920s and 1930s, businesses such as department stores and insurance companies hired psychiatrists to deal with their employees and their organizations. Although the economic depression witnessed a decrease in activity in the field, the trend was rapidly reversed during World War II, as psychiatry became actively involved in the armed forces and industrial settings. Although there was some decrease in growth after World War II, the 1950s and 1960s continued to demonstrate a rapid growth in the field, with similar developments evident in England, Sweden, and other countries. Since the 1970s, greater attention has been paid to occupational stress, drug abuse among employees, employee assistance programs, and mental health benefits utilization. It is also recognized that the focus should not only be on the individual but on the organization as well (McLean, 1974).

BASIC PRINCIPLES

As mentioned earlier, several disciplines are part of the occupational category. As a result, a variety of theoretical principles have been discussed in each discipline, depending on the emphasis given to theory over practice. However, similar issues and concepts have been addressed across all these disciplines and the relevant points that have implications for psychological health have been collected and organized in the discussion presented below. The basic principles are described under two headings: occupational functioning through development, and occupational dysfunction. A developmental perspective is necessary before one can appreciate the significance of dysfunction in this area. This will also provide the reader with a method of conceptualizing this area so that it can be applied to individual cases.

Occupational Functioning Through Development

The concept of occupation does not simply refer to one's work, but to a broad range of activities an individual engages in on a regular basis. These include play, work, leisure, and recreation (Creek, 1990). All three activities are interrelated and can be understood from a developmental point of view. According to Kielhofner (1980a; 1980b) work and play are not by-products of our day to day existence, but the essence of human experience. Work and play although seemingly involving very separate activities, have important effects on each other. Their interrelationship has been described across four developmental stages: childhood, adolescence, adulthood, and old age and retirement (Kielhofner, 1980a; 1980b).

Childhood

In childhood the primary activity is play. This is evident from infancy when the child is seen to repeat actions that are pleasurable, such as touching a toy that makes a noise or shaking a rattle. As development progresses the child is much more able to interact with the environment, increasing the opportunity to engage in a variety of playful activities. Imitation of adults and their activities becomes another important feature of children's play (Kielhofner, 1980b).

All these playful activities are important for future cognitive, social, and vocational development. Through play the child acquires skills that can be learned and rehearsed (Kielhofner, 1980a; 1980b; Creek, 1990). Play also teaches the child social rules and social norms that are important for later occupational functioning. The child learns about competitiveness, cooperation, and how to organize time—all important lessons for the future "working world." The play of childhood also becomes the leisure and recreation of adulthood, important for the adult's psychological well being (Kielhofner, 1980b; Creek, 1990).

Entry into school imposes further demands, with increased expectations to follow rules, behave appropriately, and maintain a certain level of performance. The child now adopts the more formal role of student and learns the responsibilities associated with that role such as being punctual, maintaining regular attendance, conforming to rules, obeying authority figures, completing homework assignments, and working with peers. All these skills become important in later adult occupational roles (Kielhofner, 1980b). Successful school performance is a significant contributor to positive self-esteem and is therefore an important contributor to future personality development.

Adolescence

As the child moves into adolescence there is pressure to develop further competency in adult roles. During this period, serious consideration is given to occupational choice as the adolescent explores different possibilities. Selecting an occupation begins in adolescence, and is partially completed in early adulthood with the first employment. This process, however, may continue throughout adulthood, with varying degrees of success.

Kielhofner (1980b) describes three periods that are part of this process: fantasy, tentative and realistic. In the pre-adolescent period idealized occupations are considered that may be based on parental occupation and social values. In adolescence, occupational choice is determined by more subjective factors such as sense of personal capability, interest, and values. This outlook changes to a more realistic view in adulthood when compromises are made between dreams and desires and what is actually attainable.

Adulthood

In early adulthood more time and energy are expended to pursue occupational choices. The drive for achievement and success and a sense of efficacy will motivate some to consider certain occupations or professions, while economic realities may prevent others from further exploration of interests. In most societies a working adult contributing to society is valued over a nonworking adult. Although this is traditionally referred to as "paid employment," recent acknowledgment has been granted to unpaid work (carried out by a housewife, or househusband) as equally important occupations that contribute to society by maintaining effective family functioning and family roles.

In adulthood an occupation can fulfil many needs, depending on the meaning given to this role. Daily work provides structure and organization, and keeps the individual occupied. It provides a social role and a sense of identity. For some (especially if a great deal of time, effort, and training have been expended to ensure appropriate occupational choice), occupational activities can provide a sense of purpose, a place to experience a sense of mastery, meet self-esteem needs, and provide an important medium for continued self-exploration and growth (Creek, 1990; Young & Quinn, 1992). Work environments can also provide opportunities for social interaction, social stimulation, and in some cases social support, an important factor discussed at length in the next chapter. Nevertheless, it is important to remember that for many, an occupation may simply be a means of livelihood with economic realities determining occupational choice, rather than personal ambition or aspirations (Young & Quinn, 1992). For others, leisure, hobbies, and other recreational activities may be more important in contributing to a sense of productivity than a job that has been acquired for purely economic reasons. Therefore, it is the meaning given to the occupational role that is important to consider, rather than the job itself.

In addition to work, adults continue to play during leisure time with a variety of recreational activities. The role of play changes through development from a preparatory role for work in childhood, to a supportive role in adulthood. Leisure and recreation are regenerating activities essential for the maintenance of psychological well-being, for they promote further exploratory behavior and provide energy to maintain the work role (Kielhofner, 1980b). Recreational activities gain more importance in retirement and are therefore essential to develop in adulthood (Young & Quinn, 1992).

Old age and retirement

Occupational activities change significantly in old age when many are forced to retire and leave their occupational roles. This change can be a very difficult time for some elderly persons, especially if self-esteem needs and a sense of productivity and well-being were obtained from participating in a form of vocation. There is a disengagement from the "working-world" during this period, and many factors can influence how an individual will adapt to this transition (Kielhofner, 1980b: Young & Quinn, 1992; Creek, 1990). Cultures that respect and value the elderly will continue to encourage their involvement as experienced, valued advisors to society. Societies that perceive the elderly as unproductive and unable to contribute will fail to provide a positive environment for these individuals in retirement.

Involvement in hobbies, leisure, and recreational activities may soften the negative effects of this transition for some elderly by offering them alternative outlets to maintain a certain activity level and functional capacity. Part-time or volunteer work often can continue to fulfil some of the needs that were once obtained from more full-time, regular work. Many organizations such as hospitals, daycare centers, and various community organizations can provide these experiences for the retired adult. Active involvement in some occupations, whether through leisure and recreation, volunteer work, or part-time work, will be a significant determinant of psychological well being in the retirement years.

Occupational Dysfunction

Having presented a developmental model of occupational functioning and its relationship to psychological health, we can now turn to occupational dysfunction and how it influences mental health problems. Several areas have been identified in the occupational literature, the ones selected for discussion have important implications for the mental health professional. These include (a) dysfunctions in play, (b) poor school performance, (c) job dissatisfaction/job stress, or occupational stress, (d) unemployment, and (e) inadequate leisure and recreational activities.

Dysfunctions in play

Having discussed the importance of "play" in occupational development, any obstacle to a child's involvement in play activities may impair the early learning of skills and rules that are useful in later occupational role functioning. A child who is physically handicapped and unable to actively explore the environment may have less opportunity to engage in a variety of play. This lack of experience would attenuate the acquisition of skills and produce less opportunity for the child to gain a sense of mastery. If there are additional problems that prevent interactions with other children, either through physical or mental handicaps or through socially impairing disorders such as autism, then there will be limited opportunities to experience social rules, cooperation, and competitiveness, all necessary pre-occupational experiences. Therefore any condition that interferes with a child's successful capacity to play will prevent the learning of various skills, habits and social rules in childhood, necessitating the teaching of some of these skills at a later stage of development (Kielhofner, 1980b; Creek, 1990).

Poor school performance

Performance at school has a significant impact on the child's sense of worth and self-esteem (Licht & Kistner, 1986; Perry & Bussey, 1984). School performance also influences parental perceptions of their children, which in turn influences the child's perception of him- or herself. Poor school performance then will have a significant impact on later occupational functioning. Poor school performance can be attributed to individual and school factors. Some individual factors are (1) physical illness—especially chronic diseases such as asthma, diabetes, arthritis, and others, (2) psychiatric conditions—such as depression, anxiety, psychosis, and attention deficit disorder, (3) learning disorders - such as a specific reading or arithmetic learning disability, (4) family problems, and (5) motivational problems that include emotional and self-esteem problems. School factors include socially disadvantaged schools, poor teachers, and lack of resources for special education and tutoring.

Although all these are important contributing factors towards poor school performance, one of the most common reasons for referral to mental health professionals is learning disabilities. Children with learning disabilities can have repeated experiences of academic failure, which have profound effects on their self-esteem, social interactions, and later occupational functioning (Licht & Kistner, 1986). They learn over time to attribute their failures to their abilities, and any successful experiences to luck. This attribution of failure to abilities is in keeping with their developmental stage, because most of these children are not truly identified until after age eight. It has been shown that children do not have an accurate perception of their abilities until age seven, and prior to this they overestimate their abilities, seeing themselves in the top of the class. By age seven, social comparison becomes an important factor, and children begin to see that they need to perform better than their peers in order to receive a high performance evaluation. That is, they experience their intellectual ability as fixed, and not amenable to great change. Therefore younger children are less vulnerable to academic failure than older children, who by age 10, view intelligence as a stable limiting factor in their overall performance. Therefore, increased awareness of the importance of ability and the identification of learning problems that occur around this time make a learning disabled child vulnerable to self-damaging self-attributions (Torgesen & Wong, 1986).

Learning-disabled children have been found to have beliefs that interfere with work, and they are in danger of generalizing their perceptions of academic "failure" to other areas in their life. They are also described as having poor social skills and receive negative and deprecating comments from their peers, teachers, parents, and even strangers (Lict & Kistner, 1986). These perceptions may be due to behavioral problems which tend to co-occur with learning disabilities. Specific processing deficits may make it difficult to learn social rules and norms, and contribute to organizational difficulties, an important skill necessary for future successful occupational functioning. Therefore, by understanding the academic and social consequences of being identified as a learning disabled child, one can see how important school performance is to later occupational functioning. Such an early experience of failure, unless treated successfully, may circumvent future vocational and occupational planning and decrease motivation to pursue any academic or career aspirations.

Occupational stress

Occupational stress has been given considerable attention in recent years as is evident by the development of employee assistance programs in many occupational settings (Creek, 1990). Stress at work can result from individual factors, or the interaction of them. Individual factors include control of job selection, satisfaction with job or career choice, and perception of the present occupation. Individuals who have been pressured into a form of employment for economic or other reasons and are unhappy with their selection, may experience chronic levels of frustration and unhappiness at work. There may be feelings of bitterness, unfairness, or regret that they were unable to select the job of their choice. Unless other activities can buffer this chronic level of dissatisfaction, the individual will be under significant stress on a daily basis. Chronic dissatisfaction at work could affect functioning in other social roles as a spouse, parent, or friend. If the individual experiences too many demands, feels overworked, underpaid, and is pessimistic about future advancement or improvement, then chronic levels of stress will be experienced at work, and the individual's capacity to alleviate these effects through other activities or social support will become important. Therefore perception of one's occupation, whether this is positive or negative, will influence general psychological well being.

Environmental occupational factors that contribute to job dissatisfaction or job stress include poor physical working conditions (e.g., space, lighting, ventilation, esthetics, etc.), difficult interpersonal relationships with colleagues, managerial and bureaucratic problems, poor wages, and cuts in salaries. Most of these factors may be outside the individual's control leading to chronic feelings of frustration and helplessness that can over time affect psychological functioning (Creek, 1990).

An occupational factor can by itself produce psychological symptoms and be the focus of a presenting problem, or it can precipitate a psychiatric or psychological problem such as depression or anxiety in a vulnerable individual. Having a psychological or psychiatric disorder that impairs occupational functioning can also lead to occupational stress as a result of performance difficulties and absenteeism. The cause and effect chain when considering all these factors is not always clear. A significant occupational stressor may precipitate a major depression in an individual predisposed towards this disorder. The depressive symptoms will impair occupational functioning and increase occupational stress, which may worsen the depressive symptoms and diminish any benefit from medication, if an occupationally focused intervention is not included in the treatment. Therefore identifying the occupational stressor as an antecedent, concomitant, or maintenance factor may not be as important as simply attending to it as an important variabe in the understanding and treatment of psychological and psychiatric disorders.

Unemployment

Losing a job has always been considered a significant stressful life event. It is number six on the Holmes and Rahe Scale of stressful life events (Holmes & Rahe, 1987). Being unemployed has economic, social, and personal consequences. Financial instability is the obvious and immediate concern especially if one is single, a sole supporter of a family, or a member of a dual income family that necessitates that both partners work—a common phenomenon in today's world. The availability of financial resources through personal savings, parents, banks, and other sources will likely influence the anxiety experienced over the immediate financial loss.

The financial implications will no doubt affect self-esteem and a sense of self-worth, depending on the individual's personality and vulnerabilities. The effect of job loss has been discussed by Kates and associates (Kates, Grieffe, & Hagen, 1990), who present a review of the current literature and provide an integrated model for conceptualizing and treating the psychological effects of job loss. They view unemployment as a predisposing, precipitating, or perpetuating factor in its temporal relationship to mental health problems. They stress the importance of considering multiple factors when dealing with patients who have become recently unemployed.

One of the first factors to consider is the cause of unemployment. If job loss is secondary to a plant closure and involves many workers, it will have less personal meaning than if the individual is the only one to lose a job, especially if firing is related to poor job performance. Therefore, the attribution given to unemployment will influence the actual response to the loss. Individuals who derive significant self-esteem needs from their work, may be more vulnerable to job loss, unless these needs are met in other areas. Job loss has also been found to contribute to marital and family problems, and these difficulties can further exacerbate psychological symptoms (Kates et al., 1990).

Although few studies have systematically assessed psychiatric disorders in the unemployed, some findings are noted (Kates et al,. 1990). The unemployed have been found to (1) have a higher mortality than their employed controls, (2) visit their general practitioners more often, (3) be more inactive, (4) report increased depressive symptoms with about 25% meeting the criteria for a major depressive episode, (5) have increased rates of divorce and marital problems, (6) experience more child behavior problems at home, and (7) have a greater likelihood of suicide (Pritchard, 1992). Whether it is unemployment per se or the effects of poverty that contribute to these issues is unclear.

Social support has been found to decrease the incidence of depressive symptoms in the unemployed (Bolton & Oatley, 1987). Most of these symptoms appear to improve once the individual returns to work. Older workers and women are at a higher risk of remaining unemployed for longer periods of time. Persistent unemployment is much higher for blacks and individuals with disabilities. It is probably not surprising that psychiatric patients will also have difficulties with unemployment due to social stigma, poor work history, and lack of skills, especially in conditions such as schizophrenia that have an early onset that preempts further skills training (Kates et al., 1990; Parkson & Pendegrass, 1993). These are important issues to consider when planning a comprehensive treatment. Unemployment can lead to psychological and physiological symptoms in many individuals. Those most vulnerable may be at greater risk whether this vulnerability is biological or psychological. Psychiatric illness can also lead to unemployment and needs to be considered as an important variable in the long term management and outcome of any case.

Inadequate leisure and recreational activities

The final area to consider is that of leisure and recreation. Many patients who present with symptoms of anxiety, depression, or general psychological distress tend to be inactive and uninvolved in any leisure activities. They may be overloaded with responsibilities at work and at home and have very little time for recreation. Such a lifestyle can contribute to chronic fatigue, lethargy, and chronic feelings of being "overwhelmed." Because leisure and recreational activities relax and reenergize the individual, the absence of such activities may contribute to poor functioning in other areas (Creek, 1990).

For the elderly, remaining active is very important since a greater amount of time may be spent in leisure pastimes. The lack of such activities and hobbies results in inactivity and a low rate of positive experiences that may make this group vulnerable to depression, lethargy, and general social withdrawal. Positive self-experiences that were previously obtained through work or some other role (mother, wife, husband) may no longer be available, necessitating the search for alternative activities to provide these experiences. In addition to leisure or recreational activities, some elderly participate in community work and maintain involvement with others through this process.

ASSESSMENT

Assessment of the significant occupational issues can be carried out through the clinical interview and with the aid of a variety of instruments. The focus of the assessment will depend on the presenting problem and the age of the patient. For an adult the important occupational factors to assess are educational history, employment history, career, job selection, job satisfaction, meaning of the job to the individual, and job stress. Any recent changes at work such as decrease in pay, relocation, new supervisors, new co-workers, and any new demands may be especially important to assess because these factors alter a person's working environment in a positive or negative direction. If unemployment is an issue, assessment of skills and other employment possibilities based on past experiences need to be assessed.

In the case of a child, assessment is usually aimed at assessing intelligence and identifying any learning difficulties and is usually carried out by the school or through a private consultation with a psychologist. In high school, vocational assessment can identify interests, areas of strength, and personal aptitude, to help an adolescent make career choices. Vocational assessments and career counseling can also be carried out in colleges, universities, and community centers that offer employment assistance to out-of-work individuals. Adults considering a career change may also pursue a vocational assessment to help them explore other opportunities.

Instruments are also available to assess occupational stress. The easiest to administer is the Occupational Stress Inventory, which assesses six stress-inducing work roles, namely role overload, role insufficiency, role ambiguity, role boundary, responsibility, and the physical environment (Osipow & Spokane, 1987).

FOUR PS

Significant ***predisposing*** occupational factors that can contribute to psychological difficulties in certain situations include a learning disability, limited intellectual ability, lack of opportunity to explore vocational abilities, and economic limitations (see Table 11.1). Any individual trouble (such as a personality disorder) that may create interpersonal problems and lead to difficulties in the work place with supervisors and authority figures, may also predispose an individual to occupational problems. Chronic dissatisfaction with work and chronic occupational stress may also predispose vulnerable individuals to developing a psychiatric disorder. All these occupational factors predispose an individual toward experiencing distressing psychological symptoms either directly or indirectly in the vulnerable individual.

Occupational factors that may ***precipitate*** a crisis or a psychological disorder or distress include failing a grade, test or exam, being diagnosed as learning disabled, changing schools, changes at work that stress the individual such as decrease in pay, physical relocation, loss of supportive co-workers, and most of all, loss of work.

Occupational factors that ***perpetuate*** psychological conditions can be any chronic stressful situation at school or at work. In a child these include chronic learning problems with poor academic performance, and chronic difficulties with a teacher. For an adult, any ongoing occupational stressor such as chronic unemployment can perpetuate psychological symptoms and maintain a major psychiatric disorder. Lack of hobbies and poor participation in leisure and recreational activities can also perpetuate occupational stressors by not providing the individual with an outlet for rest, and a chance to recharge.

Occupational factors that are ***protective*** contribute to psychological well-being and may buffer the individual from other stressors. In a child, good academic performance, high achievement, and positive teacher and peer relations at school can all contribute to a positive sense of self-worth, and boost self-esteem. Positive reinforcement at school is especially beneficial if there are family problems at home, because the school will provide a positive distraction from these family conflicts. Good performance at school will also invite positive responses from parents, teachers and peers, all contributing to a positive sense of self.

For an adult, satisfaction with work is a significant protective occupational factor for it can give personal meaning to life, boost self-esteem, and provide an experience of mastery and productivity that can contribute to psychological well-being. A financially lucrative, stable, enjoyable job is certainly an ideal that many strive for. If work is perceived as stimulating, exciting, and generally positive, this can be psychologically protective especially if other areas such as one's personal, marital, and family life are perceived more negatively. A positive work environment that is aesthetically pleasing, furnishes good working conditions, promotes good relationships between co-workers and between workers and supervisors, fosters autonomy and encourages creativity in employees,

Table 11.1
Occupational/School System

Predisposing	* learning problems in school * underachievement in school performance * limited intellectual ability * economic limitations * individual psychopathology * chronic dissatisfaction with work and occupational choice * poor parental modeling of occupational behavior
Precipitating	* failure at school * receiving diagnosis of learning disability * changes at school (new teacher) and work (new employer) * loss of supportive co-workers/peers * loss of employment
Perpetuating	* repeated failure at school * chronic stress at work * chronic difficulities with teacher/employer/co-worker/peer/ * ongoing unemployment * lack of leisure/recreation
Protective	* good academic achievement in school * positive teacher, peer, employer-employee relationship * satisfaction at work * work provides ++ self-esteem

and offers a chance for advancement, will provide protective occupational factors that enhance the well-being of the individual and the organization. Given the amount of time an individual spends at work, these factors can significantly influence mental health.

COPING-RESPONSE STYLE

Although an individual's occupation can be a source of stress, it can also be an escape from stress, especially if the job is perceived as very satisfying. Many individuals who enjoy their work may find it a convenient distraction from other problems such as marital and family conflicts. Loss of work for these individuals can be even more significant if their coping-response style was restricted to this area.

In addition to work, leisure and recreational activities also supply opportunities for relaxation and tension reduction. An individual who uses hobbies and recreational activities as a method of coping can be described as having an occupational coping-response style, although it may be more appropriate to refer to this as a recreational coping-response style.

For children and adolescents school can also be an escape from family problems, especially if this is a positive experience academically and socially. For some children and adolescents, participation in sports and extracurricular activities can offer distracting, positive experiences that may help them cope with academic or family problems. These outlets provide diversion from other problems and also counteract any negative feelings generated from stressful life events. An occupational coping-response style then involves active engagements in work or leisure and recreational activities, for the prime purpose of escaping from or buffering current stressful life experiences.

TREATMENT

Treatment in the occupational area involves many therapeutic interventions given the variety of problems that contribute to occupational dysfunction. Many mental health professionals including social workers, psychologists, and psychiatrists deal with occupational problems and utilize a variety of individual and systemic approaches in the treatment of clinical cases. However, the therapist most devoted to enhancing an individual's occupational functioning is the occupational therapist. Therefore, a brief discussion about the principles of occupational therapy will be presented prior to addressing specific interventions for individuals with specific occupational problems.

Occupational Therapy

Occupational therapists engage in a therapeutic relationship with clients to help them attain a certain level of healthy occupational functioning. Since engagement in meaningful and productive activity is equated with physical and psychological health, interventions are aimed at returning the individual to a normal level of functioning. If this is not possible, alternative activities will be sought to promote optimal occupational functioning.

Patients or clients are usually referred to an occupational therapist after some physical, psychological, or psychiatric disturbance is diagnosed. In general hospitals, psychiatric inpatients may be referred to the occupational therapist for an assessment of their functioning and/or treatment. In chronic institutions, occupational therapists are also involved in helping more severely impaired individuals attain a more meaningful level of functioning. The methods used to return an individual to a more adaptive level of functioning are quite variable, depending on the problems identified and the therapist's skills. Occupational therapy borrows from many other psychotherapies including psychodynamic, cognitive, behavioral, client centered, supportive, and others. Group therapy is also a popular method of treatment and many forms of group therapy (supportive, art, drama, music, social skills), are used to deal with a variety of problems (Creek, 1990; Young & Quinn, 1992; Stockwell, 1988; Hewitt, 1988).

Any therapy is preceded by an activity analysis, which examines the various components of the activities individuals are required to carry out in their occupational roles, daily functioning, and in leisure and recreation (Creek, 1990). The individual's ability to carry out these activities at the time of referral is assessed. Once this analysis is completed, more appropriate activities are considered that contain some of the desired components of previous activities that can no longer be performed.

Occupational therapists work collaboratively and supportively with their clients and set short-term, intermediate, and long-term goals. Short-term goals are realistic and meaningful. Long-term goals focus on what is ultimately desired in terms of overall level of functioning given existing limitations. Part of the treatment involves the learning of skills in order to improve physical, cognitive, psychological, and interpersonal functioning (Creek, 1990). Motivation is an important factor in therapy because the client is required to participate in many activities that are aimed at change. Many of these activities require effort, work, interactions with others, and an expectation to perform at a certain level. A good working relationship between the occupational therapist and the client is necessary because both will struggle together to reach short- and long-term goals.

Specific Occupational Problems

Having presented a discussion on the basic approach to occupational therapy, I will now turn to the application of some of these principles to specific occupational problems mentioned earlier. Not all occupational problems are treated by occupational therapists; occupational and general psychiatrists, industrial, clinical and educational psychologists, social workers, and family physicians all see individuals or organizations (school, businesses, etc.) with occupational problems. Some problems may require more specialized services that are only carried out by one of the disciplines represented in this group. For example, assessing academic performance and making recommendations for special education are usually carried out by psychologists.

Some of the interventions that have been used to treat the occupational dysfunctions presented earlier will be briefly discussed here. These include dysfunctions in play, poor school performance, job stress, unemployment, and lack of leisure and recreation.

Dysfunctions in play

Because a child's capacity to play is important for future healthy development and adaptive occupational functioning, any child unable to engage in active play requires specific interventions. Many factors limit a child's capacity to play. Some of these are severe physical and mental disabilities, physical illnesses, depriving environments, and psychological disturbances such as depression, anxiety, autism, and many others. Treating the underlying condition is the first step, for this alone may return the child to his or her previous level of functioning. If there is a delay in returning the child to a functional level of play, or if there is some resistance to conventional treatment, play therapy can be considered to help the child to resume this normal activity. Play therapy, like psychotherapy, is guided by a variety of models such as the psychoanalytic, client centered, developmental and others (Jeffrey, 1990). The major focus of therapy in this situation is to resume "function," to enable the child to return to a previous level of functioning, or to encourage the most optimal level possible in the current situation. Play therapy provides the child with a safe, stimulating environment that is specific to the child's needs. The therapist encourages and guides the child to explore and engage in a variety of play behaviors. Depending on the specific problem, a structured play approach with designated tasks may be organized to help the child move towards an optimal level of functioning. With each step the child experiences a sense of mastery and acquires a set of skills necessary for future development and successful performance in school.

Play therapy is only one of many interventions used by the occupational therapist when working with children. Many other interventions are utilized depending on the specific problem, and the child (Clancy, Clark & Michele, 1990). Occupational therapists have also been involved with developmentally handicapped children who require intensive programs that stimulate sensory, perceptual, and motor development.

Poor school performance

Poor performance in school requires specific interventions that are carried out by teachers, educational psychologists, and less frequently, occupational therapists. Other allied professionals who may be involved are speech and language therapists. Many factors can influence a child's academic performance in school, and this performance will in turn effect self-esteem and future motivation. Identifying the cause of the problem is the first step to treatment. As was mentioned earlier, learning problems can be secondary to other psychological problems such as childhood and adolescent depression, anxiety disorder, family problems and others. Treating these problems may improve performance at school; however, if the primary problem is a learning problem, then additional interventions are necessary.

Treating a child with a learning disability is complicated and requires several steps (Torgeson & Wong, 1986). Usually a child is identified as having some learning problem in grade two or three. An educational assessment carried out by a psychologist will identify whether the child has a specific learning disability. Once a specific problem is identified, the child will receive specialized instructions from a special education teacher in a small self-contained classroom for children with learning disabilities, or through resource withdrawal, where the child will be removed from the classroom for a brief period of time during the day to work with a special education teacher. A variety of techniques have been used with children with specific learning problems that are philosophically and empirically based. Different interventions have stressed different areas, such as memory, sensory deficits, sensory integration, communication and direct instruction (McCallion, 1990; Torgesen & Wong, 1986). Medications have also been used effectively to treat children with attention deficit disorders, a co-morbid condition commonly associated with learning disabilities (Pelham, 1986). Behavioral and cognitive-behavioral techniques have also been used to teach learning disabled children to gain control of their cognitive capabilities (Koorland, 1986; Ryan, Weed, & Short, 1986). More recently attention has been focused on the social skills deficits of learning disabled children, and social skills training has been added to help them develop better social relationships (Pearl, Donaghue & Brian, 1986).

Job stress

Before treating an individual suffering from occupational stress, a complete occupational assessment is necessary in order to identify the specific area of difficulty. A supportive, exploratory therapeutic approach will encourage the individual to examine their current occupational difficulties in an open, nonthreatening environment. More direct questioning may reveal hidden feelings about the job, the meaning of the job to the individual, and overall job satisfaction. If there is complete dissatisfaction at work, analyzing the various components that comprise one's work can help identify the area that is creating the greatest distress. If interpersonal problems are an issue with supervisors or co-workers, identifying the important psychodynamic, cognitive and behavioral factors that contribute to these difficulties may help in some situations. In this case helping the individuals understand their own issues and contributions to interpersonal difficulties may help them change their behavior. Teaching specific skills such as organizational and time management skills, social skills and assertiveness training may help some individuals feel more effective at work. Some individuals may be overworked, spending most of their time working or worrying about work-related issues. In this case, teaching the importance of a balanced life that includes leisure and recreational activities will be important. If the work situation cannot be improved, then considering an alternative occupation may be another possibility. Helping someone explore their interests and abilities in order to select the most appropriate choice is the job of the vocational counselor who is trained to help in this area (Kahn, 1993).

Unemployment

Unemployment is a significant occupational stressor that may bring an individual to a mental health professional. The effects of unemployment are so widespread that a variety of interventions may be required. Kates and others (Kates et al., 1990) discuss the importance of using an integrated model that considers individual and systemic factors when dealing with the psychological impact of job loss. The first step is to deal with the acute effects of job loss which is likely to generate a variety of feelings such as fear, anxiety, anger, shame, depression and many others. The ability to explore these feelings in a supportive environment is essential.

Attention then should be given to how the individuals perceived their jobs prior to unemployment. Whether the job contributed to meeting basic psychological needs such as positive self-esteem and a sense of productivity will be important to explore. Such a loss may trigger unresolved individual issues (e.g., inability to tolerate failure), that may contribute to additional negative feelings and conflicts. After individuals are given an opportunity to explore their immediate reaction, attention is given to teaching adaptive coping skills to help them manage their acute reactions, and making long-term plans regarding alternate employment opportunities. Attention is also given to improving the quality of their day-to-day life by (1) teaching stress reduction techniques, such as relaxation exercises, (2) encouraging financial planning, (3) providing vocational assistance, (4) activity scheduling, and (5) maintaining good physical health (Kates et al., 1990).

In addition to the above, systemic interventions are also utilized in the overall management of unemployment, in order to help the spouse and children cope with the loss, and to encourage supportive family behaviors. Social agencies can also be accessed in the acute management of unemployment problems, and in planning long-term goals. Obtaining information about community-based interventions such as support groups is an important component of treatment. These groups can offer support, and help individuals feel less alone with their problems. Therefore, when treating the recently unemployed, a variety of interventions at multiple levels should to be considered and carefully planned by the mental health professional (Kates et al., 1990).

Leisure and recreation

Interventions aimed at increasing leisure and recreational activities in order to improve physical and mental health are frequently ignored by many mental health professionals. Individuals who engage in very few leisure and recreational activities may be encouraged to explore these areas by helping them identify their own unique interests. Occupational therapists are probably the best trained to help someone examine their lack of leisure or recreational activities. Participation in these activities can be very helpful for individuals suffering a psychiatric disorder such as schizophrenia, depression, or anxiety. These activities can also be relaxing and energizing for those who overwork. For those individuals who are unable to work, leisure, recreation, and hobbies become even more important, and are significant for the retired elderly who need to remain active (Revetz, 1988).

The goal here is to find activities that are enjoyable and provide a sense of well-being as a result of increasing functional capacity, activity level, and a sense of productivity. Leisure and recreational activites can also facilitate social relationships as some of these activities can be shared with others. The occupational therapist is probably the best trained to assess these areas and offer possible suggestions.

SUMMARY

Occupational factors are important determinants of psychological well-being, because it is the area in which individuals spend the greatest amount of time. How we experience our work, school, leisure, play, and recreational activities can affect overall psychological functioning. These factors can be primary in contributing to psychological distress or they can be secondarily affected by other physical and psychological problems. Mental health professionals need to be alert to this important area by developing a perspective that attends to occupational factors in the assessment and treatment of psychological and psychiatric disorders. A more thorough assessment and comprehensive treatment plan can be obtained through a referral to an occupational therapist, vocational counselor, occupational psychiatrist or psychologist, or other professionals that specialize in this area.

REFERENCES

Bolton, W., & Oatley, K. (1987). A Longitudinal Study of Social Support and Depression in Unemployed Men. *Psychiatric Medicine, 17,* 453–460.

Clancy, H., Clark, M. J., & Michele, J. (1990). *Occupational Therapy with Children.* London: Churchill Livingstone.

Creek, J. (Ed.). (1990). *The Development of a Paradigm in Occupational Therapy and Mental Health: Principles, Skills and Practice.* London: Churchill Livingstone.

Hewitt, C. (1988). Training and Social Skills. In M. Wilson, (Ed.), *Occupational Therapy in Short Term Psychiatry* (2nd ed.). London: Churchill Livingstone.

Holmes, T. H., & Rahe, R. H. (1987). The Social Readjustment Rating Scale. *Journal of Psychosomatic Research, 11,* 213–218.

Jeffrey, L. (1990). Play Therapy. In J. Creek, (Ed.), *Occupational Therapy and*

Mental Health: Treatment, Planning and Implementation. London: Churchill Livingstone.

Kahn, J. (1993). *Mental Health and the Workplace. A Practical Psychiatric Guide*. New York: Van Nostrand Reinhold.

Kates, N., Grieffe, B. S., & Hagen, D. Q. (1990). In J. H. Gold, (Ed.), *The Psychosocial Impact of Job Loss*. Washington: American Psychiatric Press.

Kielhofner, G. (1980a). A Model of Human Occupation: Part I. Conceptual Framework and Content. *American Journal of Occupational Therapy, 34,* 572–581.

Kielhofner, G. (1980b). A Model of Human Occupation: Part II. Ontogenesis from the Perspective of Temporal Adaptation. *American Journal of Occupational Therapy, 34*(10), 657–663.

Koorland, M. A. (1986). Applied Behavior Analysis and the Correction of Learning Disabilities. In J. K. Torgesen, & B. Y. L. Wong, (Eds.), *Psychological and Educational Perspectives on Learning Disabilities*. San Diego, CA: Academic Press.

Licht, B. G., & Kistner, J. A. (1986). Motivational Problems of Learning Disabled Children: Individual Differences and the Implication for Treatment. In J. K. Torgesen, & B. Y. L. Wong, (Eds.), *Psychological and Educational Perspectivies on Learning Disabilities*. San Diego, CA: Academic Press.

McCallion, S. (1990). Sensory Integration. In J. Creek, (Ed.), *Occupational Therapy and Mental Health: Principles, Skills and Practice*. London: Churchill Livingstone.

McLean, A. A. (1974). *Occupational Stress*. Springfield, IL: Thomas.

McLean, A. A. (1993). Psychiatry and the Organization: A Brief History of Occupational Psychiatry. In G. Kahn, (Ed.), *Mental Health in the Workplace: A Practical Psychiatric Guide*. New York: Van Nostrand Reinhold.

Morrison, E. (1990). The History of the Profession. In J. Creek (Ed.), *Occupational Therapy and Mental Health: Principles, Skills, Practice*. London: Churchill Livingstone.

Osipow, S. H., & Spokane, A. R. (1987). *Occupational Stress Inventory*. Odessa, FL: Psychological Stress Resources.

Parkson, W., & Pendegrass, P. (1993). Rehabilitation in Schizophrenia: The Vocational Component. *Issues in Schizophrenia, 1*(3), 4–7 & 15.

Pearl, R., Donaghue, M., & Brian, T. (1986). Social Relationships of Learning Disabled Children. In J. K. Torgesen, & B. Y. L. Wong, (Eds.), *Psychological and Educational Perspectives on Learning Disabilities*. San Diego, CA: Academic Press.

Pelham, W. E. (1986). The Effects of Psychostimulant Drugs on Learning Academic Achievement in Children with Attention Deficit Disorders and Disabilities. In J. A. Torgesen, & B. Y. L. Wong (Eds.), *Psychological and Educational Perspectives on Learning Disabilities*. San Diego, CA: Academic Press.

Perry, D. G., & Bussey, K. (1984). *Social Development*. Englewood Cliffs, NJ: Prentice Hall.

Pritchard, C. (1992). Is There a Link between Suicide in Young Men and Unemployment? A Comparison of the U.K. with Other European Community Countries. *British Journal of Psychiatry, 160,* 750–756.

Revetz, C. (1988). Leisure. In M. Wilson, (Ed.), *Occupational Therapy in Short Term Psychiatry* (2nd ed.). London: Churchill Livingstone.

Ryan, E. B., Weed, K., & Short, E. J. (1986). Cognitive Behavioral Modification: Promoting Active Self-Regulatory Learning Styles. In J. K. Torgesen, & B. Y. L. Wong, (Eds.), *Psychological and Educational Perspectives on Learning Disabilities.* San Diego, CA: Academic Press.

Stockwell, R. (1988). Creative Therapies. In M. Wilson, (Ed.), *Occupational Therapy in Short Term Psychiatry* (2nd ed.). London: Churchill Livingstone.

Torgesen, J. K., & Wong, B. Y. L. (1986). *Psychological and Eduacational Perspectives on Learning Disabilities.* New York: Academic Press.

Wilson, M. (1987). *Occupational Therapy in Long Term Psychiatry* (2nd ed.). London: Churchill Livingstone.

Young, M. E., & Quinn, E. (1992). *Theories and Principles of Occupational Therapy.* London: Churchill Livingstone.

CHAPTER 12

THE SOCIAL SYSTEM

THE PERSPECTIVE

The social perspective is represented by several disciplines that include sociology, social work, social psychology, social psychiatry, and subfields of anthropology. All these fields place emphasis on the social context as an important determiner of individual and group behavior. An individual's social system includes a spouse, family, friends, neighbors, a community, a specific geographic area, and society. Since the marital and family systems are discussed in chapters nine and ten, this section will focus on the other social systems. According to this perspective, psychological distress, although experienced by the individual, is influenced by the social environment. Social factors are considered important in the onset, maintenance, outcome, and prevention of psychological distress and psychiatric disorders. The focus of study is on the quality of the individual's social environment and the interaction between the individual and the environment. Social factors such as the perceived availability of social support, social integration, community resources, sociodemographics, and social and cultural roles are all considered to influence an individual's psychological functioning.

In this perspective there is a shift in emphasis from individual factors such as intrapsychic dynamics, to the larger social environment. Interventions are aimed at changing the social environment, or changing how the individual interacts with the environment. Although several disciplines have discussed the effect of the social environment on human behavior, it is the field of social work that has given the greatest attention to this area. Social psychiatry has similarly placed significant emphasis on social factors in the understanding and treatment of psychiatric disorders. Sociology's focus has been on the impact of mental illness on society, the influence of society on mental illness, and the consequences of labeling "deviant" behavior. The relationship between illness and society is also explored in medical sociology. Social psychology studies the effects of attitudes and beliefs of groups on individual behavior, with emphasis given to "normal" behaviors, social norms, and rules that influence individual and group behavior. There is less emphasis given to clinical conditions and abnormal behavior, while more attention is paid to how social roles, gender roles, and sociocultural factors influence behavior. Other related fields such as developmental social psychology studies the development of friendships in children, and future adult social relationships.

This chapter will attend to the important social variables that effect psychological functioning. Attention given to this area early in treatment may have important implications for the course and outcome of a particular condition or diagnosis. It is therefore a very important area to consider in any treatment plan.

BRIEF HISTORY

The historical development of this perspective has its roots in several disciplines, making it difficult to trace a unifying theory. Therefore, I will discuss the development of this perspective through the fields of social work, sociology, social psychology, and social psychiatry.

The social work movement can be traced to the Middle Ages when the church assumed responsibility for taking care of the poor and disadvantaged. A Scottish minister, Thomas Chalmers, was able to obtain relief for the more disadvantaged by collecting contributions from wealthier parishioners. He is also credited with having developed the "casework methodology" used extensively in social work (Macht & Quam, 1986). In the late 1800s, more organized services developed to supply financial and material assistance to the poor, needy, and disadvantaged. One of the well-known organizations that offered this aid was the Charity Organization Society (COS) (Breakwell & Rowett, 1982). Many other services developed in the 1900s and two additional groups, hospitals and criminals, became part of the disadvantaged.

In the early 1930s state funding was provided for social workers. In 1948 with the passing of the Children's Act, social workers for the first time functioned autonomously, directing services offered by government agencies (Breakwell & Rowett, 1982). The movement to unify social workers into one federation developed in Britain in the late 1930s, which influenced a similar development in the United States. The emphasis on improving the social environment for children, the elderly, the poor, and the mentally ill was pioneered by the social work movement and continues to be the focus of this profession. Social worker involvement in multidisciplinary teams in hospitals, clinics, social agencies, government services, and many other organizations has provided a valuable input that has improved the quality of care given to many vulnerable individuals.

A discipline somewhat related to social work that also emphasizes the social environment, is the academic discipline of sociology. Sociology is the scientific study of society, its organization, structure, and influence on individual behavior (Singer & Fuhr, 1980). Sociology's historical roots can be traced to the two great revolutions in Europe. The impact of industrialization forced attention on social institutions that continued over two centuries (Giddens, 1987). The term "sociology" was coined by Auguste Comte in the mid-1800s. According to Comte the study of sociology is to seek universal laws governing human society by adopting the methods of natural science. This position was also adopted by Emile Durkheim, considered the most influential sociologist (Giddens, 1987).

As a social science, sociology covers human behavior with special attention paid to the individual's position in society, to social status, socioeconomic class, and other social variables. More recently sociology has focused on deviant behavior and mental disorders, and has offered intriguing yet controversial ideas on these topics (Cockerham, 1989). Medical sociology, a subfield of sociology, has also examined the importance of social factors in health and disease and is a rapidly growing area in the sociomedical field (Mechanic, 1978).

The two remaining fields that have contributed to this perspective are social psychiatry and social psychology. Social psychiatry is a recent discipline that has borrowed principles from sociology and has focused on the social influence on mental health. Social psychology, a subfield within academic psychology, studies social influences on behavior. It is also a relatively recent discipline developing formally in the 1950s with the introduction of attribution theory and other social psychology principles (Hilgard, Atkinson, & Atkinson, 1975). Therefore, some common roots are shared between certain disciplines, with all disciplines converging on the basic idea that social factors are significant in determining human behavior and psychological well-being.

BASIC PRINCIPLES

Trying to delineate the important principles advocated by the social perspective is difficult, because few if any resources are available that integrate the relevant concepts from the fields of social work, sociology, social psychiatry, and social psychology. These separate disciplines attend to different aspects of the social system and how it influences human behavior. Since the theme and basic purpose of this book is on formulating psychological and psychiatric disorders, only those concepts that offer a special perspective on the understanding and treatment of psychological problems will be presented. Although there are many intriguing theories and concepts represented by the disciplines under this perspective, only two will be highlighted within the context of formulation and treatment planning. These include the concept of social support, and sociodemographics and social roles. Greater emphasis will be given to the area of social support, as it has been extensively studied and is considered an important social variable in maintaining psychological health.

Social Support

The concept of social support and its relevance to mental health was first discussed in the 1970s (Caplan, 1974; Cassel, 1974; Cobb, 1976). Since then this area has flourished with numerous articles and books having been written on the topic. Caplan (1974) defined social support as an enduring pattern of social ties that have the potential to play a major role in ensuring that psychological and physical integrity are maintained in the individual. There have been many definitions of this concept, including the recent emphasis on the individual's *perception* of the availability of social support (Pierce, Sarason, & Sarason, 1991). A variety of terms have been used to define and measure social support. A "structural index" of social ties that includes marital status, close family and friends, and participation in group, church, and religious activities has been called social integration (SI) (Cohen, 1988) and has been one of the more common measures used in assessing social support.

The term social network has also been used in the literature, and has been described in structural and functional terms (Mitchell & Trickett, 1980). The structure refers to the size, density, and kinship components of the network. The functional characteristics have been called reciprocity, accessibility, homogeneity, multiplexity, and others. Network theory provides a conceptual model to understand how social support networks function. The concept of social network has been utilized to examine the social field an individual belongs to and includes the family, neighborhood, church or social organizations, self-help groups, and other organizations.

The first to use this term was Barnes (Mitchell & Trickett, 1980), a British social anthropologist who studied the social networks of a Norwegian fishing village. Since then several attempts to operationally define the term have been evident in the literature (Mitchell & Trickett, 1980; Wenger & Shahtahmasebi, 1991). Although differences exist, there are similarities with respect to the type of support social networks can provide. These can be divided into four types of support: emotional, instrumental, material, and informational.

Emotional support refers to the availability of others to provide comfort and reassurance during times of distress (Wenger & Shahtahmasebi, 1991; Coyne & Downey, 1991). Such support could be offered by a spouse, family member, friends, neighbors, or the community. Although a marriage may provide this when needed, those in unsatisfactory relationships may seek out others for emotional support when necessary. Whether a family member is contacted will depend on the relationship among family members. Despite close ties with parents and sibs, some individuals may find it difficult to confide in family members about certain issues. If a spouse or family is unavailable for support, then reliance on friends and the community increases. An individual with at least one friend to confide in who will furnish emotional support, may feel less isolated and alone during times of crisis. Those who have more than one confidant may be additionally protected, given the increased probability of available confidants. In addition to emotional support, individuals who are actively involved in social relationships and belong to a peer group, may experience a sense of belonging and develop a stronger social identity. The development of friendships and belonging to a peer group have been found to contribute significantly to children's self-esteem (Macoby, 1980) and may protect against the development of childhood psychiatric disorders (Links, 1987). Being a member of a social group that meets regularly, either through the community or through personal friendships, enhances an individual's perception that emotional support is available if needed.

Instrumental support refers to the availablity of individuals or services to supply assistance with a variety of duties and daily activities that individuals perform (Mitchell & Trickett, 1980; Wenger & Shahtahmasebi, 1991). Common examples include help with household chores, child care, car pooling, buying groceries, emergency transportation, and many others. Once again spouses and families (both nuclear and extended) can provide assistance and support in these areas. However, for single parents, unsupported spouses, and individuals separated by emotional or physical distance from their families, obtaining instrumental support may be difficult. Those who are financially secure may be able to obtain services through various community agencies or private businesses. Others may rely on neighbors and friends to help in certain situations when necessary. Neighbors can provide an instrumentally supportive network by sharing in tasks such as child care, grocery shopping, and transportation, and they can also provide emergency assistance in times of crisis. The perception that one's neighbors or friends are available, especially in an emergency, may contribute to a general sense of safety and security in the neighborhood. Community services may also give instrumental aid especially for those in need such as single parents, low socioeconomic groups, the elderly and disabled, and those with psychological and psychiatric difficulties. The importance of community groups to assist individuals with serious psychiatric disabilities such as schizophrenia has been discussed in the literature (Wasylenki, James, Clark, Lewis, Goering, & Gillies, 1992).

Material help is given by supplying products and financial assistance (Mitchell & Trickett, 1980; Wenger & Shahtahmasebi, 1991). This type of support is especially important to those in financial need who are unable to obtain these goods for themselves. Once again families may be availabe for this type of support, and if so, the individual may feel less anxious and afraid during financial crises, such as loss of employment that significantly affects financial resources. Outside of the family, there may be friends to turn to for material support in a crisis situation. Friends and neighbors may be more likely to offer food, clothing, and shelter, rather than financial aid. Outside of the immediate network are the social agencies such as welfare that provide financial assistance to the needy. Various community agencies such as the Salvation Army and other shelters donate material services for disadvantaged individuals for a brief period of time.

Informational support equips an individual with comfort through knowledge of available resources (Mitchell & Trickett, 1980; Wenger & Shahtahmasebi, 1991). Community resources and agencies disseminate information regarding the array of services available to the citizens. Neighbors may sometimes assist an individual with some of this information, although this knowledge may at times be limited. In any community one should be aware of the various support services available for the general public as well as specific services available for specific groups. General services include social clubs, shelters, social service agencies, and daycare. Specific services include self-help groups such as Friends of Schizophrenics, Families of Manic-Depressives, Incest Survivors, and Victims of Sexual Assault and Rape.

Having presented some of the different types of social support one can receive, it is important to consider two questions concerning this area: how does social support work?, and what determines a successful support experience?

How does social support work?

With respect to the first question, a variety of theories have been offered to explain how social support promotes health. In reviewing the existing literature, House, Landis & Uniberson (1988) conclude that despite past methodological difficulties, recent research indicates that the lack of social supportive relationships is a major risk factor for physical and psychological health. Two models have been proposed to explain this relationship: the buffering model and the main effect model (Cohen, 1988; Cohen & Wills, 1985; Cohen, Mermelstine, Kamarack & Hoberman, 1985; Rodin & Salovey, 1989; Cohen & Hoberman, 1983; Joseph, Williams, & Yule 1992; Wilcox, 1981). The buffering model, as the name implies, views social support as a "buffer" or protector during stressful life events. Therefore, social support is considered an important factor in promoting health during these stressful periods. The main effect model argues that social support has a constant effect on the individual's well-being, regardless of whether there are stressful life events. Therefore, social support is seen as having a constant effect on health, not just during periods of stress. Arguments have been presented in favor of each model. However, it is plausible that both models operate with social support buffering the individual during acute events, as well as maintaining support in between events.

Both models offer hypotheses regarding the mechanisms by which social support promotes health. According to the buffering hypothesis, support circumvents or prevents the biological and behavioral responses to stress that contribute to poor psychological and physical health. Biologically, this is believed to work because the neuroendocrine and immune systems dampen the neuroendocrine stress response and enhance immune function. Enhancement of immune functions in the presence of social support has been documented in primates and humans (Baron, Cutrona, Hicklin, Russell, & Lubaroff, 1990). Psychologically, the perception that social support is accessible may reduce the stress appraisal response and increase the individual's perception that they will be able to cope. This may decrease initial affective reactivity, increase problem-solving ability, and facilitate additional adaptive behaviors.

According to the main effect model, social support's influence on health is independent of stressful events. This model advocates that social support promotes social integration, one's perceived connected experience with a social group (Cohen, 1988). Social support promotes the experience of social integration by (1) providing the individual with a sense of identity, (2) enhancing self-esteem, (3) promoting healthy behaviors, (4) increasing access to social services (economic, informational, emotional), and (5) promoting a sense of well being, as a result of an increased sense of belonging and perception of control over the environment. Evidence for both models have been discussed in the literature (Cohen, 1988).

What determines a successful social support experience?

The second question addresses the determiners of a successful social support experience. Two factors contribute to whether social support will be effective: the availability and quality of social support, and the individual's capacity to access social support. Both are important factors that interact to produce a positive or negative social support experience. As mentioned earlier, spouses, families, friends, neighbors, community resources, and society are all potential support givers. The availability of any one of these, and the quality of the support offered will determine if support can be provided in a particular instance. Some supports such as neighborhood and community resources may not be available due to poor government funding, a factor not in the individual's control.

However, even if good support services exist an individual must be able to access them in order to experience their full benefits. Many individuals with serious psychiatric disabilities (e.g., schizophrenia), who are isolated as a result of poor social skills, fearfulness, or general apathy may be incapable of seeking help. Individuals without serious disabilities but who are not "social-seeking" may not consider social contacts for support. Instead they may rely on self-soothing capacities, or they may socially withdraw in order to cope. Therefore, an individual's propensity toward social support in times of stress, whether determined by individual disposition, personality style, coping style or social skills deficits, will heavily influence their ability to use social support in times of stress (Holahan & Moos; Souls & Fletcher, 1985). Helping individuals to access social supports has become part of the long-term treatment of chronic psychiatric disorders.

Sociodemographics/Social Roles

In addition to social support, sociodemographic factors have also been identified as playing an important role in psychological health. Sociodemographic factors and their influence on the prevalence, onset, and course of psychiatric disorders has been the focus of study of sociology and social psychiatry. The significant variables considered to have an important influence on mental disorders include social class, gender or sex roles, marital status, urban versus rural living, migration, and race (Cockerham, 1989; Henderson, 1988). Each of these will be briefly discussed below.

Socioeconomic class

Social class differences have been apparent in the prevalence of psychiatric disorders. Schizophrenia and personality disorders are more prevalent in the lower socioeconomic groups, while the mood and anxiety disorders show a higher prevalence in the middle and upper-middle socioeconomic groups (Henderson, 1988). Two hypotheses have been suggested to explain these differences. First, individuals in lower socioeconomic groups are viewed as more deprived and exposed to chronic levels of stress, making them more psychologically vulnerable. If an individual living in such an environment is also biologically vulnerable towards a particular disorder, the depriving environment will likely increase the chances of precipitating the disorder. Another explanation, referred to originally as the "downward drift hypothesis," states that individuals with schizophrenia or other serious psychiatric disorders move down into the lower socioeconomic groups as a result of their disabilities, impeding opportunities for successful employment and adaptive functioning in society. In schizophrenia, the early onset of the disorder prevents the individual from pursuing career and occupational opportunities. Because mood and anxiety disorders are regarded as less chronically disabling and have a later age of onset, they are less likely to interfere with successful social and occupational functioning (Cockerham, 1989).

Gender, social roles, and marital status

In addition to socioeconomic class, gender, social roles, and marital status are three sociodemographic variables that interact to influence mental health, and these will be discussed together. There are sex differences in the prevalence of psychiatric disorders, with mood and anxiety disorders being more common in women, and personality and substance abuse disorders being more frequent in men. No sex differences are evident in the incidence of schizophrenia (Henderson, 1988). Some have argued that sex roles have contributed to some of these gender differences in psychiatric disorders. Men and women are believed to have different social roles in society with women taking greater responsibilities for child care, household activities, and overall functioning of the home, while men have traditionally had the role of financial provider and have been less involved in the home. These roles have been challenged recently, as more women work outside the home, take more financial responsibility, and share in some of the more traditional male roles. Men have also been pressured to take on more of the household chores and child care activities, thereby sharing the traditional female role. However, despite some sharing of roles, women still tend to take care of 70% of the household and child care duties when both spouses work outside the home (Blumstein & Schwartz, 1983).

Despite some of these concerns, women who enjoy their careers seem to be the most psychologically adjusted (McLanaghan & Glass, 1985; Cockerham, 1989). These findings and others have pointed to the increased burden faced by many women who occupy several roles: wife, mother, and career woman. Occupying all these roles simultaneously has been equated with having two full-time jobs. The added stress has been implicated in the higher depressive and anxiety symptoms observed in women. A woman's risk for these disorders is thought to increase if she is unable to confide in her spouse, or does not have at least one supportive relationship (Beach, Sandeen & O'Leary, 1990; Rutter, 1985). Marriage has also been regarded as more protective for men than for women with respect to depressive disorders (Beggington, 1987). A single mother living with more than two young children in a low socioeconomic environment is believed to be at higher risk for emotional disorders (Brown & Harris, 1978; Cockerham, 1989). For those women who remain at home and whose social role is that of mother and caretaker, an increased risk of depression is noted when the last child leaves home. Loss of the maternal role may lead to a loss of identity, sense of purpose, and feelings of emptiness and depression (Cockerham, 1989).

The social roles or expectations placed on men also make them vulnerable to certain conditions. The socialization process that makes it unacceptable for men to freely express their feelings may explain why they are less likely to visit a professional for affective symptoms such as depression or anxiety (Henderson, 1988). Even though men may experience these symptoms they may be more likely to drink alcohol or use other substances to treat themselves. Their social role and socialization history may make it difficult for them to acknowledge psychological symptoms, considered part of a "weak" constitution. Men are also known to have more recreationally or socially based relationships rather than confiding-supportive relationships, except with their spouses. Men may therefore be less likely to seek social support, and more likely to deal with their difficulties themselves, possibly increasing the chance of alcohol or other substance abuse.

Urban versus rural living

The third sociodemographic factor examines the social environment where the individual lives. Differences have been noted in the prevalence of certain psychiatric disorders with schizophrenia, anxiety, and personality disorders more prevalent in urban settings, and mood disorders more prevalent in rural settings (Henderson, 1988; Cockerham, 1989). Prescribing tranquillizers in rural settings is double that of urban settings. Some have referred to a "rural malaise," a general apathy evident in this population as a result of low economic opportunities, low social stimulation, and isolation (Cockerham, 1989). Urban living on the other hand, although offering better socioeconomic, cultural, and social opportunties, has its own problems with pollution, crime, and overcrowded housing; stressors that are not experienced by rural dwellers. It is unlikely that the rural versus urban distinction itself influences health, but rather the individual's satisfaction with their living arrangements. There are many variables that influence satisfaction with living arrangements that need to be considered. For example, Gove, Hughes, & Galle (1979) found that overcrowding in the neighborhood was not as important as overcrowding in the home, and this was more important for women (Booth & Edwards, 1976; Cockerham, 1989). Therefore, how individuals experience their living environment is probably more important than the appearance of their living arrangements.

Immigration

The fourth sociodemographic factor important to consider is immigration, which is especially important in cities that have a high immigrant population. Immigration can have positive and negative effects depending on the circumstances and reasons for immigration (Cockerham, 1989). Those individuals leaving a country where there is intense sociopolitical conflict, war, poor living conditions, and few economic opportunities may experience positive effects from immigrating to a country that is free of such adverse conditions. Despite the positive influences, immigration is still stressful, leading to feelings of social isolation, loss of identity, poor social integration and assimilation, role change, cultural conflicts and language difficulties. Negative immigration effects can be ameliorated if these individuals are connected with similar ethnic social organizations. Because individuals who have recently immigrated have also left their extended families, they may be in need of support from these services.

Race: culture

The final sociodemographic factor to be discussed is that of race and culture. Although there is no support for racial differences in the incidence of mental disorders, an individual's race or cultural background is important because it can influence affective expression, comfort with psychological distress, health seeking behavior, and feelings of stigmatization. For example, in some cultures it may be acceptable to cry when one is feeling depressed and to seek professional help for psychological problems. Other cultures may have unspoken prohibitions against the open expression of certain affects, and may believe seeking professional help for psychological problems is unneccessary and indicative of weakness or failure. Other cultures may rely on spiritual beliefs or folklore to deal with physical and psychological problems and may be more uncomfortable with mental health professionals. These must be taken into account when treating individuals from different cultural backgrounds.

Depression, anxiety, schizophrenia, and other disorders occur in individuals from a wide range of ethnic backgrounds. Culturally based attitudes towards mental health professionals will influence the development of a therapeutic alliance and compliance with treatment. Clinicians who are aware of and sensitive to these issues may be more likely to obtain a good therapeutic alliance with patients from diverse cultural backgrounds, increasing the chance of a successful treatment outcome.

ASSESSMENT

Assessment within the social perspective involves assessing the social supports available to the individual and the important sociodemographic factors that influence psychological well-being. A careful clinical assessment can identify the quality, accessibility, and perceived availability of a variety of social supports. First, the quality of the marital and family relationships can be assessed with respect to their ability to provide social support. Assessment of these two systems is discussed in chapters nine and ten and will not be discussed here. Other potential supports that should be assessed are friends, neighbors, and the community.

The assessment can begin with an evaluation of the individual's immediate social circle, including the number of friends available for recreational and social activities as well as confiding relationships. The presence of at least one confidant with whom the individual can share a more intimate relationship is important to note. If there are no friends or confidants, the individual's social skills and capacity to access social contacts need to be assessed. Shyness, social phobia, introversion, and extreme sensitivity to rejection can inhibit social-seeking behaviors. Socially disabling conditions such as schizophrenia can severely affect the development of social skills as well as impair the individual's capacity to consider the context when interpreting social situations. These individual factors determine one's ability to access social support and are very important to assess so that treatment can focus on improving these areas.

The second area to assess is the individual's immediate surroundings, specifically this involves assessing the quality of the living conditions, neighborhood, housing, and supportive capacity of the neighbors. Is there a sense of safety and security one feels at home? Can neighbors be called upon during times of crisis? Are other mothers available to talk to about child care and community resources? The individual's perception of the availability of neighborhood support and the actual quality of that support is important to assess. If very little support has been obtained through this system and other supports (family or spouse) are deficient, then interventions aimed at improving the supportive capacity of this network may be important to consider in treatment.

The final area to assess is the community resources available to an individual. Social workers are probably the most knowledgeable about this area, psychiatrists and psychologists the least. Community support groups are especially important for individuals (and their families) suffering from major psychiatric disorders. Several community resources have been developed for certain diagnostic groups such as schizophrenia, bipolar disorders, anxiety disorders and others. Support groups and self-help groups may also be available for other psychological conditions, and the availability of these services, as well as the individual's utilization of them should be assessed. In addition to therapeutically oriented groups, social groups or organizations in the community for immigrants, singles, and other individuals who feel isolated may be important to ascertain so that these individuals can be directed to these support networks if it is appropriate.

The assessment of the individual's social support network, and their own individual capacity to access and utilize this network is important because these systems can sometimes provide the necessary support that may decrease the need for mental health professionals. Their buffering effects and influence on the outcome of many psychological conditions/ disorders cannot be overemphasized.

In addition to clinical assessment several assessment instruments have been developed to assess social support. Some of these are the People in Your Life Scale (Marziali, 1987), the Social Adjustment Scale (Weissman & Bothwell, 1976), the Social Support Questionnaire (Sarason, Levine, Bashum, & Sarason, 1983), the Social Provisions Scale (Cutrona & Russell, 1987) and the Interpersonal Support Evaluation List (Cohen & Wills, 1985).

THE FOUR PS

Table 12.1 presents the four Ps important to the social perspective. Significant ***predisposing*** social factors that make an individual vulnerable to a psychological or psychiatric condition include low socioeconomic conditions, social or geographic isolation, poor neighborhood conditions, unavailability of a spouse or family, few friends, and a poor social support network. An individual may be predisposed toward social isolation if they have poor social skills, suffer from social anxiety, and are generally mistrustful about others' social support giving capabilities. There is an interaction between the individual and the social environment that determines overall social vulnerability. Those who have limited social supports and difficulty accessing them when needed are the most vulnerable during times of stress.

Precipitating social factors are acute events that change the individuals' social support network or social role in society, making them more psychologically vulnerable. Significant social precipitants that affect the availability of social support include loss of a spouse through death, separation or divorce, loss of family support, loss of a close friend or friends, geographical relocation, loss of community supports through withdrawal of government funding, changes in neighborhood support, changes in schools, and any other changes in the structure or availability of an existing social support network that was buffering the individual, or at least had the potential to do this in times of stress. Precipitating events that can affect one's social role in society include a change in socioeconomic class as a result of financial losses, change in role as spouse, parent, or companion, or change in position in society as a result of immigration, race, or culture. These precipitants are viewed as having a negative effect on the individual, in that it places the individual in a less

Table 12.1
Social System

Predisposing	* low socioeconomic living conditions * social or geographic isolation * poor neighborhood conditions * unavailability of spouse, family, friends * poor social skills * individual psychopathology * race, culture, immigration
Precipitating	*Events that change availability of social support –loss of spouse (death, separation, divorce) –loss of family –loss of friends –loss of support network (moves, etc.) *Change in social role –change in socioeconomic class –change in role as parent, spouse, –change in position in society (immigration, etc.)
Perpetuating	* chronic social isolation * poor living conditions * poverty * frequent moves * chronic social skills deficits * chronic social anxiety
Protective	*strong available social support via –spouse, family –friends –neighbors –community * good social skills * stable social role, socioeconomic class

favorable social role in society, making him or her more vulnerable to experiences of low self-esteem, and other psychological symptoms.

Perpetuating social factors can be important in maintaining psychological distress or preventing therapies or treatments from being effective. Chronic marital and family stress were already discussed as important perpetuating factors that can maintain distressing psychological symptoms. Chronic social isolation, difficult living situations, poverty, chronic lack of community resources, and frequent moves are all significant perpetuating social factors that can affect an individual's psychological well being. Other factors are chronic physical disabilities, social skills deficits, and social anxiety that prevent an individual from accessing social support, thereby perpetuating social isolation.

Protective social factors buffer the individual during stressful times by providing social support. Some of these protective factors include a supportive spouse and family, availability of friends and confidants, helpful and supportive neighbors, safe and secure neighborhoods, and involvement in community support groups. In many cases it may be the *perception of availability* and not the actual involvement in social support networks that is protective. There may be a main protective effect provided by the knowledge that support is available if needed. For individuals with psychological and psychiatric disorders community offered programs may offer some protection by promoting health and well being through a variety of measures. Some individual social factors can also be protective in that they increase the chance of the individual receiving social support. These include physical attractiveness, extroversion, good social skills, and good listening and empathic skills. All these factors make an individual more attractive to others, thereby increasing the frequency of social contact and increasing the probability of receiving social support when needed.

Sociodemographic factors that can be seen as protective include higher socioeconomic class, racial or cultural privileges, marital status, good living conditions, and satisfaction with existing social roles.

COPING-RESPONSE STYLE

An individual with a socially oriented coping-response style can be described as someone who seeks social contact during times of stress. The ability to confide in someone during these times may have beneficial effects on the individual. They may see a friend, a spouse, a family member, a support group, or a mental health professional for help. They could be described as having a coping-response style that is socially oriented, in that a social relationship is sought after and utilized to lessen the experience of distress. If there has been a recent loss of a significant supportive figure or network, the individual may be more vulnerable and more likely to seek professional help.

Tapping this coping-response style may be helpful when planning treatment. These individuals will probably respond to a variety of forms of therapy that involve a therapeutic relationship including individual and group therapy, as long as therapy provides some "supportive function." Because the support is experienced through a relationship these individuals may be less motivated to use self-help books or other individual self-directed methods of treatment that do not involve a supportive relationship.

For those individuals who rarely seek social support during difficult times, therapy could help them overcome barriers to accessing social support, so that they too can benefit from its effects. Therefore, having a social support network and a coping-response style that readily accesses these resources is adaptive for the individual and should therefore be reinforced in therapy.

TREATMENT

The focus of treatment according to this perspective is based on the theory that social support has beneficial effects on mental health. The goal is to attend to individual factors limiting access to social support and to improve existing resources that provide social support.

Enhancing Individual Access to Social Support: Social Skills Training

Individual therapy can help remove the intrapsychic, cognitive, and behavioral barriers to accessing social support. Individual factors such as shyness, introversion, social phobia, and fear of relationships may all be treated by individual therapy. Psychodynamic therapy may help the individual deal with a variety of conflicts, defenses, and relational patterns that act as barriers to accessing and utilizing social supports. Behavioral and cognitive-behavioral therapists focus on avoidance behaviors and skills deficits and use various techniques such as exposure and skills training to decrease anxiety, and specifically performance anxiety associated with social contact. The major focus of treatment is to improve an individual's ability to access social support.

Social skills are usually learned in childhood and adolescence through a variety of processes that include teaching and modeling by parents and teachers and reinforcement and punishment by peers. These same principles that contribute to the natural development of social skills have been used in social skills training groups. Modeling, behavioral rehearsal, and social reinforcement are the three most common techniques used in social skills training groups (Becker, Heinberg, & Bellack, 1987). Most social skills groups involve specific diagnostic groups (e.g., schizophrenia, depression) or individuals with a similar problem (shyness). The format of the group and the specific skills focused on will differ depending on the specific deficits that are identified. Most social skills groups conduct an assessment prior to instituting treatment so that specific social skills assets and deficits can be identified. Following the assessment, specific skills will be targeted based on the assessment.

If significant deficits exist in initiating and maintaining any social interaction, then attention will be focused on this area. Three different sets of skills are taught that are considered essential in order to carry out effective social interactions: receiving skills, processing skills, and sending skills (Becker et at., 1987). The first skill requires attending to the social environment and social context and reading interpersonal cues. This skill is significantly impaired in individuals with a diagnosis of schizophrenia. This difficulty of interpreting social contextual cues has been explained by the information processing deficit associated with this disorder (Dawson, Munroe-Blum, & Bartolucci, 1983). Social skills training with this group involves teaching methods of attending to the social context, with specific attention given to identifying social cues (Lieberman, Neucaterline, & Wallis, 1982). Social skills training programs have also helped children and adolescents with behavioral disorders to form better social relationships with their peers (Zaragosa, Vaugh, & MacIntosh, 1991; Mathur & Rutherford, 1991).

Processing skills involve problem-solving and being able to select the most appropriate skill for the situation. Different situations, and the desire for different outcomes call upon different problem-solving skills. Individuals with a schizophrenic illness may also be hampered in this area because of their inability to process, organize, and select alternative skills in different situtations. Some individuals with a diagnosis of personality disorder may also have deficits in this area due to a rigid limited behavioral repertoire in social situtations. Those who suffer from excessive shyness or social anxiety may be able to interpret social cues, but may have limited problem-solving abilities and a limited repertoire of skills to select from as a result of anxiety induced behavioral inhibition that prevents these individuals from engaging in social behaviors.

The final set of skills are the "sending skills." This refers to the verbal and nonverbal behaviors of social communication. Focusing on content is just as important as how the message is sent. Individuals with deficits in this area can be taught these skills through modeling, role playing and practicing.

Many of these skills are necessary to some degree in order for one to develop a social network. These skills increase the chances that an individual will be able to access the available social supports. Those deficient in these skills may have greater difficulty developing a social support network, thereby increasing the chance that they are socially isolated and vulnerable during stressful periods.

Availability of Social Support

Once an individual is able to access social supports, the next issue concerns the availability of social support networks. There has been an increase in the number and variety of social support groups available in the community. Most of these groups have become specialized, and are aimed at specific populations. Support groups exist for individuals with certain disorders such as schizophrenia, bipolar disorder, phobias, panic disorders and nonpsychiatric medical conditions such as cancer, AIDS, multiple sclerosis, and many others (Sauer & Coward, 1985; Stevens, 1992; Wasylenki et al., 1992; Leserman, Perkons, & Evans, 1992). Individuals identified with specific conditions should be informed of available support groups in the community.

In addition to diagnostic groups, support groups or group therapy is available for individuals who share common traumatic life events. Groups have been developed for survivors of incest, sexual assault and rape victims, recent widows or widowers, and separated and divorced individuals. These groups can often provide significant support to individuals by means of (1) a social tie to combat feelings of loneliness and isolation, (2) a safe place to vent feelings and develop coping strategies, and (3) a place to normalize reactions or feelings related to the specific issue (Rodin & Salovey, 1989; Sauer & Coward, 1985). Support groups provide the individual with a personal experience of being part of a community, and decrease any isolation effects that may have been caused by their negative experiences (Cohen, 1988).

The experience of seeing others with similar emotional responses to a similar event, can be very comforting, and can provide not just support but a place to work through many unexpressed feelings and individual issues. Individual therapy in combination with active participation in a support group may be a superior treatment to either therapy alone. Alternatively, a group experience may be sufficient and superior to individual therapy, particularly if the active ingredient of change or therapeutic impact comes from being in the presence of others who are perceived to truly understand the psychological effects of a particular significant event. How groups and group therapy affect individual change has been described by Yalom (1985) and others (Sampson & Marthas, 1981), and these principles can be applied to many group experiences.

In addition to locating groups for the "identified patient," it is important to remember significant others that live with the patients, or are at least in frequent contact with them. This includes spouses, children, extended families, and friends. How individuals perceive their significant others, and how these significant others react to the individuals and their condition may have an important effect on course and recovery, which has become especially evident in the major psychiatric disorders where the family's reaction to the patient's illness or condition is considered important in preventing relapse and admission to hospital (Keitner & Miller, 1990; Goering, Lance, & Freeman, 1992; Strachan, 1986). In addition, family members and close friends experience their own distress in reaction to their friend's or family member's illness. They are some times confused as to "what to do" and "how to react," so as not to worsen the situation. Family members may feel guilty or angry about the illness, and may express these feelings indirectly in more destructive ways to the patient.

As a result of these factors several support groups have been developed for families and friends who live with or have frequent contact with someone suffering from a major psychiatric disorder or psychological condition. Examples of existing groups that have successfully provided support to families and friends include Families of Schizophrenics, Friends of Schizophrenics, Families of Manic-Depressives, Al-Anon, and many others. Information regarding the availability of such groups should be given to family and friends of patients even when not requested or perceived as needed at the time of initial presentation. During the initial phases of assessment and treatment families and friends may deny the illness, making it difficult for them to access support groups. Only after the diagnosis has been accepted will family members be more receptive to such options.

In summary, support groups can be extremely useful in the treatment of many psychological conditions. Therefore, it is important to remain informed of such services in the community. Their preventative and therapeutic effects can contribute greatly to the outcome of many disorders. Group treatments are also cost effective in that the ratio of patient to therapist is higher than individual therapy, and in many cases paraprofessionals and volunteers can be trained to conduct such groups. The availability of better resources may also decrease the use of mental health services. If cost effective and therapeutically effective support groups can provide the first line of treatment, this can circumvent the need for mental health professionals, freeing them to offer services to those who are unable to use support groups.

SUMMARY

Social factors are important in the onset, course, and maintenance of psychiatric and psychological disorders. Adopting a social perspective forces one to consider some of the important variables that influence general psychological well-being. Although spouses and families are the first line of potential support givers, friends, neighbors, and a variety of community resources can also be considered as part of the wider social support network. In some cases this latter group may be the only available source of support. Helping individuals access these resources is an important component of a comprehensive treatment plan. In addition to considering an individual's social support network, sociodemographic factors and social roles are additional variables that can influence the development and course of a variety of psychological problems. Individual and group therapies that strengthen social support networks, encourage role flexibility, and buffer against adverse sociodemographic conditions may have a significant effect on the short- and long-term outcome of psychiatric and psychological disturbances.

REFERENCES

Baron, R. S., Cutrona, C. E., Hicklin, D., Russell, D. W., & Lubaroff, D. M. (1990). Social Support and Immune Function Among Spouses of Cancer Patients. *Journal of Personality and Social Psychology, 59,* 344–352.

Beach, S. R. H., Sandeen, E., & O'Leary, D. K. (1990). *Depression in Marriage.* New York: Guilford Press.

Bebbington, P. E. (1987). Marital Status and Depression: A Study of English National Admission Statistics. *Acta Psychiatria Scandinavica, 75,* 640–650.

Becker, R. E., Heinberg, R. G., & Bellack, A. S. (1987). *Social Skills Training Treatment for Depression.* New York: Pergamon Press.

Blumstein, P., & Schwartz, P. (1983). *American Couples.* New York: Simon and Schuster.

Booth, A., & Edwards, J. (1976). Crowding and Family Relations. *American Psychological Review, 41,* 308–321.

Breakwell, G. M., & Rowett, C. (1982). *Social Work: A Social Psychological Approach.* United Kingdom: Van Nostrand Reinhold.

Brown, G. N., & Harris, T. (1978). *Social Origins of Depression.* London: Tavistock.

Caplan, G. (1974). *Support Systems and Community Mental Health.* New York: Behavioral Publications.

Cassel, J. (1974). Psychosocial Processes and Stress: Theoretical Formulation. *International Journal of Health Services, 4,* 471–482.

Cobb, S. (1976). Social Support as a Moderator of Life Stress. *Psychosomatic Medicine, 38,* 300–314.

Cockerham, W. C. (1989). *Sociology of Mental Disorders,* (2nd ed.). Englewood Cliffs, NJ: Prentice Hall.

Cohen, S. (1988). Psychosocial Models and the Role of Social Support in the Etiology of Physical Disease. *Health Psychology, 7,* 269–297.

Cohen, S., & Wills, T. A. (1985). Stress, Social Support, and the Buffering Hypothesis. *Psychological Bulletin, 98,* 310–357.

Cohen, S., Mermelstine, R., Kamarck, T., & Hoberman, H. (1985). Measuring the Functional Components of Social Support. In I. G. Sarason & B. R. Sarason, (Eds.), *Social Support: Theory, Research and Applications.* The Netherlands: Dordrecht.

Cohen, S., & Hoberman, H. M. (1983). Cognitive Events and Social Supports as Buffers of Life Change Stress. *Journal of Applied Social Psychology, 13,* 99–125

Coyne, J. C., & Downey, G. (1991). Social Factors in Psychopathology: Stress, Social Support and the Coping Process. *Annual Review of Psychology, 42,* 421–425.

Cutrona, C. E., & Russell, D. (1987). The Provisions of Social Relationships and Adaptating to Stress. In W. H. Jones, & D. Perlman, (Eds.), *Advances in Personal Relationships.* Vol. 1, Greenwich, CT: JAI Press.

Dawson, D., Munroe-Blum, H., & Bartolucci, G. (1983). *Schizophrenia in Focus. Guidelines for Treatment and Rehabilitation.* New York: Human Science Press.

Giddens, A. (1987). *Sociology. A Brief but Critical Introduction,* (2nd ed.). New York: Harcourt Brace Jovanovich.

Goering, P. N., Lance, W. J. & Freeman, S. J. J. (1992). Marital Support and Recovery in Depression. *British Journal of Psychiatry, 160,* 76–82.

Gove, W. R., Hughes, M., & Galle, O. R. (1979). Overcrowding in the Home: An Empirical Investigation of Its Possible Psychological Consequences. *American Sociological Review, 44,* 59–80.

Henderson, A. S. (1988). *An Introduction to Social Psychiatry.* Oxford: Oxford University Press.

Hilgard, E. R., Atkinson, R. C., & Atkinson, R. L. (1975). *Introduction to Psychology,* (6th ed.) New York: Harcourt Brace Jovanovich.

Holahan, C. J., & Moos, R. H. (1990). Life Stressors, Resistance Factors, and Improved Psychological Functioning. An Extension of the Stress Resistance Paradigm. *Journal of Personality and Social Psychology, 58,* 909–917.

House, J. A., Landis, C., & Uniberson, D. (1988). Social Relationships in Health. *Science, 241,* 540–545.

Joseph, S., Williams, R., & Yule, W. (1992). Crisis Support, Attributional Style, Coping Style and Post-Traumatic Symptoms. *Personality and Individual Differences, 13,* 1249–1251.

Keitner, G. I., & Miller, I. W. (1990). Family Functioning and Major Depression: An Overview. *American Journal of Psychiatry, 147*(9), 1128–1137.

Leserman, J., Perkons, D. O., & Evans, D. L. (1992). Coping with the Threat of

AIDS. The Role of Social Support. *The American Journal of Psychiatry, 149,* 1514–1520.

Lieberman, R. P., Neucaterline, K. H., & Wallis, C. J. (1982). Social Skills Training and the Nature of Schizophrenia. In J. P. Curin & P. M. Montei, (Eds.), *Social Skills Training: A Practical Handbook for Assessment and Treatment.* New York: University Press.

Links, P. S. (1987). *Social Supports and Child Psychiatric Disorders.* Unpublished Master of Science Thesis for Design Measurement and Evaluation, McMaster University, Hamilton, Ontario.

Macht, M., & Quam, J. (1986). *Social Work: An Introduction.* Columbus, OH: Merrill Publishing.

Macoby, E. E. (1980). *Social Development: Psychological Growth and the Parent Child Relationship.* New York: Harcourt Brace Jovanovich.

Marziali, E. A. (1987). People in Your Life: Development of a Social Support Measure for Predicting Psychotherapy Outcome. *The Journal of Mental and Nervous Disease, 175,* 327–338.

Mathur, S. R., & Rutherford, R. B. (1991). Peer Mediated Interventions Promoting Social Skills of Children and Youth Behavioral Disorders. *Education and Treatment of Children, 14,* 227–242.

McLanaghan, S. S., & Glass, J. L. (1985). A note on the trend in Sex Differences in Psychological Distress. *Journal of Health and Social Behavior, 26,* 328–336.

Mechanic, D. (1978). *Medical Sociology: A Comprehensive Text,* (2nd ed.). New York: Free Press.

Mitchell, R. E., & Trickett, E. J. (1980). Task Force Report: Social Networks as Mediators of Social Support. An Analysis of the Effects and Determinants of Social Networks. *Community Mental Health Journal, 161*(1), 27–44.

Pierce, G. R., Sarason, I. G., & Sarason, B. R. (1991). General and Relationship Based Perceptions of Social Support: Are Two Constructs Better than One. *Journal of Personality and Social Psychology, 61,* 1028–1039.

Rodin, J., & Salovey, P. (1989). Health Psychology. *Annual Review of Psychology, 40,* 533–579.

Rutter, M. (1985). Resilience in the Face of Adversity. Protective Factors and Resistance to Psychiatric Disorder. *British Journal of Psychiatry, 147,* 598–611.

Sampson, E. E., & Marthas, M. (1981). *Group Process for the Health Professions,* (2nd ed.). New York: John Wiley and Sons.

Sarason, I. G., Levine, H. M., Bashum, R. B., & Sarason, B. R. (1983). Assessing Social Support: The Social Support Questionnaire. *Journal of Personality and Social Psychology, 44,* 127–139.

Sauer, W. J., & Coward, R. T. (1985). The Role of Social Support Networks in the Care of the Elderly. In W. Sauer & R. T. Coward (Eds.), *Social Support Networks in the Care of the Elderly.* New York: Springer Publishing.

Singer, L., & Fuhr, M. (1980). *Sociology: A Student's Introduction.* Washington, DC: University Press of America.

Souls, J., & Fletcher, B. (1985). The Relative Efficacy of Avoidant and Non-

Avoidant Coping Strategies: A meta Analysis. *Health Psychology, 4*(3), 249–288.

Stevens, E. S. (1992). Reciprocity and Social Support: An Advantage for the Aging Family. *Families in Society: The Journal of Contemporary Human Services, Nov,* 533–541.

Strachan, A. (1986). Family Intervention for Rehabilitation of Schizophrenia: Toward Protecting and Coping. *Schizophrenia Bulletin, 12,* 678–698.

Wasylenki, D., James, S., Clark, K., Lewis, J., Goering, P., & Gillies, L. (1992). Clinical Care Update. Clinical Issues in Social Network Therapy for Clients of Schizophrenia. *Community Mental Health Journal, 28,* 427–440.

Weissman, M. M., & Bothwell, S. (1976). Assessment of Social Adjustment by Patient Self-Report. *Archives of General Psychiatry, 36,* 1011–1015.

Wenger, G. C., & Shahtahmasebi, S. (1991). Survivors: Support Network Variation and Sources of Help in Rural Communities. *Journal of Cross Cultural Gerontology, 6,* 41–82.

Wilcox, B. L. (1981). Social Support, Life Stress, and Psychological Adjustment. Test of the Buffering Hypothesis. *American Journal of Community Psychology, 9,* 371–386.

Yalom, I. D. (1985). *The Theory and Practice of Group Psychotherapy,* (3rd ed.). New York: Basic Books.

Zaragoza, N., Vaughn, S., & MacIntosh, R. (1991). Social Skills Intervention, and Children with Behavior Problems: A Review. *Behavioral Disorders, 16,* 260–275.

CHAPTER 13

CASE ILLUSTRATION

In order to illustrate the application of the multiperspective model, a case will be presented that was assessed, formulated, and treated according to this model. The patient's name and various demographic information have been changed to maintain anonymity.

CASE PRESENTATION

Susan is an 18-year-old, single, attractive young female, who presented with a two-year history of daily vomiting. The vomiting occurred mainly when she was away from home, and was associated with anxiety symptoms that included palpitations, sweaty palms, dizziness, shortness of breath, and nausea. Most of these symptoms came on suddenly in new social situations and when she was out of the house by herself; they were least likely to occur at home. At the time of presentation she was vomiting 2–3 times a day and was avoiding almost all outside activities except her part-time work located close to her home. Her main fear was that she would vomit in public and embarrass herself. Several episodes of vomiting in public had left her feeling "devastated," and had resulted in her running home. These events led her to avoid large social gatherings and increased the time she spent with her mother and boyfriend.

There were no associated symptoms of depression or substance abuse, and there was no indication that she had an eating disorder. She had been medically investigated extensively for her symptoms with negative results. After much discussion the consulting physician had recommended a psychiatric consultation which Susan initially rejected. However, as her symptoms continued she initiated the referral herself, feeling that it was her last chance to "get rid of the vomiting."

She had been prescribed an anxiolytic by her family physician, which she found marginally effective and rarely took due to her dislike of medications. At the time of presentation she complained that she was "at the end of her rope," and was willing "to do anything" to improve her symptoms. On her own initiative she had begun to take walks by herself and had engaged in an exercise program, hoping that it might distract her from her symptoms. She had on occasion received some relief because of these activities, but the effects were not long lasting and they did not generalize to other situations.

Significant events surrounding the onset of her symptoms include the termination of a two year relationship with a married man that she had kept secret from her family. Her attraction to this man was to some extent based on the intense interest he showed in her, something she said she had never really experienced. His excitement in her, excited her, and she found this very hard to give up. She noticed the beginning of gastrointestinal problems such as stomachaches and nausea just prior to the breakup of this relationship. During this period she had experienced a great deal of distress, being overwhelmed by feelings of guilt and ambivalence over her affair with the married man. Although she refrained from intercourse, she was sexually intimate with this man. She described feeling very uncomfortable with any form of sexual intimacy except for kissing, but tolerated it for him. She did not see any connection between the onset of her symptoms and this past relationship. As far as she was concerned it was in the past and she had "gotten over" the entire ordeal.

At the time of presentation she was living with her parents, and working part-time as a cashier, a job she found unstimulating but maintained as a result of a supportive employer. She had no career aspirations and felt lost with respect to any future plans. Her parents were also described as supportive, although the support came mainly from her mother who took care of her when she returned home after her episodes of vomiting. Her father worked in a retail business and her mother was a homemaker. She described spending very little time with her father and a significant amount of time with her mother who was her most frequent companion. Mother and daughter seemed to spend more time together than mother and father. She acknowledged chronic marital tension between her parents, and described father as being distant from the rest of the family. Her older sister was married with two children and lived close to the family. Her brother had recently moved out of the home to live with his girlfriend, an action that had ostracized him from the rest of the family.

At the time of presentation she was involved in a relationship with a young man, who lived close to her. This relationship had begun almost immediately after she had terminated the affair with the married man. This current boyfriend, who worked in the same business as her father, was described as supportive and understanding, especially concerning her vomiting. He was always willing to take her home whenever she had an "attack" when they were out together. She described this as a good relationship with no major difficulties except for "occasional" sexual problems that she did not wish to discuss in the initial assessment. In the second assessment session, she did admit to feeling bored at times in the relationship. Socially her life was very limited. She had only two girlfriends she described as acquaintances with whom she spent very little time. She did not have any close friends in whom she could confide, and described her mother as being her best friend.

Although she did not have a formal psychiatric history, she did endorse symptoms of separation anxiety and school refusal when she first went to kindergarten. Family history revealed no psychiatric admissions or contact with mental health professionals; however mother showed evidence of long standing agoraphobia of a mild-to-moderate degree, evident by her need for a companion whenever she left the home. Her father suffered from multiple somatic complaints that included stomachaches, headaches, and backaches.

Despite few memories of her childhood, Susan described this as a basically "happy" time. She did remember her mother taking care of her when she was ill, but had no memories of any special moments or experiences with her father. She had always felt that her father was uninterested in her and in the family. Her memories of him were that he was always busy in the garage or somewhere outside of the house, returning only at mealtimes and in the evenings to sleep. As she got older she became more involved in helping her mother with the household duties. Much of this helping behavior was motivated by pity that her mother was neglected by her husband.

Socially, Susan maintained friendships as a child and as an adolescent, but did not have any significant confiding, intimate relationships. She had boyfriends from late adolescence, although none of these relationships were described as emotionally significant. She had always felt uncomfortable sexually, and had not been sexually active until her relationship with the married man.

With respect to her school performance, she describes performing in the average range. She felt she could have worked harder to improve her grades, but never felt motivated to do so. She had considered a career as a nurse or veterinarian, but had never seriously pursued either of these occupations. Following the completion of grade 12, she worked in a variety of clerical jobs, purely for financial reasons. Her lack of motivation and uncertainty about the future had made it difficult for her to pursue any career plans, something she continued to struggle with.

ASSESSMENT

The information presented above was obtained in the first two sessions. Additional assessments were carried out to obtain a complete picture of the vomiting behavior. In between the two sessions Susan was instructed to keep a record of her vomiting, and her anxiety symptoms, and any thoughts and feelings associated with her vomiting. A family assessment was recommended; however, she rejected the idea, stating that she did not wish to have her family involved. In order to respect her wishes for autonomy (considered important early in therapy), a tentative family assessment was made based on the information obtained in the individual session. This was sufficient to arrive at a formulation.

DIAGNOSIS

Based on the initial assessment the patient received a DSM-III-R diagnosis of: Axis I: panic disorder with agoraphobia-moderate.

FORMULATION

The initial assessment provided sufficient information to make a preliminary formulation. Figure 1 presents the multiperspective grid for this patient that was completed after the initial assessment. The formulation is that of an 18-year-old girl with a primary complaint of vomiting in the context of a panic disorder with agoraphobia. The formulation needs to explain the development of these symptoms and why they are being maintained. I hope that this understanding will suggest possible treatment interventions.

It is important to keep in mind that the initial formulation is a hypothesis and needs to be tested and modified as additional data is uncovered over the course of therapy. When using the multiperspective grid to formulate it is not necessary to repeat the four Ps for each category, but rather to describe these factors by integrating them into the theoretical model chosen to understand the patient. At times it may be important to indicate which factors are predisposing or perpetuating, etc., but this is unnecessary for each case. The purpose of the grid is to provide a framework for formulation. What is chosen to be included in the formulation depends on which model you feel will be the most applicable in terms of understanding, and more important, in treatment. In formulating this case several columns of the grid can be explored and then integrated to provide a comprehensive, coherent theory that explains why this individual is presenting with this problem at this particular time (see Table 13.1).

PERSPECTIVE FORMULATIONS

From a *biological perspective,* Susan may be vulnerable towards developing a panic disorder, given the similar agoraphobic symptoms seen in her mother. This biological predisposition may contribute to a low threshold for experiencing anxiety symptoms. Her vulnerability to gastrointestinal symptoms may be related to an inherited vulnerability in that system, given chronic gastrointestinal symptoms experienced by her father, who may express emotional distress through this system. There was no evidence of any biological precipitating or perpetuating factors that could be identified that may have brought on or maintained the disorder. Her good health may be seen as generally protective from a biological point of view.

The *behavioral perspective* offers an alternate view of the problem. Gastrointestinal symptoms began in association with the married man who became a conditioned stimulus for anxiety. Therefore, being with the married man made her anxious and anxiety made her vomit. Over time anxiety became generalized to any time she was outside the house and may have precipitated the vomiting in other situations. Other situations that made her anxious may have also triggered the vomiting, an effect of generalization. Staying at home was not associated with the married man, and therefore became a discriminative stimulus for "not vomiting"; however, any anxiety experienced at home would likely precipitate vomiting. Over time, anxiety was relieved if she stayed at home or came home after having an "attack." Consequently, avoidance behaviors were reinforced by anxiety reduction. Secondary reinforcers such as attention from family and significant others maintained her vomiting and avoidance behavior as was evident by the supportive gestures she received from her mother, boyfriend, and employer during these times. Because the reinforcement history revealed an inadequate frequency and variety of reinforcers predating the disorders, social attention may have become a significant reinforcer that maintained her vomiting behavior. Her work although limited, can be viewed as a behavioral protective factor because it is the only activity that gets her out of the house.

Cognitively, she was also vulnerable towards psychological difficulties given the likelihood that she developed early maladaptive schemas centering around worthiness (feeling defective, unlovable, incompe-

Table 13.1
Multiperspective Grid—Case of Susan

	INDIVIDUAL FACTORS			
	BIOLOGICAL	BEHAVIORAL	COGNITIVE	PSYCHO-DYNAMIC
PREDISPOSING	• Fam history - anxiety - agoraphobia - gastrointestinal vulnerability	• Classical conditioning married man (CS) ↓ anxiety→ vomiting • poor* R history	• EMS - worthlessness - autonomy • NAT - failure	• arrest in oedipal stage • attchm't to bad objects • ↓ mirror/ideal fun'c • insecure attachment
PRECIPITATING		• loss of *R - rel'ship • generalization of CR to "out of house"	•affair/loss of ↓ activate EMS ↓ ↑ NAT	• affair/loss of ↓ guilt/unresolved issues ↓ anxiety/vomitin • time to individuate
PERPETUATING		• *R of avoidance via ↓ anxiety • *R of vomiting via ↑ attention	• NAT → EMS self-perpetuating • ↓ challenging environment	• repression/ suppression • poor self-objec • attachment to bad objects
PROTECTIVE	• good health	• work ↓ ↓ avoidance	• perceives self as attractive	• ? current objec choice (boyfriend)
COPING-RESPONSE STYLE	• somatizer • anti-meds	• action-oriented • "do-er"	• not reflective • not introspective	• not reflective • not introspecti • no insight
TREATMENT	• anti-dep • anti-anx ↓ but • anti-med	• Relaxation/ systematic desensitization • exposure	?	• currently unavailable ↓ not initial approach

*R = reinforcement; P = punishment; ↑ = increase; ↓ = decrease; tx = therapy; hx = history; NAT = negative automatic thoughts; beh = behavior; EMS = early maladaptiv schemas; dysf'nc = dysfunction; rel'ship = relationship; CR = conditioned response mi = mirroring; ideal = idealizing; func = functions; attachm't = attachment; CS = conditioned stimulus

SYSTEMIC FACTORS			
COUPLE	FAMILY	OCCUPATIONAL/ SCHOOL	SOCIAL
• relationship with father • difficulties with intimacy	• dysf'nc structure • poor affective communication • triangulation • intergenerational family dysf'nc	• underachiever in school • poor occupational hx • no career aspiration • poor family modeling	• poor social hx • shyness • poor social support
• ? ↑ demands for intimacy (sexual) in current rel'ship	• impending separation from family ↓ leaving mother alone	• need to develop career plans	• loss of rel'ship • loss of friends after "affair"
• collusive projective identification interaction • ongoing ambivalence re: relationship	• chronic dysf'nc system • triangulation • parental marital discord	• *R of illness behavior at work • no work demands	• avoidance of social situations
• Supportive rel'ship	• good instrumental functioning	• good relationship with employer	• attractive • good verbal skills
• Rel'ship gives some support	• support from mother for "vomiting" • not a familial coper	• not an occupational coper	• not a social-support seeker
• Not as initial approach ↓ ? later	• unavailable for intervention (? Reassess)	• vocational counseling	• social skills • exposure • ↑ support

tent, guilty, ashamed and embarrassed unrelenting standards and autonomy (difficulty being alone, inability to individuate). Her early childhood suggests that she received very little encouragement and positive feedback about her abilities. It is possible that these early maladaptive schemas made her vulnerable towards developing an anxiety disorder. Her affair triggered these schemas and precipitated a series of automatic thoughts about her "badness," and these thoughts led to intense feelings of guilt, shame, and anxiety. Once these thoughts were activated, they maintained the anxiety and vomiting symptoms. She also had persistent thoughts about failure that made it difficult for her to take risks and venture into new career opportunities. She did, however, see herself as reasonably physically attractive and competent at her work, a positive self-perception that may have cognitively protected her from depression, in that it contributed to some experience of positive self-esteem.

Psychodynamically, several models can be utilized to understand her symptoms. Her vomiting can be viewed as a manifestation of her guilt over her affair with the married man. Since these symptoms began during this relationship this is not an unlikely hypothesis. Her casual rejection of this possibility may also illustrate that she had repressed some aspects of this relationship, and these unresolved issues may have been surfacing through the vomiting. The vomiting allowed her to purge her feelings of disgust and temporarily gave expression to the repressed material. The ongoing repression mechanisms may have perpetuated the vomiting in that it did not allow the feelings of guilt to be addressed. Repressed guilt by itself does not explain all her symptoms, however. Her involvement with a married unavailable man suggests two intrapsychic conflicts: unresolved oedipal issues and attachment to bad objects. Her attraction to a married man suggests the lack of resolution of the oedipal phase given her wish to become involved with another woman's husband. His unavailability and yet exciting aspect points to her attraction to "bad" objects. In many ways she is repeating the same dynamics of her relationship with her father, a man who was unavailable to her and yet was someone she longed to be close to. This longing, although repressed, is likely to express itself through an attraction to unavailable men, for through these relationships she may sustain the "false" sense of hope of satisfying some of her early unmet needs. Her attraction to the married man was also fueled by her experiencing herself as an exciting object, something she never experienced before, especially from her father. It is therefore possible that this idealized forbidden man became the object and container of her good parts. Having projected the good parts on to him, losing him would in a sense destroy the goodness in her. This hypothesis also suggests that she lacks a good internalized object that can allow her to contain her own anxiety, by providing her with an internal sense of safety and comfort. Without an internalized good object she will be vulnerable to experiences of anxiety and panic during periods of separation. This may also indicate inadequate mirroring and idealizing experiences in the early developmental years, making her more vulnerable towards self-objects that can provide this for her, even if only for a brief period of time. She is therefore vulnerable towards fragmentation when these functions are no longer provided, which is likely what happened when her relationship with this man ended. Because she was unable to internalize these functions adequately in the early years, she will continue to be vulnerable unless she is provided with these functions through another self-object, or is able to internalize these functions through a successful therapeutic experience.

The history also suggests an insecure attachment based on the difficulty she had separating from her mother in the early years. Developmentally she is at an age where separation and individuation from the family of origin is being seriously considered, something she is likely struggling with, and, therefore she is maintaining her vomiting and anxiety symptoms. An inability to separate and differentiate from her family would create difficulties for her in becoming autonomous and developing a sense of identity. This would then lead to difficulties with intimacy, given that a sense of identity precedes the capacity to be intimate in relationships. Evidence in the history suggests difficulty with identity issues as is seen in her inability to separate from her parents, her difficulties with occupational choices, her chronic sense of emptiness and boredom, and her difficulties with her own sexuality. However, her capacity to engage in a relationship that is supportive, can be viewed as a protective psychodynamic factor in that it indicates the ability to select an object that is nurturing.

The dynamic theories most useful in formulating this case are those that deal with the issues of attachment, separation, individuation, self-other differentiation, and her relationship with her internalized good and bad objects.

Systemically there are significant issues in the couple, family, occupational, and social areas. In examining the couple factors it is important to consider those relationship issues that may have contributed to her present condition, and those that are at the present time maintaining her symptoms. Significant *couple* issues that impact on her present overall level of functioning and the future also need to be considered. Her relationship history suggests that she was able to engage men in relationships, although they seemed to lack any form of intimacy. Given her relationship with her father, one may predict that she might have some difficulties in her relationships with men. Her relationship with the married man seemed to precipitate her symptoms.

Other couple issues that may be relevant include her boredom in her present relationship. Her motivation for getting involved with her present boyfriend is questionable, given that she became involved with him right after her breakup with the married man. It is possible that she has always been ambivalent about this relationship but is unable to give it up because of her separation fears and the possibility that it distracts her from her previous relationship. Other possibilities include an increase in demand for emotional, physical, and sexual intimacy in the present relationship, something that she is unable to give or receive, and can avoid through her vomiting. On a protective note, her current relationship does provide support and companionship and the occasional opportunity to leave the house. There is also some question about the boyfriend's motives for being involved in a relationship that is more platonic than romantic and that is socially and recreationally quite limited. It is possible that as a couple they collude with each other's projective identification patterns which keep them from developing a more intimate relationship. As conflict avoiders they may interact on a superficial level with very little reinforcement exchanged between them. Yet despite their limited reinforcing capabilities as a couple, this relationship may be more reinforcing than their own independent lives. It is also possible that at the present time Susan is experiencing ambivalent feelings about committing to the relationship, in that doing so would precipitate a separation from mother, something that is likely to generate a great deal of anxiety.

Family factors are also important in this case. Family history suggests a closer relationship between the patient and her mother than between father and mother. There appears to be a rigid boundary between mother and father and between father and the rest of the family. Mother acts more like one of the children and her boundaries with them appear diffuse. There is also evidence of a coalition between mother and the children against the father. It is possible that as the children tried to separate, their mother became symptomatic, and she may have been experiencing this threat as the patient, her youngest, was trying to leave home. This suggests that Susan was and probably still is an attachment figure for her mother.

Alternative explanations include a triangulation phenomenon whereby the parental marital conflict that had remained unattended to while the children were home, became activated as the parents faced the possibility of being alone. Triangulating the daughter and keeping her symptomatic, keeps her at home, preventing the parents from dealing with their relationship. The guilt that Susan experiences when she goes out and leaves her mother alone supports this hypothesis. These chronic perpetuating factors then contribute to a dysfunctional family system. Father's uninvolvement and mother's agoraphobia suggest parental difficulties in their own families of origin, hence transmitting these dysfunctions across generations.

Therefore, all these factors predispose these parents to parenting difficulties, leading to a dysfunctional family system. In such a system members do not feel safe and secure, affective expression is inhibited, and they are unable to successfully individuate and differentiate from the family without emotional cutoffs. One protective factor may be this family's ability to deal well instrumentally with the day-to-day chores of family life; this may have provided some sense of order in the household at least on an instrumental level.

Occupationally there were important issues relevant to her case. Her school performance indicated that she had been an underachiever and appeared to lack the interest or motivation to pursue any career opportunities. This attitude was also reinforced by her family who did not model any occupational behaviors that may have stimulated her interest. She also had a poor work history in that she selected jobs that were safe yet unstimulating for her, and, therefore, unable to provide certain self-esteem needs. She had some idea of what she wanted to do, but would always question her confidence or her interest. She did, however, have a good relationship with her employers, which could be viewed as a protective factor for her in that she was able to maintain employment despite her disinterest. There were no specific occupational precipitants noted that coincided with her disorder except her awareness that in order to leave home she had to obtain gainful employment, and she was unsure as to what type of work she wanted to pursue. This chronic struggle led her to consider the possibility of remaining home. She was, however, aware that she might not be able to do this indefinitely, and this possibility likely maintained her anxiety symptoms. It is possible that her employer's support over her vomiting reinforced this behavior, thereby perpetuating this symptom.

Socially the patient was rather limited, having very few friends, no confiding relationships, and a poor social support network. The history suggests that she might always have felt somewhat shy and inadequate in social situations, fearful of rejection by her peers. There was no evidence of a significant social precipitant except the loss of the relationship with the married man, and a feeling of being ostracized by the few friends that knew about her affair. Her chronic lack of social relationships could maintain her symptoms in that friends were unavailable to encourage her outside the home and to help her eventually individuate. The absence of friendships also deprived her of the opportunity to share common experiences with her same-age peers, especially in the area of romantic relationships and sexual behavior, an important context for young adults to develop their own sense of identity. Protective social factors include some success in high school with friends and boyfriends, good verbal skills, and her physical attractiveness that may increase her opportunity for further social relationships.

INTEGRATED FORMULATION

Having presented a brief formulation according to each perspective, it is now necessary to combine these areas in order to arrive at a comprehensive, integrated formulation. Susan is biologically and psychologically vulnerable to experiencing specific psychological difficulties given certain precipitants. She has a biological predisposition towards anxiety that expressed itself at a very early age. Psychological factors such as an anxious mother and distant father made it difficult for Susan to experience a secure attachment with a primary caretaker, making her vulnerable to separation anxiety. In addition, she was unable to internalize a sufficient good object as well as adequate mirroring and idealizing functions, which contributed to further vulnerabilities in that she needed someone to accept her projected good parts and to provide her with the necessary self-object functions. All these factors contributed to a negative self-view and led to the formation of an early maladaptive schema that she was unworthy and incapable of functioning independently. These schemas likely contributed to her limited occupational aspirations and social relationships.

As she developed into adolescence she seemed motivated to pursue relationships with men, probably due to her longing to repair her distant relationship with her father, which may have made her attracted to unavailable men, leading to the relationship with the married man. This relationship and its termination were the major precipitants of her symptoms. While involved in the relationship, her unworthiness schema was triggered and so were her hopes to finally fulfil the unmet needs from her rejecting father. This man was also the first person to show significant interest in her, making her feel that she was an interesting and exciting person to be with. All these issues came to the surface when she became involved in this relationship and were difficult to suppress after the relationship ended.

Behavioral factors contributed to her symptoms developing into a disorder. Other factors also maintained these symptoms; however, for at the same time she was faced with the major developmental task of separating and individuating from her family, something that was very difficult for her because of her own insecure attachment, triangulation in her family, and poor development of a sense of identity. Pressure to become more intimately involved in a mature relationship also maintained her symptoms.

Therefore, biologically and psychologically Susan was vulnerable to develop these symptoms given the right precipitant that could activate and trigger intrapsychic, cognitive, and family issues. Once these symptoms developed her family structure, couple relationship, her own psychological makeup, current developmental tasks, and pressure to move forward into adulthood maintained her symptoms, because without these symptoms she would have seriously to consider separating, individuating, developing her own sense of identity, and being available for a mature relationship.

Her seeking therapy at this time probably indicated that part of her wanted to move on, even though she only requested symptom relief. She has, nevertheless, managed to work, is initiating some activities on her own, and is bright and motivated to improve her symptoms. All these are protective factors that will help her in therapy.

COPING-RESPONSE STYLE

Please see Table 1 which illustrates the coping-response style for this patient. From the initial assessment it became apparent that Susan was not interested in taking medications and had not used them in the past to cope with physical or psychological difficulties, suggesting that she was not a biologically oriented coper. However, she did attribute her symptoms to a medical illness, suggesting a somatizing coping-response style similar to her father's.

At the initial presentation she did not appear to be very psychologically minded in that she did not attribute any of her symptoms to anxiety and was unable to connect her anxiety symptoms to any issues in her life. She was not introspective, did not explore her feelings or her thoughts, and did not make any connections between her symptoms and past and present experiences in her life. She seemed quite psychologically naive and did not appear to be motivated for deep self-exploration, but she was willing "to do" things to help improve her symptoms. She had already engaged in certain activities to help her overcome her vomiting symptoms.

She did not use her family for support, except after she vomited, indicating that illness seemed to be the only way in which she could access family support. Her relationship with her boyfriend was supportive in that he tolerated her symptoms, and she was occasionally able to talk to him about her problems. Emotional support, however, was lacking in this relationship and in any other relationship that she had. Occupationally, her work provided the only escape from home, and in this sense it was a distraction for her. However, work was also unstimulating and unchallenging and did not provide her with any experience of a sense of mastery, productivity, or creativity. She also engaged in very few recreational and leisure activities that provided her with any relaxation and enjoyment. Her social support network was significantly limited. She had no friends to confide in or to share experiences with, an important area for successful social development and for accessing future social support. Therefore, her most frequent coping-response style could be described as behavioral, with very limited coping skills in other areas, something to consider developing in treatment.

TREATMENT

After arriving at a comprehensive formulation and considering the patient's coping-response style, decisions can be made regarding treatment. A variety of independent treatment options can be considered for this case. Therapists practicing one or two forms of therapy would consider their approach as probably the most appropriate. A purely biologically oriented clinician might consider giving Susan medication for her panic disorder, such as an antidepressant or long-acting benzodiazepine, both known to be effective in treating such cases. A behavior therapist might implement a behavioral program that includes relaxation exercises and exposure and response prevention. A clinician who practices both forms of therapy might administer medications and institute a behavioral program. A cognitive or cognitive-behavioral therapist would explore her thought processes more carefully to challenge early maladaptive schemas and the automatic thoughts associated with her anxiety and vomiting. A psychodynamic therapist might not see the patient if she is considered psychologically unavailable for psychodynamic therapy or psychoanalysis. Couple issues and specifically the sexual problems might be pursued through couple therapy. The family triangulation and dysfunctional structure may have been altered through family therapy. A variety of individual or group therapies might be used to help Susan develop friendships and a social support network. Vocational counseling could also be considered to help her explore occupational and career opportunities.

It is apparent that a variety of therapies can be offered to help Susan with her symptoms and general difficulties. Not all therapists would consider all these approaches, and the decision regarding which approach to select will more than likely depend on the therapist's orientation. However, the grid covers all these approaches, and, therefore, alerts the clinician to consider a variety of options. Based on the grid for this patient (see table 13.1), the following treatment was carried out.

At the initial interview Susan presented with a behavioral coping-response style, in that she wanted "to do" anything to improve her symptoms. She was opposed to taking medications, did not wish her family involved, and did not, at least initially, present as a very psychologically minded individual. As a result, a behavioral approach was considered first, even though psychodynamic and family issues were regarded as important in this case. Because the patient's goals for treatment were respected, the intervention that could give her efficient symptom relief, with documented evidence of effectiveness, was chosen.

Weekly sessions were held, and Susan was taught relaxation exercises, which she practiced daily, and a gradual exposure program was carried out. She was instructed to keep a daily record of her relaxation exercises, her exposure, anxiety level, and the thoughts and feeling associated with her vomiting. She was very compliant in keeping these records, and although she struggled with some of the exposure exercises, she continued to work hard at decreasing her avoidance behavior.

After three months of relaxation exercises and exposure and response prevention, her symptoms began to improve from vomiting three times a day (at initial presentation), to just two to three times a week. As she kept behavioral records of her symptoms and her progress, she became more aware of her feelings. Her behavioral records revealed that her vomiting was usually preceded by uncomfortable feelings, feelings she had difficulty describing. With time she began to see that her vomiting was related to feelings of anxiety, and sometimes the anxiety was associated with ambivalence regarding sexual contact with her boyfriend. This seemed to reactivate feelings of guilt and shame regarding her affair with the married man. While exploring these feelings she started to make connections between a variety of feelings and the vomiting. Behavior therapy continued to help her deal with her avoidance behaviors and psychodynamic therapy helped her explore her inner experiences. The therapies were integrated. Behavioral exposure made her more aware of her feelings, and these were explored through psychodynamic therapy.

In six to nine months her vomiting symptoms had decreased to about once a week, and she began to spend more time by herself outside the home. Despite significant symptomatic improvement, she seemed unsettled and struggled with many issues. During this time the behavior therapy was monitored less often. At this point in therapy she began to deal with her disappointment in herself about her inability to leave home, her sense of boredom with her relationship, her discomfort with sex, her feelings of inadequacy, and her uncertainty about her future. These issues were explored over the next two years in a supportive, exploratory, dynamically oriented therapy. She became much more aware of her feelings as she experienced them, and as she explored some of these issues, she began to talk about her family. She experienced rage and disappointment that her father had never been available to her and her mother. While exploring her relationship with her father she began to see her own attraction to unavailable men and her own fears of being rejected by them. Any man who showed any interest in her was easily idealized, and she began to recognize this. She became aware of angry feelings toward her mother who she felt had never been there for her unless she was ill. She also realized that she had always taken care of her mother and had always been worried about leaving her alone. This realization made her see that her difficulty in leaving home was partly related to her guilt over leaving mother alone with a distant husband.

This was a very difficult time for her in therapy and her vomiting symptoms returned, although not with the same intensity. Vomiting was also noted whenever I was away on holidays and this connection was interpreted to her as her fear of losing me and being abandoned. Her ambivalent attachment to me was also explored and although this was initially difficult for her, she was able to examine our relationship, and her feelings toward me.

As the transference relationship was explored and worked through, so were some of her feelings towards her parents. By now she was going out by herself, vomiting once a month, and starting to enjoy her relationship with her boyfriend. Family of origin work was integrated into the therapy to help her individuate and differentiate from her family. This process required that she no longer align herself with her mother against her father, and that she develop a separate relationship with each, leaving them to sort out their own marital problems. She was then able to relieve herself from the guilt she felt regarding leaving her mother alone. In developing a separate relationship with her father she became surprised at her father's positive response and interest in her. At the same time her relationship with her boyfriend was explored, and individual sensate focus exercises were recommended to help her overcome her sexual anxieties.

Occupational and vocational interests were also explored in therapy and it was recommended that she pursue formal vocational counseling, which she eventually did. Social relationships with girlfriends were also encouraged, and she began to initiate them with much success. After three years of therapy she was going out regularly, alone and with friends, feeling more sexually comfortable with her boyfriend and enjoying their relationship, enrolling in a night course, and considering a variety of occupational choices. She was virtually free of her panic disorder symptoms and her vomiting had all but disappeared. As we worked through termination she began to explore her feelings toward me and her experience in therapy. She had some mild symptoms of nausea as we discussed termination, but these quickly subsided, and she herself was able to interpret the meaning of the brief return of her symptoms. As we worked through the process of termination she began for the first time to entertain the idea of leaving home.

CASE SUMMARY

This case illustrates several points:

1. It could be formulated multiperspectively, individually, and systemically.
2. The formulation lead to specific interventions.
3. Interventions were matched according to the patient's coping-response style and it was used as a guide to decide when and how to intervene that best followed the patient's needs.
4. The patient became more available for dynamic therapy as behavior therapy was carried out.
5. Other systemic issues that at first were not available for exploration, such as the family, couple and social area, were gradually explored over time.

This is not to say that three years should be required to achieve these results. Symptom relief was achieved within six months, but the patient's goals in therapy changed as symptoms improved, and she became more interested in understanding herself. This case strongly challenges the belief of many psychodynamic therapists that the presence of distressing symptoms is required to motivate an individual in therapy. In this case symptom relief was the motivating factor to seek other answers. Symptom improvement stimulated a greater need for understanding inner experiences, and in fact the large percentage of psychodynamic work was done when the patient was free of symptoms.

Family therapy was never an option, and I wonder if it might have produced faster results. Medications could also have been used to speed the recovery process. However, the patient was opposed to medications and family interventions, so effective treatments congruent with her coping-response style had to be found in order to enhance a better therapeutic alliance and compliance in treatment. Once improvement was noticed using these other modalities, it was unnecessary to push the patient into these areas. As the formulation changed when more information was revealed in the sessions, different directions were taken based on the process occurring in therapy.

It is difficult to present all aspects of the treatment. The transferential and counter-transferential phenomena were very important in this case and were dealt with as the specific issues arose. These issues are important in all therapies whether or not the therapist decides to use them. In this case they were very helpful and were utilized throughout the therapy process, regardless of the specific intervention used at the time.

Therefore, in this case, the multiperspective grid served as a guide in all phases of management, assessment, formulation, and treatment. It encouraged the consideration of a variety of perspectives, and exploring all these areas provided a much richer formulation. This formulation and the patient's coping-response style, were helpful in considering the initial treatment. As therapy progressed, other therapies were integrated that were based on the formulation and the process in therapy. This approach to formulation encourages a broader view of the *person* who is presenting with a particular problem, and I hope will increase the chance of a better therapeutic outcome—the ultimate goal of this model.

CHAPTER 14

FROM FORMULATION TO TREATMENT INTEGRATION

The major purpose of this book as mentioned in the introductory chapter is to provide learners with a clinical tool that systematically encourages the consideration of a variety of perspectives in order to arrive at a comprehensive formulation and treatment plan. The purpose of the multiperspective grid is to serve as a framework or working schema that can accommodate multiple treatment options. The grid can potentially suggest interventions in eight areas; however, in reality, only one or a few of these therapies may be initiated with alternate therapies being considered as treatment progresses. Therefore, the grid is a first step towards treatment integration and how this process can be carried out will be described in this chapter. Prior to examining the integrative capacity of this model a brief discussion of the psychotherapy integration literature will be presented to furnish the reader with the relevant background in this area so that the model can be assessed within this context.

THE PSYCHOTHERAPY INTEGRATION MOVEMENT

Historically, psychotherapy developed within individual schools beginning with the psychoanalytic movement. Subsequently, similar independent movements developed their own brand names of psychotherapy such as behavioral therapy, cognitive therapy, humanistic and experiential therapy, systemic therapy, and many others. For a considerable period of time these separate schools maintained their distinctiveness and competed for superior status in the general area of psychotherapy. However, several developments began to diffuse these energetic debates and a new movement emerged, a movement that discouraged ideological segregation and encouraged theoretical and clinical integration. Although the formal psychotherapy integration movement is about 15 years old, initial integrative developments can be traced to the early 1930s when French (1933) discussed combining learning and psychoanalytic principles at the Annual American Psychiatric Association meeting. Freud himself acknowledged the importance of exposure in treating phobias although he did not refer to specific behavioral principles. Other individuals who continued to explore this area include Dollard and Miller (1950) and Alexander (1963). Dollard and Miller's translations of psychoanalytic concepts into learning theory principles is considered one of the first attempts at theoretical integration between two major schools of psychotherapy. Alexander (1963) studied the process of change in both therapies and argued against an "unidirectional approach," stating that insight often followed behavioral change rather than the other way around as advocated by psychoanalysis.

These initial attempts to integrate psychoanalytic and behavioral schools led to the merging of other schools. From the 1950s to the 1970s behavior therapy flourished and its documented success led other schools to integrate some of these interventions. Behavior therapists also considered psychodynamic, humanistic, cognitive, and systemic issues as they began to expand and deal with more complicated psychological problems (Gold, 1993). The most well-known initial model that integrated psychotherapy and behavioral therapy was Wachtel's (1977) Cyclical Psychodynamic model (Gold & Wachtel, 1993) one of the first truly integrative models of psychotherapy. Since then there has been an explosion in the field with numerous integrative models now discussed in the literature. Some of these include the Cognitive-Analytic Model (Ryle & Low, 1993), the Cognitive-Interpersonal-Experiential model (Reeve, Ink, & Safran, 1993), Multimodal Therapy (Lazarus, 1981; 1992), the Transtheoretical model (Prochaska & DiClemente, 1992), and many others (see Stricker & Gold, 1993; Norcross & Goldfried, 1992).

The rapid development of the psychotherapy integration movement was influenced by many factors. In the 1970s and 1980s increasing pressure from insurance companies and government agencies demanded that the field of psychotherapy be held more accountable by demonstrating that psychotherapy was beneficial. This led to an outpouring of articles in psychotherapy research and soon major conclusions were drawn. First, with a few exceptions, all psychotherapies were found to be equally effective across a variety of problems, with no school of psychotherapy demonstrating superiority over another (Smith, Glass, & Miller, 1980; Shapiro & Shapiro, 1982). Others, however, have challenged this statement arguing that the quality of the research did not permit a definitive conclusion (Stiles, Shapiro, & Elliott, 1986). Despite this debate, the original conclusion made by Smith and others (1980) had its effect on the general psychotherapy community; differences between therapies were deemphasized and the search for common ingredients across all therapies directed future research (Gold, 1993; Lambert, 1992).

In addition to changes in the general psychotherapy movement, sociopolitical changes in the 1960s and 1970s such as the challenge of traditional roles, governments, civil rights, the women's liberation movement, and the sexual revolution all promoted a "desegregation" movement, considered by some to have influenced similar developments in psychotherapy (Gold, 1993).

All these developments led to a strong interest and movement toward psychotherapy integration. In 1983 this movement was formalized with the development of the Society for the Exploration of Psychotherapy Integration (SEPI), a professional organization that has a rapidly growing membership. In addition, there are at present three journals solely devoted to psychotherapy integration: the *Journal of Psychotherapy Integration,* the *Journal of Integrative and Eclectic Psychotherapy,* and *Integrative Psychiatry* (Norcross & Newman, 1992). The integrative movement was also supported by a recent NIMH workshop (Wolfe, & Goldfried, 1988; Goldfried & Newman, 1992), that advocated the integration of the best elements from independent schools of psychotherapy in order to produce a more efficient, effective, and safer treatment. Despite the enthusiasm and energy generated, the psychotherapy integration movement is in its infancy and therefore lacking in empirical outcome research. It has yet to be demonstrated that integrative therapies are equal to or superior to pure forms of psychotherapy, although some suggest that there may be fewer dropouts and faster results with integrative approaches (Glass, Victor, & Arnkoff, 1993).

A variety of models and methods for integration have been discussed in the literature. These include (1) integrating techniques from pure forms of psychotherapy, (2) integrating theories of disorders, (3) prescriptive matching of client to treatment based on client characteristics and the presenting problems, (4) integrative models of therapy change, and (5) generic models of integration (Glass et al., 1993). All these models or approaches to integration have been discussed in two recent comprehensive sources (Norcross & Goldfried, 1992; Stricker & Gold, 1993) and will not be extensively described here. The models differ with respect to their emphasis on theory versus technique, on integrating two or more theories or therapies, on integrating multiple variables common to all therapies, and on the attention given to individual client variables. Some models are more comprehensive, examining multiple factors (e.g., multimodal therapy [Lazarus, 1981; 1992], and Systemic Treatment Selection [Beutler & Clarkin, 1990]) while others integrate two or three approaches (e.g., cognitive-analytic therapy [Ryle, 1990; Ryle & Low, 1993]).

In addition to the development of a variety of integrative models, there has been a shift in emphasis from eclecticism to integration. *Eclecticism* refers to the borrowing of a variety of techniques across approaches based on what is considered most effective without adhering to any particular theory. *Integration* refers to the blending of two or more theories in order to produce a unified, coherent, superior theory, essential to the development of integrative techniques (Mahoney, 1993). Integrative psychotherapy is defined as a particular approach while psychotherapy integration is viewed as a process. Norcross and Prochaska (1988) argue that this movement has shifted from "eclecticism by default" to "integration by design." Therefore, integration appears to be the more popular term, and its definition implies the importance of both theoretical and technical integration, even though the former is given greater emphasis.

THE MULTIPERSPECTIVE MODEL—A STEP TOWARDS INTEGRATION

The model presented in this book can be viewed as an integrative model in that it (1) systematically encourages the consideration of a variety of theoretical models, (2) offers the formulation as the vehicle to conceptual integration, (3) identifies individual characteristics for prescriptive matching of patient to treatment, and (4) offers a framework to consider sequential or simultaneous treatment integration.

The Grid Encourages the Learning of a Variety of Perspectives

Norcross and Newman (1992) pointed out that the second ranked obstacle to integration is the lack of commitment and training of students in multiple theories and interventions. In order for students or clinicians to consider integrative therapies, they must first acquire a sufficient knowledge base in a variety of theoretical models or therapies including the biological model. This approach understandably requires greater effort and motivation from the student because a wide knowledge base and broader theoretical background are demanded, but it is not an impossible task since most mental health professional training programs require a minimum of four years to complete (and some even more), providing ample time to learn and be exposed to a variety of theoretical perspectives. Current training programs, however, are still inadequate in their ability to provide such wide coverage with some schools offering psychotherapy training in only one approach.

The fundamental principles of some of the major models of treatment have been presented in chapters 5–12. A basic understanding of these principles is sufficient for one to develop a reasonable conceptual model of each theoretical approach. It is a starting point, and more sophisticated analyses of these concepts can be obtained through further readings. What has been presented is sufficient for the beginner to consider applying these theories to actual clinical problems.

Before integrative therapies can be considered, it is essential to have a theoretical knowledge base in a variety of perspectives, which will also permit one to carry out a comprehensive assessment—a prerequisite to considering integrative approaches. The therapist's capacity to assess the client from a variety of perspectives will determine the specific model(s) of therapy that will eventually be chosen. Therefore, the first step to practicing integrative therapy is to develop a wide theoretical knowledge base in a variety of treatment models, and to then develop assessment capabilities in each area. This is also the first step in completing the multiperspective grid.

The Formulation as the Vehicle for Conceptual Integration

Psychotherapy integration involves blending concepts and ideas from two or more theoretical approaches to create a unifying whole that is different from the sum of its parts. A variety of models have been presented in the literature that carry out this process. A good example is cognitive analytic therapy which integrates object-relations principles and cognitive theory to produce an integrated object-relations-cognitive therapy (Ryle, 1990; Ryle & Low, 1993). It is probably easier to integrate two theories than it is to integrate three or more theoretical frameworks. The multiperspective model permits one to integrate several models through a coherent formulation. The formulation brings together the relevant theoretical principles and blends them into a unified theory that can account for a variety of individual and systemic factors. Before a unifying theory is developed, each perspective is applied separately so that a careful theoretical analysis of the pure forms precedes any attempt at integration, promoting a sophisticated theoretical approach to integration rather than a "mishmashing" of poorly understood concepts. This approach, of course, requires a more thorough understanding of each perspective. Once a perspective formulation is considered under each column of the grid, the most useful models are chosen based on the patient and the presenting problem. The most useful theoretical models are then integrated to produce a more comprehensive sophisticated formulation that is truly a theoretical integration of a variety of perspectives. There will be some difficulty initially in selecting the models most appropriate for the formulation. This procedure can be guided by research, the disorder, and the patient. With experience the clinician will develop an intuitive method of selecting models for integration that can later be articulated and empirically investigated. Therefore, the grid is a first step for the systematic and comprehensive exploration of psychotherapy integration because it offers the clinician a framework for formulation—a means to conceptually integrate a variety of theoretical models.

The formulation, like psychotherapy integration, is a process. The formulation will change as time and therapy progress and should, therefore, be repeatedly examined, modified, and challenged. This model also integrates the biological perspective, usually missing in many integrative models of therapy. Therefore, it is an integrative treatment model, the specific treatment or treatments implemented being determined by the formulation. How the formulation can be viewed as a means to theoretical integration was illustrated in the case example presented in the previous chapter.

Prescriptive Matching of Patient to Treatment

Specific integrative models were discussed that identify patient characteristics and then match them to specific treatment approaches. Certain patient characteristics such as aptitude, coping, reactance, and personality styles, have been identified and used to match patient to pure or integrative forms of psychotherapy (Glass et al., 1993). With respect to this variable the multiperspective formulation model examines individual patient factors when considering treatment options. Coping-response styles were described that can be used to clinically identify patient characteristics that may be useful in matching patient to treatment. As discussed in chapter 3, individuals can be described as having a variety of coping-response styles that may suggest integrative approaches. For example, an individual may have a cognitive and behavioral coping-response style, suggesting a cognitive-behavioral approach, or a cognitive and self-exploratory coping-response style, suggesting a cognitive-analytic approach.

Similarly individual and systemic coping-response styles could be matched with an integrative therapy of the respective approaches. For example, a depressed woman with marital problems may have an individual coping-response style that suggests a cognitive-behavioral therapy. She may have also utilized her marital relationship as a source of support, but marital discord may have diminished the use of this system as a coping resource, thereby suggesting the need for marital therapy. Whether to first pursue individual cognitive-behavioral therapy and then marital therapy, or marital therapy alone, using a cognitive-behavioral approach, will depend on the formulation and the severity of the depressive symptoms. However, as mentioned earlier, the lack of a specific coping-response style does not mean that the associated treatment should not be considered, especially if sufficient evidence exists for a particular approach with a given problem. In the example cited above, if the woman's depressive symptoms were severe, pharmacological treatment could be considered and integrated with an individual cognitive-behavioral approach followed by marital therapy.

The coping-response style simply acts as a guide and suggests a place to begin so that the maximum therapeutic alliance can be obtained, and a smoother therapy with greater compliance and chance for improvement is possible. Individual characteristics could be important determiners of pure or integrative forms of therapy. It is not the only factor determining treatment selection, but it is an important variable that may have significant implications for integrative therapy.

Sequential versus Simultaneous Integration

Once the formulation is completed and the coping-response style is considered, a variety of treatment options may be evident. As mentioned above the formulation explores the possible theoretical explanations for the presenting problem according to a variety of perspectives. Working through this process will highlight those theories that seem the most applicable in explaining the individual's difficulty and in suggesting treatment. Once the specific models are chosen that best explain the difficulties, an integrated formulation will point to the best treatment options. The decision to choose one approach first, and to add others as therapy progresses, or integrating two or more approaches simultaneously, will depend on the presenting problem, the individual's coping-response style, the available evidence for a particular approach, and the patient's capacity to use the therapy. For example, a patient suffering from an anxiety disorder may initially benefit from a cognitive-behavioral approach. Later, as symptomatic relief is obtained, an exploratory approach might help uncover more deep seated problems that are contributing to the anxiety disorder. At this point the cognitive-behavioral therapy (CBT) could be phased out and the therapy could shift to a psychodynamic approach, or CBT and dynamic therapy could be carried out concurrently as discussed in cognitive-analytic therapy. Behavior therapy and psychodynamic therapy have also been practiced concurrently with the former changing maladaptive behavioral patterns and the latter modifying character structure (Wachtel, 1977). Behavioral change is also known to produce insights indicating the complementary and synergistic capability of psychodynamic behavioral approaches.

The grid suggests a place to begin, but also highlights additional areas to explore either simultaneously or sequentially. Because formulation is viewed as a dynamic process, it will change as therapy progresses requiring periodic updating of the grid.

An additional method of selecting particular therapy either sequentially or simultaneously can be determined by *process markers* that may identify behavioral, cognitive, intrapsychic or systemic issues that are relevant at a particular point in time. The concept of markers in therapy has been discussed in the literature (Rice & Greenberg, 1984; Greenberg & Safran, 1987) and can be useful in considering the integration of various treatments. For example, while conducting behavioral therapy for an anxiety disorder, exposure therapy or self-monitoring may reveal underlying feelings regarding unresolved developmental issues. This "access to unresolved feelings," could be a marker for either an experiential or dynamic therapy. Other examples of markers include intensive "focus on thought processes" that suggest a cognitive intervention, "patient-therapist relational issues" that suggest transference interpretations, and "unfinished business" from the past involving a significant other (parent, sibling, ex-spouse, etc.) that indicates gestalt–empty chair intervention. The marker guided approach deals with technical integration in that specific interventions are utilized at choice points to enhance therapeutic effectiveness. This method can help integrative therapists make treatment decisions regarding the introduction of a new intervention. The grid can be used as a guide to monitor therapy and to prepare therapists for possible markers in therapy as they emerge, which can be evaluated with respect to the current formulation to determine whether it may be appropriate to implement a specific intervention. If the formulation and coping-response style suggest that the marker be followed then a specific intervention can be utilized that should be consistent with the formulation.

The approach to treatment integration described above was illustrated in the case example presented in chapter 13. The suggestions are to be viewed as a first step towards integration. It is a working model that has not as yet been empirically investigated with respect to treatment outcome, and is being offered as a clinical tool to consider methods of integration.

SUMMARY

The multiperspective grid provides a framework that encourages the therapist to consider a clinical problem from a variety of perspectives. The grid encourages a comprehensive assessment and formulation within each perspective before an integrated formulation is attempted. Once this is completed the grid provides a method for considering individual differences through the assessment of the coping-response style. Following this the grid assists the therapist in considering a variety of therapies. Pure forms based on a perspective formulation, or combined therapies based on an integrated formulation, can be considered. The initial formulation, the coping-response style, the availability of an effective treatment, and the therapeutic process that identifies markers for specific interventions, can all aid in selecting the best treatment or treatments for an individual case.

As therapy progresses additional data may modify the original formulation necessitating an alteration in the treatment plan, which illustrates the dynamic nature of the formulation, making the point that a formulation is a hypothesis about causation based on the *current available data.* Therefore, the original formulation should be constantly challenged by the therapist, who needs to remain *open* to alternative interpretations as therapy progresses, so that more effective therapies that are consistent with the current formulations are considered. The multiperspective grid presented in this book guides the therapist through this process. The rules for considering specific therapies and integrating a variety of therapies have been described. However, a more systematic process for integrating therapies is still missing, and the model presented in this book is offered as a "first step" towards this process.

In addition, empirical data is necessary to evaluate the usefulness of this model. It will be important to demonstrate that the model (1) can be utilized by students in clinical cases, (2) encourages the learning of a variety of perspectives, (3) increases the chances that clinical cases will be viewed multiperspectively, (4) encourages the consideration of a variety of treatment options, and (5) leads to a better therapeutic outcome. Preliminary data with a small group of psychiatry residents indicates that they are able to utilize the model, that it "forces" them to view the patient from different perspectives, and that learning these perspectives increases their ability to consider a variety of therapeutic options

(Weerasekera & Linder, 1994). Nevertheless, the model still needs to be evaluated on a larger scale and its relationship to outcome still needs to be investigated. At this point in time the focus is on demonstrating the usefulness of this model as a teaching tool. Following this will be an evaluation of its usefulness as an integrative model of therapy, and its relation to outcome. I hope future research will explore these areas.

REFERENCES

Alexander, S. (1963). The Dynamics of Psychotherapy in the Light of Learning Theory. *American Journal of Psychiatry, 120,* 440–448.

Beutler, L. E., & Clarkin, J. F. (1990). *Systematic Treatment Selection: Toward Targeted Therapeutic Interventions.* New York: Brunner/Mazel.

Dollard, J., & Miller, N. E. (1950). *Personality and Psychotherapy.* New York: McGraw-Hill.

French, T. M. (1933). Interrelations between Psychoanalysis and the Experimental Work of Pavlov. *American Journal of Psychiatry, 89,* 1165–1203.

Glass, R., Victor, B. J., & Arnkoff, D. B. (1993). Empirical Research on Integrative and Eclectic Psychotherapies. In G. Stricker, & G. R. Gold, (Eds.), *Comprehensive Handbook of Psychotherapy Integration.* New York: Plenum Press.

Gold, G. R. (1993). The Socio-Historical Context of Psychotherapy Integration. In G. Stricker, & G. R. Gold, (Eds.), *Comprehensive Handbook of Psychotherapy Integration.* New York: Plenum Press.

Gold, G. R., & Wachtel, P. L. (1993). Cyclical Psychodynamics. In G. Stricker, & G. R. Gold, (Eds.), *Comprehensive Handbook of Psychotherapy Integration.* New York: Plenum Press.

Goldfried, M. R., & Newman, C. F. (1992). History of Psychotherapy Integration. In J. C. Norcross, & M. R. Goldfried (Eds.), *Handbook of Psychotherapy Integration.* New York: Basic Books.

Greenberg, L. S., & Safran, J. D. (1987). *Emotion in Psychotherapy: Affect, Cognition and the Process of Change.* New York: Guilford Press.

Lambert, M. J. (1992). Psychotherapy Outcome Research: Implications for Integrative and Eclectic Therapists. In J. C. Norcross & M. R. Goldfried (Eds.), *Handbook of Psychotherapy Integration.* New York: Basic Books.

Lazarus, A. A. (1981). *The Practice of Multimodal Therapy.* New York: McGraw-Hill.

Lazarus, A. A. (1992). Multimodal Therapy: Technical Eclectisism with Minimal Integration. In J. C. Norcross, & M. R. Goldfried (Eds.), *Handbook of Psychotherapy Integration.* New York: Basic Books.

Mahoney, M. J. (1993). Diversity and the Dynamics of Development in Psychotherapy Integration. *Journal of Psychotherapy Integration, 3*(1), 1–13.

Norcross, J. C. (1992). *Case of Eclectic Psychotherapy.* New York: Brunner/Mazel.

Norcross, J. C. & Goldfried, M. R. (Eds) (1992). *Handbook of Psychotherapy Integration*. New York: Basic Books.

Norcross, J. C., & Newman, C. F. (1992). Psychotherapy Integration: Setting the Context. In J. C. Norcross, & M. R. Goldfried (Eds.), *Handbook of Psychotherapy Integration*. New York: Basic Books.

Norcross, J. C., & Prochaska, J. O. (1988). A study of eclectic (and integrative) views revisited. *Professional Psychology: Research and Practice, 19,* 170–174.

Prochaska, J. O., & DiClemente, C. C. (1992). The Transtheoretical Approach. In J. C. Norcross, & M. R. Goldfried (Eds.), *Handbook of Psychotherapy Integration*. New York: Basic Books.

Reeve, J., Ink, T. A., & Safran, J. (1993). Toward an Integration of Cognitive, Interpersonal, and Experiental Approaches to Therapy. In G. Stricker, & G. R. Gold (Eds.), *Comprehensive Handbook of Psychotherapy Integration*. New York: Plenum Press.

Rice, L. N., & Greenberg, L. S. (1984). *Patterns of Change: Intensive Analysis of the Psychotherapeutic Process*. New York: Guilford Press.

Ryle, A. (1990). *Cognitive-Analytic Therapy: Active Participation in Change*. Chichester: Wiley.

Ryle, A., & Low, W. J. (1993). Cognitive-Analytic Therapy. In G. Stricker, & G. R. Gold, (Eds.), *Comprehensive Handbook of Psychotherapy Integration*. New York: Plenum Press.

Shapiro, D. A., & Shapiro, D. (1982). Meta-analysis of Comparative Therapy Outcome Studies: A Replication and Refinement. *Psychological Bulletin, 3,* 581–604.

Smith, M. L., Glass, G. V., & Miller, T. I. (1980). *Benefits of Psychotherapy*. Baltimore: Johns Hopkins University.

Stiles, W. B., Shapiro, D. A., & Elliott, R. (1986). Are All Psychotherapies Equivalent? *American Psychologist, 41,* 165–180.

Stricker, G., & Gold, J. R. (Eds) (1993). *Comprehensive Handbook of Psychotherapy Integration*. New York: Plenum Press.

Wachtel, P. L. (1977). *Psychoanalysis and Behavior Therapy: Towards an Integration*. New York: Basic Books.

Weerasekera, P., & Linder, B. Evaluating the Effectiveness of the Multiperspective Grid in Teaching Psychiatry Residents Psychotherapy Integration. Paper presented at the Annual Meeting of the Canadian Psychiatric Association, September 23, 1994. Ottawa, Canada.

Wolfe, B. E., & Goldfried, M. R. (1988). Research on Psychotherapy Integration: Recommendations and Conclusions from an NIMH Workshop. *Journal of Consulting and Clinical Psychology, 56,* 448–451.

APPENDIXES

APPENDIX I

Guide to Writing an Integrated Formulation

This patient is a (age) (sex) who presents with a diagnosis of (DSM-IV),
e.g., a major depressive episode, panic disorder with agoraphobia-moderate, generalized anxiety disorder, etc.,

In formulating this patient's case it is important to consider the multiple factors responsible in leading (him/her) to present with (diagnosis) at this particular point in time. The history reveals that the patient is biologically vulnerable toward (diagnosis) as a result of having a positive family history for this disorder. The patient's (specify relative/s) also appears to have suffered from (diagnosis). Other biological factors that may have contributed include (specify other biological factors),
e.g., prenatal, postnatal complications, developmental conditions, inherited temperament, illnesses, etc.

Given this biological predisposition, certain psychological factors also may have contributed to increasing this patient's vulnerability toward this condition. The patient's early developmental years suggest a primary caretaker who was (specify predisposing psychodynamic variables here),
e.g., unable to contain projections, unable to provide an adequate holding/containing environment, inadequate in providing mirroring and idealizing functions, unable to provide good object experiences, an insecure attachment figure, etc.

This likely led to a (describe psychodynamically),
e.g., insecure attachment, infantile-dependent, self-object dependent, traumatic, etc.
relationship with the primary caretaker.

This would result in the patient (specify psychodynamic state),
e.g., being fixated or arrested in a specific psychosexual stage or paranoid-schizoid position, excessively using primitive, immature defenses (splitting), lacking good object experiences, being vulnerable to attachment to bad objects, being vulnerable to destructive projective-identification interactions, etc.

thus experiencing (himself/herself) as (specify psychodynamic variable/s),
e.g., internally bad, vulnerable to fragmentation and disintegration, chronically dependent on self-objects for mirroring and idealizing functions, anxiously attached, longing for the exciting-rejecting object, inadequate, worthless, destructive, etc.
and others as (specify psychodynamic variable/s).
e.g., persecutory, idealized objects, unavailable, essential for self-object functions, etc.

This initial experience would lead to the development of early maladaptive schemas such as those related to (specify early maladaptive schema),
e.g., autonomy, connectedness, worthiness, or unrelenting standards

These schemas would be maintained by certain cognitive distortions such as (specify cognitive distortions),
e.g. generalization, catastrophizing, minimizing, personalizing, etc.
leading the patient to perceive (his/her) world as (describe cognitively),
e.g., threatening, dangerous, frightening, defeating, etc.

These psychodynamic and cognitive precursors would generate certain maladaptive behaviors such as (specify maladaptive behaviors),
e.g., avoidance, skills-deficits, etc.

The behavioral history also suggests that these behaviors were (reinforced/punished), by (describe how or who did this) thus (increasing/decreasing) the chance that they will (continue to/no longer) occur. This behavioral history does suggest (specify behavioral variables),
e.g., a low rate of reinforcement, inadequate reinforcers, inability to access reinforcers, high rate of punishment, poor modeling history, etc.
indicating a further vulnerability toward (diagnosis or problem).

These early developmental factors were reinforced by a family environment that was (specify family predisposing factors),
e.g., chaotic, disorganized, lacking in intimacy, lacking in structure with clear boundaries and hierarchies, lacking in good communication, abusive, etc.

Such a family atmosphere likely (aggravated/attenuated) this patient's difficulties by (elaborate on how family factors contribute that is unique to this case). The family's main difficulties seemed to have been (specify family pathology),
e.g. affective communication, instrumental communication, parental psychopathology, a closed system, etc.

In addition to this, the family had to struggle with (specify social context),
e.g., low socioeconomic status, social or geographic isolation, poor neighborhood conditions, immigration, racial problems, etc.
which (has continued to be/no longer is) a problem for the patient, as (he/she) seems to be living in (the same/a different) social climate as indicated by (specify patient's current social situation). This early social and familial climate likely led to the development of (specify social skills),
e.g., good/poor social skills, chronic social anxiety,
and can be perceived as (buffering/exacerbating) the patient's disorder given the (numerous/lack of) social support figures in (his/her) life.

Significant relationships appear to be (adaptive/maladaptive) suggesting (specify couple predisposing factors),
e.g., a dysfunctional/functional interactional style, a destructive projective identification interactional style, poor/good communication and problem-solving skills, poor/good self-other differentiation, etc.
that may (attenuate/exacerbate) the patient's current condition.

The patient's family and social history has also lead (him/her) to have (limited/a variety of) occupational experiences as a result of
e.g., poor/good occupational modeling, economic disadvantages/advantages

This in conjunction with the patient's (specify occupational predisposing factors),
e.g., learning disabilities, exceptional learning ability, underachievement, limited intellectual ability, high intelligence, poor/good work history, etc.
has made it (difficult/much easier) for (him/her) to succeed occupationally. This has further contributed to (his/her) personality development by (specify how).

Given this developmental course and underlying biological vulnerability, the recent occurrence of (specify recent event),
e.g., illness, drugs, loss of relationship, death, failures, changes in jobs, relationships, social situation, family, etc.
may have precipitated the disorder.

Other precipitants occurring concurrently with this main event include (specify and elaborate on other precipitants). All these events may have interacted leading to the development of this patient's disorder. This disorder has been maintained by (specify and elaborate on all perpetuating factors),

e.g., chronic illness, chronic substance abuse, chronic use of maladaptive defenses, chronic dependence on others for self-object functions, chronic use of destructive projective identification interactions, chronic low rate of reinforcement, inability to access reinforcers, chronic use of cognitive distortions, chronic relationship problems, chronic family problems, chronic financial problems, chronic social isolation, etc.

However, the (presence/absence) of protective factors such as (specify protective factors),
e.g., good health, negative psychiatric family history, capacity to relate, mature defenses, good insight, introspective capability, ability to access reinforcers, good history of variety of reinforcers, stable couple and or family relationships, good social skills and use of social support, good financial situation, etc.
will (buffer/worsen) the course of this patient's disorder, suggesting a (good/poor) prognosis for recovery.

In coping with this condition, this patient has up to now (specify how patient has coped)
e.g., used drugs, become very active, problem-solved, searched for meaning, sought family, spouse or friends for support, escaped into work, etc.
suggesting a (specify coping-response style),
e.g., biological, behavioral, cognitive, dynamic, familial, couple-focused, social support seeking, occupationally oriented,
coping-response style.

Given this coping response style and diagnosis, the available research suggests treatment begin with (specify first line of treatment),
e.g., medications, behavior therapy, cognitive therapy, psychodynamic therapy, couple therapy, family therapy, socially focused therapy, occupational therapy
or the integration of (specify one or more treatments) at different points in time depending on what is needed for immediate relief and what the patient is willing to follow. The ultimate goal of therapy is to (describe goal of treatment) and return the patient to an optimal level of functioning that will include (describe individually and systemically).

*Special acknowledgement to Dr. Stephen Allnutt for his constructive feedback concerning the organization of this section.

APPENDIX II

EMPTY GRID FOR CLINICAL USE

________________________ patient's first name)

________________________ (patient's diagnosis)

	INDIVIDUAL FACTORS				SYSTEMIC FACTORS			
	BIOLOGICAL	BEHAVIORAL	COGNITIVE	PSYCHODYNAMIC	COUPLE	FAMILY	OCCUPATIONAL/ SCHOOL	SOCIAL
PREDISPOSING								
PRECIPITATING								
PERPETUATING								
PROTECTIVE								
COPING-RESPONSE STYLE								
TREATMENT								

INDEX